ATTACHMENT

Also Available

Attachment Theory and Research:
New Directions and Emerging Themes
Edited by Jeffry A. Simpson and W. Steven Rholes

Enhancing Early Attachments:
Theory, Research, Intervention, and Policy
*Edited by Lisa J. Berlin, Yair Ziv, Lisa Amaya-Jackson,
and Mark T. Greenberg*

The Evolution of Mind:
Fundamental Questions and Controversies
Edited by Steven W. Gangestad and Jeffry A. Simpson

ATTACHMENT

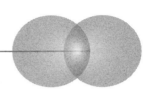

The Fundamental Questions

Edited by

Ross A. Thompson
Jeffry A. Simpson
Lisa J. Berlin

THE GUILFORD PRESS
New York   London

Copyright © 2021 The Guilford Press
A Division of Guilford Publications, Inc.
370 Seventh Avenue, Suite 1200, New York, NY 10001
www.guilford.com

Printed in the United States of America

This book is printed on acid-free paper.

Last digit is print number: 9   8   7   6   5   4   3   2   1

Library of Congress Cataloging-in-Publication Data

Names: Thompson, Ross A., editor. | Simpson, Jeffry A., editor. |
  Berlin, Lisa J., editor.
Title: Attachment : the fundamental questions / edited by
  Ross A. Thompson, Jeffry A. Simpson, Lisa J. Berlin.
Description: New York : The Guilford Press, [2021] | Includes
  bibliographical references and index.
Identifiers: LCCN 2020040264 | ISBN 9781462546022 (cloth)
Subjects: LCSH: Attachment behavior.
Classification: LCC BF575.A86 A7985 2021 | DDC 155.9/2–dc23
LC record available at *https://lccn.loc.gov/2020040264*

This volume is for those to whom we are attached . . .

to Janet, Scott and Andi, and Brian and Bekah —R. T.

to Chris and Natalie,
and Jameson, Audrey, Naomi, and Emma —J. A. S.

to Mom, Bob, and Sammie —L. J. B.

. . . and to our futures together.

About the Editors

Ross A. Thompson, PhD, is Distinguished Professor of Psychology at the University of California, Davis, where he directs the Social and Emotional Development Lab. Dr. Thompson studies the development of positive social motivation in young children, with a focus on the influence of early relationships. He also writes on the applications of developmental science to practice and policy related to children in poverty, early childhood mental health, and early education. He is an associate editor of *Child Development,* past president of Zero to Three, and a recipient of the Urie Bronfenbrenner Award for Lifetime Contribution to Developmental Psychology in the Service of Science and Society from Division 7 of the American Psychological Association.

Jeffry A. Simpson, PhD, is Distinguished University Teaching Professor and Chair of the Department of Psychology at the University of Minnesota, where he directs the Doctoral Minor in Interpersonal Relationships. Dr. Simpson's research interests center on adult attachment processes, trust, human mating, social influence, and how early developmental experiences are related to adult health, relationship functioning, and parenting outcomes. He is a past editor of *Personal Relationships* and the *Journal of Personality and Social Psychology: Interpersonal Relations and Group Processes,* and has served as president of the International Association for Relationship Research.

Lisa J. Berlin, PhD, is Professor at the University of Maryland School of Social Work. Dr. Berlin's multidisciplinary research program cuts across human development, psychology, social work, and public health. Her studies address early child–parent attachment as well as programs and policies for families with young children, including Early Head Start, child care, and home visiting. She is especially interested in the extent to which attachment-based interventions can improve publicly funded programs designed to support early parenting and child development. Dr. Berlin has been a Zero to Three fellow and in 2019 was named among the 100 most influential contemporary social work faculty.

Contributors

Lieselotte Ahnert, PhD, Department of Education and Psychology, Freie Universität Berlin, Berlin, Germany

Ting Ai, MA, Department of Psychology, University of Kansas, Lawrence, Kansas

Joseph Allen, PhD, Department of Psychology, University of Virginia, Charlottesville, Virginia

Michelle E. Alto, PhD, Mt. Hope Family Center, University of Rochester, Rochester, New York

Ximena B. Arriaga, PhD, Department of Psychological Sciences, Purdue University, West Lafayette, Indiana

Ashleigh I. Aviles, MA, Department of Human Development and Family Sciences, University of Texas at Austin, Austin, Texas

Marian J. Bakermans-Kranenburg, PhD, Clinical Child and Family Studies, Vrije Universiteit Amsterdam, Amsterdam, The Netherlands

Lisa J. Berlin, PhD, School of Social Work, University of Maryland, Baltimore, Baltimore, Maryland

Kristin Bernard, PhD, Department of Psychology, Stony Brook University, Stony Brook, New York

Cathryn Booth-LaForce, PhD, Center on Human Development and Disability, University of Washington, Seattle, Washington

Jude Cassidy, PhD, Department of Psychology, University of Maryland, College Park, College Park, Maryland

James S. Chisholm, PhD, School of Anatomy, Physiology, and Human Biology, University of Western Australia, Perth, Australia

Ann Chu, PhD, Department of Psychiatry, School of Medicine, University of California, San Francisco, San Francisco, California

Dante Cicchetti, PhD, Institute of Child Development, University of Minnesota, Minneapolis, Minnesota

Judith A. Crowell, MD, Division of Child and Adolescent Psychiatry, Department of Psychiatry and Behavioral Sciences, Stony Brook University Medical Center, Stony Brook, New York

Mary Dozier, PhD, Department of Psychology, University of Delaware, Newark, Delaware

Keely A. Dugan, BS, Department of Psychology, University of Illinois at Urbana–Champaign, Champaign, Illinois

Katherine B. Ehrlich, PhD, Department of Psychology, University of Georgia, Athens, Georgia

R. Pasco Fearon, PhD, Research Department of Clinical, Educational and Health Psychology, University College London, London, United Kingdom

Brooke C. Feeney, PhD, Department of Psychology, Carnegie Mellon University, Pittsburgh, Pennsylvania

R. Chris Fraley, PhD, Department of Psychology, University of Illinois at Urbana–Champaign, Champaign, Illinois

Cynthia A. Frosch, PhD, Department of Educational Psychology, University of North Texas, Denton, Texas

Tiffany George, BS, Department of Psychology, Texas A&M University, College Station, Texas

Omri Gillath, PhD, Department of Psychology, University of Kansas, Lawrence, Kansas

Yuthika U. Girme, PhD, Department of Psychology, Simon Fraser University, Burnaby, British Columbia, Canada

Ashley M. Groh, PhD, Department of Psychological Sciences, University of Missouri, Columbia, Missouri

Bridget K. Hamre, PhD, Center for Advanced Study of Teaching and Learning, University of Virginia, Charlottesville, Virginia

Nancy Hazen, PhD, Department of Human Development and Family Studies, University of Texas at Austin, Austin, Texas

Jeremy Holmes, MD, FRCPsych, Department of Clinical Psychology, University of Exeter, Exeter, United Kingdom

Deborah Jacobvitz, PhD, Department of Human Ecology, University of Texas at Austin, Austin, Texas

Susan M. Johnson, PhD, Department of Psychology, University of Ottawa, Ottawa, Ontario, Canada

Brenda Jones Harden, PhD, School of Social Work, University of Maryland, Baltimore, Baltimore, Maryland

Heidi Keller, PhD, Faculty of Human Sciences, Universität Osnabrück, Osnabrück, Germany

Nina Koren-Karie, PhD, Center for the Study of Child Development, University of Haifa, Haifa, Israel

Madoka Kumashiro, PhD, Department of Psychology, Goldsmiths, University of London, London, United Kingdom

Michael E. Lamb, PhD, Department of Psychology, University of Cambridge, Cambridge, United Kingdom

Alicia F. Lieberman, PhD, Department of Psychiatry, School of Medicine, University of California, San Francisco, San Francisco, California

Linxi Lu, EdM, Department of Applied Developmental and Educational Psychology, Boston College, Boston, Massachusetts

Fiona Maccallum, PhD, School of Psychology, University of Queensland, Brisbane, Australia

Jody Todd Manly, PhD, Mt. Hope Family Center, University of Rochester, Rochester, New York

Antina Manvelian, MA, Department of Psychology, University of Arizona, Tucson, Arizona

Judi Mesman, PhD, Centre for Child and Family Studies, Leiden University, Leiden, The Netherlands

Mario Mikulincer, PhD, Baruch Ivcher School of Psychology, Interdisciplinary Center Herzliya, Herzliya, Israel

Joan K. Monin, PhD, Department of Chronic Disease Epidemiology, Social and Behavioral Science Division, Yale School of Public Health, New Haven, Connecticut

Gilda Morelli, PhD, Department of Applied Developmental and Educational Psychology, Boston College, Boston, Massachusetts

Mirjam Oosterman, PhD, Clinical Child and Family Studies, Vrije Universiteit Amsterdam, Amsterdam, The Netherlands

David Oppenheim, PhD, Center for the Study of Child Development, University of Haifa, Haifa, Israel

Nickola C. Overall, PhD, School of Psychology, University of Auckland, Auckland, New Zealand

Margaret Tresch Owen, PhD, Center for Children and Families, University of Texas at Dallas, Dallas, Texas

Ramona L. Paetzold, PhD, Department of Management, Texas A&M University, College Station, Texas

K. Lee Raby, PhD, Department of Psychology, University of Utah, Salt Lake City, Utah

W. Steven Rholes, PhD, Department of Psychology, Texas A&M University, College Station, Texas

Glenn I. Roisman, PhD, Institute of Child Development, University of Minnesota, Minneapolis, Minnesota

David A. Sbarra, PhD, Department of Psychology, University of Arizona, Tucson, Arizona

Carlo Schuengel, PhD, Clinical and Family Studies, Vrije Universiteit Amsterdam, Amsterdam, The Netherlands

Phillip R. Shaver, PhD, Department of Psychology, University of California, Davis, Davis, California

Jeffry A. Simpson, PhD, Department of Psychology, University of Minnesota, Minneapolis, Minnesota

Anna Smith, BS, Mt. Hope Family Center, University of Rochester, Rochester, New York

L. Alan Sroufe, PhD, Institute of Child Development, University of Minnesota, Minneapolis, Minnesota

Howard Steele, PhD, Department of Psychology, The New School, New York, New York

Miriam Steele, PhD, Department of Psychology, The New School, New York, New York

Ohad Szepsenwol, PhD, Department of Education and Educational Counseling, The Max Stern Yezreel Valley College, Yezreel Valley, Israel

Alessandro Talia, PhD, Institute for Psychosocial Prevention, Universität Heidelberg, Heidelberg, Germany·

Anne Tharner, PhD, Clinical Child and Family Studies, Vrije Universiteit Amsterdam, Amsterdam, The Netherlands

Ross A. Thompson, PhD, Department of Psychology, University of California, Davis, Davis, California

Sheree L. Toth, PhD, Mt. Hope Family Center, University of Rochester, Rochester, New York

Marinus H. van IJzendoorn, PhD, Department of Psychology, Education, and Child Studies, Erasmus Universiteit Rotterdam, Rotterdam, The Netherlands

Jennifer Warmingham, MA, Mt. Hope Family Center, University of Rochester, Rochester, New York

Everett Waters, PhD, Department of Psychology, Stony Brook University, Stony Brook, New York

Harriet S. Waters, PhD, Department of Psychology, Stony Brook University, Stony Brook, New York

Theodore E. A. Waters, PhD, Department of Psychology, New York University, Abu Dhabi, Abu Dhabi, United Arab Emirates

Allison West, PhD, Bloomberg School of Public Health, Johns Hopkins University, Baltimore, Baltimore, Maryland

Amanda P. Williford, PhD, Center for Advanced Study of Teaching and Learning, Curry School of Education, University of Virginia, Charlottesville, Virginia

Charles H. Zeanah, MD, Department of Psychiatry and Behavioral Sciences, Tulane University, New Orleans, Louisiana

Debra M. Zeifman, PhD, Department of Psychological Science, Vassar College, Poughkeepsie, New York

Contents

TOPIC 3: THE NATURE AND FUNCTION OF INTERNAL WORKING MODELS

TOPIC 4: STABILITY AND CHANGE IN THE SECURITY OF ATTACHMENT

INTRODUCTION

CHAPTER 1

Attachment Theory in the 21st Century

Ross A. Thompson
Jeffry A. Simpson
Lisa J. Berlin

Attachment theory has held a prominent place in psychology for more than half a century. Inaugurated with Bowlby's (1951) seminal writings on the nature of the child's emotional tie to caregivers, and advanced by Ainsworth's (1967; Ainsworth, Blehar, Waters, & Wall, 1978) conceptual and methodological insights, the scope of attachment research has expanded during the last 70 years to encompass adult romantic relationships, the relational bases for social and personality development, developmental psychopathology, clinical intervention, and public policy problems in divorce and custody, child care, and child protection. At the same time, attachment theory and research have evolved in response to changes in families and family relationships, advances in developmental biology, and increasing sophistication in research methodology. Attachment theory has also progressed with seminal conceptual advances, such as the "move to the level of representation" (Main, Kaplan, & Cassidy, 1985) in the 1980s, concerted work on adult attachment and its underlying interpersonal processes in the 1990s, and increased sophistication in intervention applications in the 2000s. An expanding research literature has provided new empirical perspectives to classic issues concerning attachment and development, raising new questions about stability and change in attachment relationships, the formative influence of early attachments, and attachment in relation to culture. Taken together, these efforts have helped to make attachment theory one of the most generative and influential theories in the social and behavioral sciences.

Inevitably, and desirably, the increased research, expanded scope, and broadened applications have provoked new perspectives on classic theoretical questions and have created new debates within the field. As attachment theory moves into its eighth decade, it seems appropriate to take stock of where it stands with regard to some of these fundamental theoretical issues, many of which date back to Bowlby's seminal work. Here are some of the fundamental questions: What kinds of relationships constitute attachment relationships? What are the indicators of a secure attachment? What is the nature of the internal working models underlying secure or insecure attachments, and how do they influence behavior, thought, and emotions? How important are early attachment relationships for later behavior? What later behavior should these relationships impact, and what are the limits of their influence? How is attachment manifested in different cultures, and what are its key transcultural applications? What are the implications of attachment theory for clinical intervention and publicly funded services for children and families?

The fact that these fundamental questions continue to inspire discussion and new perspectives attests to the generativity of attachment theory. This underscores the value of considering the different perspectives that have emerged about these issues as the field moves into the future. For example, the term *attachment* originally applied in Bowlby's (1969, 1973, 1979, 1980) theory to the affectional bond between a young child and the mother. Since then, however, it has been extended to children's relationships with fathers and child care providers, relationships between adult romantic partners, and even relationships with siblings, close friends, teachers, and coaches. What do these different meanings of *attachment* have in common that distinguish them from other kinds of close, affectional relationships? Another way of understanding the defining qualities of attachment relationships is to consider how children and adults respond to separations from and the loss of their attachment figures. What are the key processes and mechanisms involved in these experiences of separation and loss, and what further insights do they provide about the nature of attachment?

As another illustration of the generativity of contemporary attachment thinking, the view that attachment relationships can affect behavior, thought, and emotions via internalized mental representations of relationships (i.e., internal working models) is shared by researchers studying attachment in childhood and adulthood. However, these researchers have very different ways of conceptualizing how internal working models are organized, how they develop and change with experience, and how they function in different social contexts. Is there a common thread among these different ways of conceptualizing working models that may provide greater precision to this central theoretical concept?

Further consideration of these fundamental issues is also required in light of new empirical advances. Longitudinal datasets including different measures of attachment have offered a new look, for example, at the question of whether early attachment remains consistent or changes over time and, if the latter, the correlates of changes in attachment. The Collaboration on Attachment Transmission Synthesis (Verhage et al., 2020) provides another powerful data-analytic approach by pooling data for individual-participant data meta-analyses. These longitudinal studies also invite reflection on early attachment as a predictor of later behavior, with evolutionary and biological models drawn from life history theory, neuroscience, and molecular genetics offering important new contributions to this question. When considered together, what can we say about which domains of later behavior should be shaped by early attachments and their associated experiences, and why?

New empirical initiatives during the past half-century have also been important in expanding the implications of attachment theory for clinical intervention and public policy. Concerning clinical intervention, what are the central mechanisms underlying the efficacy of attachment-based interventions? Concerning public policy, what can we learn about the applications (and misapplications) of attachment ideas with respect to the custody and care of children when parents divorce, the design of developmentally appropriate child care policies and effective child protection practices, as well as foster care, home visitation, and other programs?

Finally, some fundamental issues deserve further discussion because of their importance to the next generation of attachment research. A central measurement issue, for example, is whether variability in attachment security is best captured using continuous measures (which most adult attachment researchers regularly use) or with categorical measures inspired by the Strange Situation (which still predominate in the developmental study of attachment). Considering the methodological pluralism that has historically characterized attachment research, does *attachment* mean the same thing when different operationalizations and measures are used? If not, how can we interpret them? Another research question concerns attachment and culture, which has been addressed by researchers both within and outside the community of attachment scholars, often yielding strikingly divergent conclusions about suitable methodology and appropriate research generalizations. What can we learn from this debate that might inform researchers who study attachment relationships in a world with increasingly diverse family structures and social conditions?

The fundamental questions posed in this volume are clearly not *all* of the issues in attachment theory and research that could be considered "fundamental." It would require a much longer book to encompass those. Rather, the questions selected for discussion here are those that are

currently unresolved, are important to the future of attachment thinking, and are the basis for continuing discussion and (sometimes) debate
among attachment researchers. Even though these questions could have
been addressed in a single-authored book, our preference was to enlist
other attachment scholars to offer their own ideas and perspectives. After
consultation with colleagues in the field, we identified a collection of contemporary issues and, for each issue, invited prominent and emerging
scholars in the attachment field who have either addressed these issues
in prior work or, we thought, had valuable views to offer. The format we
chose is not point–counterpoint exchanges but rather a forum for articulating alternative perspectives. The overall goal of the book is to inform
the field, foster greater understanding of different perspectives, promote
greater theoretical clarity, encourage more collaboration across perspectives and disciplines, and contribute to useful new research in coming
decades. In the end, we hope that this volume will also convey to scholars
and students outside the community of attachment researchers that many
fundamental questions that undergird attachment theory still remain
open, generative, and inviting of further inquiry.

The Fundamental Questions of This Book

Nine central issues relevant to attachment theory and research constitute
this volume, as outlined below. We formulated each issue in terms of one
or two central questions to clarify the topic and guide contributors. For
each issue, we invited four to six experts to contribute short essays articulating their viewpoint and to comment about future directions for the
field. Both established authorities and emerging scholars are included
among our list of authors. Because attachment theory and research influence thinking in developmental, clinical, social/personality, and other
areas of psychology, contributors from diverse fields were invited for most
topics. We also attempted to include a diversity of theoretical and methodological perspectives to address each issue. Each author was limited to
approximately 2,200 words (and approximately 20 references) to encourage authors to profile their point of view succinctly rather than to write a
literature review or summarize their research program. This resulted in
more focused, concise, and direct essays. In addition, we provided each
author with the list of the nine fundamental questions and those who had
agreed to write about them so each author could consider their contribution within this broader context. Authors were not expected to address or
respond to any perspective other than their own, however.

   The nine sections of the book follow, and the book concludes with an
integrative commentary by us.

Defining Attachment and Attachment Security

The central questions we posed to authors are *What kinds of relationships "qualify" as attachment relationships? What are the origins and nature of security?* These questions are foundational to attachment theory and research, and as the scope and applications of attachment theory have expanded over time, answers to these questions have broadened. Developmental attachment researchers initially focused exclusively on infant–parent attachments, regarding them as developmentally formative and as prototypical of later attachment relationships, before expanding their inquiry to parent–child attachments later in childhood, adolescence, and adulthood. Adult attachment researchers in social/personality psychology expanded the scope of attachment relationships to include adult romantic relationships and relationships with relatives, friends, and even coworkers. Developmental attachment researchers, however, typically perceive *adult attachment* as the adult's current state of mind with respect to attachment based on early caregiving experiences. At all ages, an individual is likely to have multiple attachment figures, including nonparental caregivers (like child care providers) and adult partners who may have some, but perhaps not all, of the primary functions of attachment figures. Is there a compelling reason, therefore, for calling certain close, affectional relationships "attachments" and not others? If so, what do they share in common? Within these portrayals of the meaning of attachment there are also variations in what constitutes security, although an emphasis on the proximity-seeking, secure base, and safe haven functions of attachment may remain relevant throughout life. The authors we asked to profile these different perspectives are L. Alan Sroufe; Richard Pasco Fearon and Carlo Schuengel; Lieselotte Ahnert; Phillip Shaver and Mario Mikulincer; Deborah Jacobvitz and Nancy Hazen; and Ashleigh Aviles and Debra Zeifman.

Measuring the Security of Attachment

The central questions are *How should attachment security be assessed? What are the advantages and challenges of alternative measurement approaches?* As the scope and applications of attachment research have expanded, there has also been a broadening of well-established measures beyond the Strange Situation. These include narrative interviews that probe childhood representations, self-report measures that ask people how they relate to close others, attachment script-based assessments, the use of priming methodologies designed to activate representations of security, and other strategies. Some measures are relationship-specific, while others assess generalized characteristics of relational security or insecurity.

Is there a central element of attachment relationships captured by each of these diverse assessments? In recent years, there have also been efforts to directly compare alternative methodologies (such as categorical vs. continuous measures) in their psychometric and analytic strengths and weaknesses, raising the question of what should be the criteria for preferring one measure of attachment over another. The authors who were invited to profile these alternative approaches are Howard and Miriam Steele; Lee Raby, Chris Fraley, and Glenn Roisman; Theo Waters; Judith Crowell; and Omri Gillath and Ting Ai.

The Nature and Functioning of Internal Working Models

The central questions are these: *What are internal working models? How do they operate?* Bowlby's concept of mental representations deriving from attachment relationships has been one of the most generative aspects of attachment theory, but it has also produced disparate views regarding what internal working models actually are, how they operate, and their influence on personality, thinking, memory, and behavior. In some portrayals, working models are construed as relationship-specific and hierarchically organized; in others, generalized working models characterize individuals and their overall approach to relationships. Theoretical portrayals of working models also vary according to whether they are regarded as stable or dynamic over time, consciously accessible or primarily unconscious, whether they enlist well-known cognitive and social-cognitive skills (and if so, which ones), and the mechanisms by which working models are believed to influence behavior, thought, and feelings. Are there common elements to these diverse formulations that could provide a theoretically consistent portrayal of working models and their functioning? We invited Jude Cassidy; Harriet, Theo, and Everett Waters; David Oppenheim and Nina Koren-Karie; Ross Thompson; and Yuthika Girme and Nickola Overall to provide their views.

Stability and Change in the Security of Attachment

Our questions: *Should we expect attachment security to remain consistent over time? Is there evidence for stability in attachment security?* The expectation that early attachment quality leaves an enduring mark on later relationships of different types is one of the most enduring and debated elements of attachment theory, and it has been explored in many longitudinal studies. Does research support this view, and if so, how strong is the relation between earlier and later security? What conditions precipitate change in attachment? Stability and change in attachment have also been studied by attachment researchers from different disciplines within psychology. Do the dynamics of attachment relationships look different when they are examined as developmental processes or as interpersonal processes in adult relationships? We invited essays on these issues from Chris Fraley and Keely Dugan; Cathryn Booth-LaForce and Glenn Roisman; Joseph Allen; Ramona Paetzold, Steve Rholes, and Tiffany George; and Ximena Arriaga and Madoka Kumashiro.

The Continuing Influence of Early Attachment

The core questions: *What domains of later behavior should early attachment relationships predict, and why? For what domains should we not expect an association with early security? What are, in other words, the boundary conditions for the continuing influence of early attachment?* These questions are theoretically important for understanding the formative influence of early relationships on development, especially because an expanding research literature has documented a much broader range of later outcomes than Bowlby's theory initially envisioned. These questions are also significant given that new ways of understanding the impact of early experience have emerged since Bowlby's theory, including views from life history theory, molecular genetics, and developmental neuroscience. Does the cumulative body of research on this topic, combined with new theoretical models, alter or refine expectations for how and why early security is important? We invited Glenn Roisman and Ashley Groh; Marinus van IJzendoorn, Anne Tharner, and Marian Bakermans-Kranenburg; Katherine Ehrlich and Jude Cassidy; Mario Mikulincer and Phillip Shaver; and Ohad Szepsenwol and Jeffry Simpson to contribute their perspectives to this section.

Culture and Attachment

Our core questions: *How are attachment processes manifested in different cultures? How does culture manifest itself in attachment processes?* Attachment relationships develop in increasingly diverse families, contexts, and cultures, yet Bowlby's theory addressed processes underlying human adaptation that potentially have universal implications, at least according to many attachment theorists. Most attachment research to date has been conducted in Western industrialized societies, although some researchers have extended their inquiry to a wider range of non-Western contexts. Nevertheless, some researchers who study children in small communities in low- and middle-income countries have been critical of the generalization of attachment formulations and methods beyond Western contexts. How, then, do culture and attachment intersect? How should attachment be studied in a culturally appropriate manner? We invited Heidi Keller; Gilda Morelli and Linxi Lu; Judi Mesman; and James Chisholm to contribute their perspectives on this issue.

Separation and Loss

Here are the questions we posed: *How do people respond to the loss of an attachment figure? What are the key processes and mechanisms involved?* The loss of an attachment figure was of central concern to Bowlby in his *Attachment and Loss* trilogy, and it remains an important concern in both developmental and adult attachment research. Diverse perspectives on the consequences of loss have emerged from studies addressing Bowlby's concerns (a child's traumatic loss of a parent) and from research on adult romantic breakups, dysfunctional marriages and divorce, and bereavement in older adults. These studies have examined psychological and biological processes as well as normal and pathological mourning. Are there common threads in the process of loss and detachment across ages and contexts that can clarify our understanding of why attachment relationships are so significant? We invited Ann Chu and Alicia Lieberman; Phillip Shaver and Mario Mikulincer; David Sbarra and Antina Manvelian; Brooke Feeney and Joan Monin; and Fiona Maccallum to offer their perspectives.

Attachment-Based Interventions

Our core questions: *How do attachment-based interventions work? What are the key processes and mechanisms involved?* Clinical applications of attachment theory have been an enduring part of attachment thinking from the beginning, but they have expanded considerably in recent years as a range of new attachment-based interventions for children and adults have been developed and evaluated. Unsurprisingly, a focus on relationships is a shared characteristic of these interventions, but what are the processes through which relationships are repaired or strengthened? Are there common characteristics of attachment-based interventions across the lifespan? Is it possible to identify the core contributors to therapeutic efficacy and, if so, do they provide greater understanding of the nature of attachment relationships, both healthy and dysfunctional? We invited Marian Bakermans-Kranenburg and Mirjam Oosterman; Mary Dozier and Kristin Bernard; Sheree Toth, Michelle Alto, and Jennifer Warmingham; Alessandro Talia and Jeremy Holmes; and Susan Johnson to contribute essays about these issues.

Attachment, Systems, and Services

Here are the central questions: *How are attachment theory and research relevant to systems and services for children and families? What lessons can we learn from these programs?* Attachment theory has become increasingly applied to the design of public policies affecting children and families, including custody standards when parents divorce and the design of child care programs and child protection policies, as well as early home visitation, early childhood care and education programs, and foster care. Attachment theory can contribute to these policies and programs because of its focus on maintaining continuity in significant relationships for children, recognizing the importance of multiple attachment figures, and emphasizing the quality of care. Are there other lessons for attachment theory that stem from the design and evaluation of these programs? Do these lessons provide ideas for how current policies and practices can be improved in the future? We invited Margaret Tresch Owen and Cynthia Frosch; Bridget Hamre and Amanda Williford; Michael Lamb; Jody Todd Manly, Anna Smith, Sheree Toth, and Dante Cicchetti; Charlie Zeanah and Mary Dozier; and Lisa Berlin, Allison West, and Brenda Jones Harden to address these issues.

Commentary

In the final chapter, we draw together various themes and issues raised for each of the nine fundamental questions, considering the points of convergence, divergence, and what we have learned about each central issue. As we wrote to contributors, our goal was not—and is not—to offer a final position on any of the questions, nor to take sides; rather, it is to sharpen perspectives, assess where the field currently stands, and suggest how it could fruitfully proceed into the future. We also raise some additional questions for the future of attachment theory and research.

For Whom Is This Book Intended?

This is a time of widening interest in attachment theory, and this book exists alongside others that provide perspective on the field as a whole. These include a revised edition of Robert Karen's classic *Becoming Attached* (Karen, in press) and Robbie Duschinsky's (2020) *Cornerstones of Attachment Research,* among many others. This book, however, is unique in its goals and format, and we hope it has a unique contribution to attachment theory and research. Much more than reiterating perspectives that they have articulated elsewhere, the authors of these chapters have synthesized their views into fresh perspectives that, juxtaposed with others addressing the same questions, offer novel and useful insights into the current status of attachment theory and research, and perspective on its future.

Our primary audience is the community of attachment-informed scholars, researchers, and clinicians. They will find new ideas in these chapters that, we hope, will develop and extend their own thinking about close relationships and the psychological and developmental impact of close relationships throughout life. In particular, we hope that reading this volume will help our colleagues attain deeper understanding and appreciation of other views and perspectives in the field, facilitate clearer communication with those who hold different views, promote collabora- tive thinking that improves theory and research, and contribute to a gen- erative future for the field. A much broader audience for this volume is those who use the ideas of attachment theory in their research in allied fields (such as clinical psychology and developmental psychopathology, family sociology, and evolutionary biology) and in practice, whether in law and public policy, social work, education, or other fields. The format of the chapters and our selection of contributors was guided by the expec- tation that this volume would be useful to a broad audience outside the attachment field, including interested readers in the general public who find attachment theory valuable.

This volume has also been shaped by the hope that it will be used by teachers and their students in advanced undergraduate courses and graduate seminars. Indeed, such a seminar was one of the motivating rea- sons for this book—to provide a resource that did not previously exist for students. When combined with the most recent edition of the *Handbook of Attachment* (Cassidy & Shaver, 2016), this volume can be part of a thought- provoking introduction to the field. Perhaps the most fundamental lesson of these chapters is one intended for emerging scholars: After a half- century, a theory that has generated an enormous amount of research, reshaped important areas of public policy, had significant implications for therapeutic intervention, and penetrated public thinking about the developmental impact of early relationships still has many questions that remain open, interesting, and inviting of further inquiry.

And Our Thanks

When we began this project, we did not know whether our ambitious plan for a collection of more than 45 chapters by leading scholars would elicit a receptive response. Consequently, we were pleased that, with only a few exceptions, every invitation we sent to contributors was accepted. Even more gratifying was how helpfully the authors worked with us, within the contexts of their own demanding schedules and the emergence of a pan- demic, and within the constraints of length and citation count, to create thoughtful and forward-looking discussions of fundamental questions of attachment theory. Although several commented that writing with such brevity was more difficult than writing a chapter of conventional length, each author responded constructively and creatively in crafting and revis- ing their chapters. To them, our greatest thanks.

Seymour Weingarten acted as an excellent and highly supportive editor-in-chief at Guilford Press by planting the idea for the book, waiting for it to gestate, and then facilitating the introduction of three attachment researchers who had not previously met to enact the vision. We are grateful for that vision and his persistence.

Finally, we three have experienced this collaboration as a wonderful meeting of minds and generous spirits. Any one of us drafting this introduction would have thanked the other two for making this enterprise immensely enjoyable, stimulating, and enriching, so we do so now.

REFERENCES

Ainsworth, M. D. S. (1967). *Infancy in Uganda*. Baltimore: Johns Hopkins.

Ainsworth, M. D. S., Blehar, M., Waters, E., & Wall, S. (1978). *Patterns of attachment*. Hillsdale, NJ: Erlbaum.

Bowlby, J. (1951). *Maternal care and mental health*. Geneva, Switzerland: World Health Organization.

Bowlby, J. (1969). *Attachment and loss: Vol. 1. Attachment*. New York: Basic Books.

Bowlby, J. (1973). *Attachment and loss: Vol. 2. Separation*. New York: Basic Books.

Bowlby, J. (1979). *The making and breaking of affectional bonds*. London: Tavistock.

Bowlby, J. (1980). *Attachment and loss: Vol. 3. Loss, sadness and depression*. New York: Basic Books.

Cassidy, J., & Shaver, P. R. (Eds.). (2016). *Handbook of attachment: Theory, research, and clinical applications* (3rd ed.). New York: Guilford Press.

Duschinsky, R. (2020). *Cornerstones of attachment research*. New York: Oxford University Press.

Karen, R. (in press). *Becoming attached: First relationships and how they shape our capacity to love* (rev. ed.). New York: Oxford University Press.

Main, M., Kaplan, N., & Cassidy, J. (1985). Security in infancy, childhood, and adulthood: A move to the level of representation. In I. Bretherton & E. Waters (Eds.), Growing points of attachment theory and research. *Monographs of the Society for Research in Child Development, 50*(1–2, Serial No. 209), 66–104.

Verhage, M. L., Schuengel, C., Duschinsky, R., van IJzendoorn, M. H., Pasco Fearon, R. M., Madigan, S., . . . the Collaboration on Attachment Transmission Synthesis. (2020). The Collaboration on Attachment Transmission Synthesis (CATS): A move to the level of individual-participant-data meta-analysis. *Current Directions in Psychological Science, 29*, 199–206.

TOPIC 1

DEFINING ATTACHMENT
AND ATTACHMENT SECURITY

- What kinds of relationships "qualify" as attachment relationships?

- What are the origins and nature of security?

CHAPTER 2

Attachment as a Relationship Construct

L. Alan Sroufe

He spoke with tears of fifteen years
How his dog and him traveled about
The dog up and died. He up and died . . .
After twenty years he still grieves
—JERRY JEFF WALKER, "Mr. Bojangles"

The attachment theory of Bowlby and Ainsworth contains very specific propositions. First and foremost, attachment is a relationship construct. It refers to the emotional connection *between* two individuals. It is true that individuals as they mature develop particular orientations regarding close relationships. These orientations become *individual* characteristics, but attachment itself refers to relationships, not individuals. In the case of infant–caregiver attachments, which for Bowlby was the prototype, the infant not only commonly has multiple attachment relationships, but they may at times be distinctive (i.e., qualitatively different; Main & Weston, 1981). This makes clear that attachment is not a characteristic of the infant. Such a perspective opens up exciting developmental questions regarding when and how such attachments are consolidated along with other social experiences into a more unified individual stance regarding attachment. Distinguishing attachment orientation as an individual characteristic and attachment itself as a relationship construct is the starting point for this pursuit.

A second proposition is that the attachment concept refers to a special kind of relationship. Not all relationships, not even all that are important, are properly considered attachment relationships. Attachment refers to a particular kind of strong, enduring emotional connection that serves certain specific functions, and to a particular way the behavior of one individual is organized with respect to another. There is a stronger desire to share feelings with those who are attachment figures than with others, greater emotional reactions when encountering them, more distress or concern upon being separated from them, and more intense grief upon their loss. Bowlby (1973) emphasized safety and feelings of well-being as important functions of attachments, whereas Ainsworth and our group (Sroufe & Waters, 1977) additionally emphasized the provision of a secure base for exploration. In any case, attachment figures are central in the person's world. As Bowlby stated, "Intimate attachments to other human beings are the hub around which a person's life revolves, not only when he [sic] is an infant or a toddler or a school-child but throughout his adolescence and his years of maturity as well, and on into old age" (1980, p. 422).

A third proposition concerns the distinction between the presence or "strength" of attachments and their quality. In this system, maladaptive, anxious attachments are thought to be as strong as secure attachments. Especially in infancy, it is presumed that all infants who have been raised by someone will become attached to that person (or those persons), even if they have been maltreated (Cicchetti & Barnett, 1991). Developmentally delayed children become attached. Children with handicaps become attached. Attachment is a biological imperative. It is the rule, and the only exceptions—as in the case of the Romanian orphans—occur when there is no consistent caregiver interacting with the infant (Zeanah, Smyke, Koga, Carlson, & Bucharest Early Intervention Project Core Group, 2005).

Which Relationships Are Attachment Relationships?

This is a somewhat complex question. The case is easiest with infant–caregiver attachments because the attachment behavioral system is so visibly and frequently activated. According to Bowlby (1973), it is when individuals are stressed, frightened, or ill that closeness with attachment figures is especially sought. Such conditions are frequently present in infants. Likewise, infants use attachment figures as a secure base for exploration in a literal way. They do not just think about caregivers when threatened: They do things that are easily observed, such as looking at them or approaching. They range away from caregivers and return, and show things to them from a distance, continually monitoring their availability. Even blind infants who have been equipped with sonar keep caregivers central as they explore (Joseph Campos, personal communication).

All infants are more comfortable exploring novel environments when an attachment figure is present, although the clarity of this "preferential treatment" depends on the quality of the attachment (Ainsworth, Blehar,

Waters, & Wall, 1978). In the case of infants who fail to go to parents when frightened (the most clear manifestation of "disorganized attachment"), it is assumed that the attachment system was activated but is in conflict with the fear system, resulting in compromised behavior (Main & Hesse, 1990). Typically, preferential treatment is also manifest when the infant has something to share or wants reassurance ("social referencing") and when greeting caregivers upon waking or upon reunion following brief separations. Anxiety is experienced when attachment figures are unexpectedly unavailable (Bowlby, 1973, 1980).

According to these criteria, infants generally, but not always, are attached to both parents. They may also be attached to nannies, who may even be primary attachments. They may be attached to day care providers, especially where there is continuity of care, but these may not always be attachment relationships. It depends on the nature of the interaction between them, both quantity and quality. They may be attached to grandparents or other adult caregivers and, in many cases, to siblings (especially in cultures where siblings often care for young children).

Beyond infancy, it becomes more difficult to determine whether a relationship is an attachment relationship, partly because individuals have greatly expanded ways of coping and rarely are distressed in the highly visible ways infants are. Life partnerships generally are attachment relationships, as are many nonmarital adult love relationships, when individual lives are organized around each other (see Shaver & Mikulincer, Chapter 5, and Aviles & Zeifman, Chapter 7, this volume). When these are genuine attachments, the same criteria apply as with infant–caregiver attachments. One can use one's partner as a base of security and one prefers the presence of the partner when distressed, ill, or frightened. Typically, grief ensues following the loss of any attachment figure. Although rare, it is possible to have a marriage that is not an attachment relationship. Even marriages are attachments only if there is a deep emotional connection and grief following loss.

What about other relationships? Are friends attachment figures? Are teachers? What about pets? Mr. Bojangles was apparently attached to his dog, given his grief reaction and the degree to which their lives were intertwined. Each of these kinds of relationships may be attachments at times, but in many (or even most) cases they are not, even though they are important relationships. Children certainly have close friends and favorite teachers. They may prefer them to others. But they generally are not preferred figures when one is ill or frightened. These are times when children seek to be with attachment figures in particular. They may well miss these nonattachment relationship partners when they change locations or otherwise are cut off from them, but they generally will not go through the characteristic phases of grief and mourning when these people are lost.

Importantly, humans have many social motives beyond attachment. There is a general motive for social connection, for community (Smith, 2017). There are also evolutionarily based motives for joint attention, affective sharing, and cooperation (Tomasello, 2019). There are many kinds of relationships that are vital for human well-being, even when they are not attachment relationships. Close relationships with peers are an excellent case in point. Special functions of peer relationships are learning how to cooperate and to negotiate conflicts (Hartup, 1980). It is precisely because peers are equals that this is so. There is empirical evidence that close peer relationships in fact promote the capacities to work effectively on conflicts and enhance collaborative skills (Sroufe, Egeland, & Carlson, 1999). Likewise, sibling relationships have a unique place. These are often the most durable relationships. They have some of the same emotional features of parent–child relationships while being more similar to peers in terms of age. They are uniquely placed for developing capacities of leading and following, *whether or not* they are attachment relationships per se (Sroufe, 2005). Similarly, getting on well with teachers and attracting their affection supports educational attainment. All of these relationships promote development. Differentiating attachment relationships from other social relationships, though at times difficult, enables a fuller picture of the individual's development because of the unique functions served by various kinds of relationships. There is more to development than feeling secure.

Another question is whether one can be attached to an object or place. It is not possible to have an attachment *relationship* with an inanimate object because of the impossibility of the object sharing the emotional connection. Behaviorists once argued that an attachment figure was merely a "discriminative stimulus" for certain behaviors. This was inferred because a sheep would bleat a great deal when a familiarized object (a grapefruit) was removed from its pen (Cairns, 1966). By this reasoning, the sheep was attached to the object. Bowlby, too, noted the disruptive effects of being separated from one's home and community. In his 1973 book Bowlby explained why the unfamiliar was a "natural cue to danger," given that in the environment in which we evolved predation was more likely in unknown places. So things other than attachment relationships are relevant to one's sense of security, including being in circumstances learned to be safe, or being surrounded by highly familiar objects (e.g., the toddler's doll or blanket).

Decades ago, our research showed that infants are less wary at home than in the lab (Sroufe, Waters, & Matas, 1974). It is important to distinguish these other sources of security from the security derived from an attachment relationship. Even at home, the infant is more confident if an attachment figure is present. The infant is also more confident when on the attachment figure's lap (rather than at some distance) and is less wary when the caregiver introduces a novel object before unfamiliar persons do the same thing. Attachment relationships promote security beyond mere familiarity.

What Leads to Secure Attachments?

"Securely attached" is actually shorthand for "secure in this relationship." When an infant is secure, he or she is confident in the availability and responsiveness of a particular attachment figure. Such confidence derives from the cumulative interactive history of the relationship as mentally represented by the infant. Studies based on hours of observation confirm that such confidence is based in a history of attuned, sensitive responsiveness from the caregiver to infant (Ainsworth et al., 1978; Pederson, Gleason, Moran, & Bento, 1998; Posada et al., 1999). Studies with lesser amounts of observation, including those with large samples, find smaller, but still significant, links between responsiveness and security (National Institute of Child Health and Human Development [NICHD], 1997). Moreover, all studies converge in finding a minimal link between early infant temperament and later security (Vaughn & Bost, 1999).

There is reason to believe that security in adult relationships also is captured by the notion of "confidence" in the reliability and supportiveness of the partner. In this case, however, there generally is reciprocity, wherein each person can both use the partner as a secure base and also be a secure base of support for that partner (Crowell et al., 2002). When partners are confident about each other they typically have a secure attachment relationship. In contrast, the attachment relationship of other couples may be characterized by ambivalence or hostility. Negative as it was, the relationship between George and Martha in the play *Who's Afraid of Virginia Wolff?* clearly was an attachment, caustically intertwined as they were.

There are additional layers of complexity in attachment relationships beyond infancy. Development has a progressive, cumulative nature, wherein new experiences are sought and processed within previously established frameworks. At each age individuals become more active forces in their own development, as more experience is accumulated. For example, some preschoolers, because of their histories, are more doubtful about positive responsiveness from others. Such a stance can compromise their engagement and access to corrective experiences, so they may carry forward increased doubt (Sroufe, 1983). Ultimately, it is clear that some adults have more difficulty having confidence in their partner, even when their partner is generally caring and responsive. This is a place where developmental attachment theory comes together with the vast literature on adult romantic relationships and individual attachment orientations (see, e.g., Shaver & Mikuliner, Chapter 5, and Girme & Overall, Chapter 17, this volume).

Conclusion

Distinguishing attachments from other relationships is important, not just for clarifying the attachment concept but also for expanding understanding of social development. For example, our prior work shows quite clearly that those with histories of secure attachment more often have closer relationships with their teachers and peers, that attachment and peer experiences taken together much more strongly predict developmental outcomes than either one does alone, and that later relationships can alter developmental trajectories (Sroufe, 2005). Likewise, distinguishing the quality (i.e., security) of attachment from its "strength" helps us understand the power of anxious, maladaptive child–caregiver attachments. It resolves mysteries such as why maltreated children frequently want to stay with their parents and why couples like George and Martha remain together despite their mutual vitriol. It is well established that infant attachment experiences predict aspects of later functioning and also that adults have different attachment orientations regarding close relationships. One key developmental question now concerns how early attachments of varying quality combine with later attachments and the array of other important social relationships to produce these adult orientations. Pathways likely will be complex.

REFERENCES

Ainsworth, M. D. S., Blehar, M., Waters, E., & Wall, S. (1978). *Patterns of attachment*. Hillsdale, NJ: Erlbaum.

Bowlby, J. (1973). *Attachment and loss: Vol. 2. Separation*. New York: Basic Books.

Bowlby, J. (1980). *Attachment and loss: Vol. 3. Loss, sadness and depression*. New York: Basic Books.

Cairns, R. (1966). The development, maintenance, and extinction of social attachment behavior in sheep. *Journal of Comparative and Physiological Psychology, 62,* 298–306.

Cicchetti, D., & Barnett, D. (1991). Attachment organization in maltreated preschoolers. *Development and Psychopathology, 3,* 397–411.

Crowell, J. A., Treboux, D., Gao, Y., Fyffe, C., Pan, H., & Waters, E. (2002). Assessing secure base behavior in adulthood: Development of a measure, links to adult attachment: Representations and relations to couples' communication and reports of relationships. *Developmental Psychology, 38*(5), 679–693.

Hartup, W. (1980). Peer relations and family relations: Two social worlds. In M. Rutter (Ed.), *Scientific foundations of developmental psychiatry* (pp. 280–292). London: Heinemann.

Main, M., & Hesse, E. (1990). Parents' unresolved traumatic experiences are related to infant disorganized attachment status: Is frightened or frightening parental behavior the linking mechanism? In M. Greenberg, D. Cicchetti, & E. M. Cummings (Eds.), *Attachment in the preschool years* (pp. 161–182). Chicago: University of Chicago Press.

Main, M., & Weston, D. (1981). The quality of the toddlers' relationship to mother and to father: Related to conflict behavior and the readiness to establish new relationships. *Child Development, 52,* 932–940.

NICHD Early Child Care Research Network. (1997). The effects of infant child care on infant–mother attachment security: Results of the NICHD study of early child care. *Child Development, 68,* 860–879.

Pederson, D., Gleason, K., Moran, G., & Bento, S. (1998). Maternal attachment representations, maternal sensitivity, and the infant–mother attachment relationship. *Developmental Psychology, 34,* 925–933.

Posada, G., Jacobs, A., Carbonell, O. A., Alzate, G., Bustamante, M., & Arenas, A. (1999). Maternal care and attachment security in ordinary and emergency contexts. *Developmental Psychopathology, 35,* 1379–1388.

Smith, E. E. (2017). *The power of meaning.* New York: Broadway Books.

Sroufe, L. A. (1983). Infant–caregiver attachment and patterns of adaptation in preschool: The roots of maladaptation and competence. In M. Perlmutter (Ed.), *Minnesota symposium on child psychology* (Vol. 16, pp. 41–83). Hillsdale, NJ: Erlbaum.

Sroufe, L. A. (2005). Attachment and development: A prospective, longitudinal study from birth to adulthood. *Attachment and Human Development, 7,* 349–367.

Sroufe, L. A., Egeland, B., & Carlson, E. (1999). One social world: The integrated development of parent–child and peer relationships. In W. A. Collins & B. Laursen (Eds.), *Relationships as developmental context: The 30th Minnesota symposium on child psychology* (pp. 241–262). Hillsdale, NJ: Erlbaum.

Sroufe, L. A., & Waters, E. (1977). Attachment as an organizational construct. *Child Development, 48,* 1184–1199.

Sroufe, L. A., Waters, E., & Matas, L. (1974). Contextual determinants of infant affective response. In M. Lewis & L. Rosenblum (Eds.), *Origins of fear* (pp. 49–72). New York: Wiley.

Tomasello, M. (2019). *Becoming human.* Cambridge, MA: Harvard University Press.

Vaughn, B., & Bost, K. (1999). Attachment and temperament: Redundant, independent, or interacting influences on interpersonal adaptation and development? In J. Cassidy & P. R. Shaver (Eds.), *Handbook of attachment: Theory, research, and clinical applications* (pp. 198–225). New York: Guilford Press.

Zeanah, C. H., Smyke, A. T., Koga, S. F., Carlson, E., & Bucharest Early Intervention Project Core Group. (2005). Attachment in institutionalized and community children in Romania. *Child Development, 76,* 1015–1028.

CHAPTER 3

What Kinds of Relationships Count as Attachment Relationships?

R. Pasco Fearon
Carlo Schuengel

This deceptively simple question is a fundamentally important one for people studying attachment. Crucial developmental questions pivot around it, such as: To whom can a child form an attachment (siblings, teachers, foster carers, friends)? How many attachments can a child have? Is each attachment as important? How do we know when an attachment has formed and what makes that happen? What happens when attachments are broken (or fade)? Mary Ainsworth, following John Bowlby and Robert Hinde, articulated many of the key concepts needed here (Ainsworth, 1991), including what we mean by a relationship, attachment behavior, and affectional bonds. Much of what we discuss in this chapter is an elaboration of those earlier works. We first discuss Robert Hinde's formulation of relationships. We then discuss Ainsworth's conception of attachment as a type of affectional bond. We describe some promising initial studies that have applied these theoretical ideas, noting that efforts to follow up on these leads are overdue.

Hinde's (1997) seminal book provides an exceptionally clear analysis of relationships. We focus on two of Hinde's key assertions. First, Hinde considered a relationship to represent a higher-order description of more or less predictable patterns of interaction between two (or more) individuals, shaped by their past history of interactions with one another and their respective representations or expectations concerning them. Thus, per definition, a relationship cannot be directly inferred from a single interaction; it is inferred from the patterning of numerous interactions over time.

There are a number of implications that arise out of this framework that are often not made explicit in the attachment literature. A key one is that separation–reunion procedures like the Strange Situation do not provide a direct and unambiguous measure of a relationship because they involve a single, relatively short observation. Rather, we *infer* that it captures something important about a relationship, based on theory and the wider body of evidence—for example, noting that over short periods of time a child's pattern of attachment behavior seems quite stable (e.g., when tested again; see Pinquart, Feußner, & Ahnert, 2013) and is predictable from measures of parent–child interaction taken earlier and/ or at home (De Wolff & van IJzendoorn, 1997). These considerations are important because there are circumstances and populations where there is uncertainty about whether behavior in the Strange Situation reflects a relational process, such as adopted children with a history of neglect (e.g., see Rutter, Kreppner, & Sonuga-Barke, 2009), children who showed signs of neurological dysregulation as neonates (Spangler, Fremmer-Bombik, & Grossmann, 1996), and indeed infants who were overly distressed during the administration of the Strange Situation (Granqvist et al., 2016). So, although the Strange Situation is a powerful tool for understanding the quality of the parent–infant attachment relationship, we must also stay vigilant about the assumptions made when using it, particularly when we examine behaviors, circumstances, or populations that have not been the subject of much validation research.

Second, Hinde (1997) argues that relationships reflect the generalization of patterns of interactions over time and across *different forms of interaction*. As most relationships involve diverse forms of interaction, reflecting different social goals and functions, a relationship cannot usually be described as being simply of one kind or another. In that sense, the term *attachment relationship* is potentially misleading, even though it is a widely used and useful shorthand. Rather, it is probably more accurate to describe attachment as a domain within a relationship—that domain of interactions concerned with the seeking and provision of comfort and feelings of safety. This characterization reminds us that many other domains exist within relationships that may influence the attachment domain and can shape the overall structure or quality of the relationship. Play, for example, can affect attachment, attachment can affect play, attachment can affect feeding, and so on. Thus, the question posed in the title should really be "How can we tell whether a relationship has an attachment domain embedded within it or not?" Relatedly, we might ask "What are the conditions that allow a relationship to come to acquire an attachment domain?" And perhaps we could even ask "Are some relationships incapable of taking on an attachment domain at all?"

The majority of attachment research has been conducted with families where there have been no severe disruptions in the continuity of care or profound disturbances in the quality of care, and evidence suggests that in such circumstances children readily engage in attachment interactions with their caregivers, and attachment becomes a central domain of the parent–child relationship. Typically, research focuses on the *quality* or patterning of attachment, not its presence or absence. Furthermore, most research has investigated these processes comparatively late in the first year of life, meaning that the attachment domain is usually fully established by the time we study it. This kind of research has taught us much about how attachment behavior is organized within well-established parent–child relationships, but we know much less about how such relationships acquire an attachment domain in the first place, or how this emerges in the context of new relationships or rebuilds after a relationship is disrupted. We need different tools to understand these processes.

These crucial issues come to the fore in contexts where assumptions about the presence of an attachment domain within a relationship may not hold, like a newly established foster care placement or a child's relationships with teachers or nursery workers. Dozier and colleagues developed the Parent Attachment Diary (Stovall-McClough & Dozier, 2004) to monitor, through the eyes of foster caregivers, the emergence of attachment interactions day by day or week by week. Similarly, Zeanah, Smyke, Koga, and Carslon (2005) developed, in the context of the Bucharest Early Intervention Project (BEIP), an observational measure of the extent to which children show clear selective attachment behavior to caregivers. These studies lay the groundwork for studying the presence (vs. absence) and formation of attachments, which will complement the tools we use to study the organization (e.g., security vs. insecurity) of established attachments. With the availability of smart monitoring devices and experience sampling methodologies, now is a good time to push this research agenda forward.

An important related term introduced by Bowlby and elaborated by Ainsworth is *affectional bond*, of which attachment bonds form a subset (see Ainsworth, 1991). Ainsworth defined an affectional bond as "a relatively long-enduring tie in which the partner is important as a unique individual, interchangeable with none other. In an affectional bond, there is a desire to maintain closeness to the partner . . . inexplicable separation tends to cause distress and permanent loss would cause grief" (1991, p. 38). Hinde's assertion focuses on attachment relationships from an outside observer's standpoint and emphasizes their dyadic properties. Ainsworth's concept of an attachment bond, by contrast, concerns one individual's subjective experience of being in an attachment relationship—the emotions and internal representations associated with it. Attachments are a fundamentally important type of affectional bond characterized by feelings of comfort, belonging, and safety (Ainsworth, 1991), and for children especially, they are likely to be the most important bonds they have. However, more than one kind of affectional bond may exist between one individual and another. Grief reactions may, therefore, reflect more than just a loss of an attachment; these may reflect the loss of everything significant afforded by that relationship.

Why and how some relationships acquire such affectional characteristics, and how attachment bonds in particular form, are poorly understood. Presumably some determination of trust or confidence in the long-term commitment of the partner is involved. But it is striking how little we know about the minimal conditions for attachment bonds to form, other than noting that, in young children, multiple and repeatedly changing caregivers (seen in some forms of institutional care) or profound neglect almost certainly do not meet those minimal requirements (Zeanah & Gleason, 2015).

Although much of children's attachment behavior is focused on individuals with whom they have a profound affectional bond, it is likely children can show attachment behavior toward individuals where such a bond is minimal, weak, or emerging. This is because affectional bonds are presumably the product of feelings aroused during repeated interactions, and so the initial bond is likely a consequence of these interactions. And indeed, during the early phase of forming attachments, children arguably cannot wait until a lasting bond has formed before seeking the protection they need. Observations from the BEIP suggest this because children placed in foster care rapidly displayed attachment behavior to their new caregivers, typically within 2–3 months (Smyke et al., 2012). We know from other sources that children readily seek comfort from others when placed in foster care, in day care, or at school (Seibert & Kerns, 2009; Stovall-McClough & Dozier, 2004), and this does not always lead to lasting affectional bonds (see Ahnert, Chapter 4, this volume). Such transitory (or secondary/supplemental; see Ainsworth, 1991) attachments may become attachment bonds, but not necessarily. One avenue toward improved understanding may be to test transactional associations between interactions in the attachment domain of the relationship (as defined by Hinde) and the intensity of attachment-related feelings associated with the emerging bond (as defined by Ainsworth) over time.

Although we have focused primarily on attachment during childhood, these principles are just as applicable in adulthood, if not more so. An important example of transitory attachments in adulthood is seen in therapy. Both Bowlby and Ainsworth considered the importance of attachment to therapeutic relationships. While many therapeutic relationships may involve attachment behavior on the part of the client, most therapeutic relationships do not involve deep affectional bonds. For most clients, one's sense of self and one's relationship to the world and the future does not become organized in fundamental ways around the therapist, and eventual loss of that relationship is both expected and often nontraumatic. Ainsworth (1989) suggested that the relationship with the therapist does not penetrate as widely across the domains of one's life as some other relationships, which is why its loss is not perceived as an existential threat. Of course, in highly vulnerable clients, or where the boundaries of the relationship have become confused, the loss of the therapeutic relationship may be traumatic (see Talia & Holmes, Chapter 40, this volume).

The notion that attachment behavior can be deployed flexibly and should be distinguished from slow-developing attachment bonds may provide clues regarding several seemingly contradictory observations or intuitions about attachment. For example, the notion of penetrance may help to explain the observation that when given a choice, children preferentially seek contact with the caregiver who provides the most care, not the one to whom they have a secure attachment (Umemura, Jacobvitz, Messina, & Hazen, 2013). In addition, some relationships involving attachment may end without a lasting impact, whereas the ending of others may bring great grief and anxiety (see, e.g., Bifulco, Harris, & Brown, 1992).

These considerations lead naturally to the question of the kind of individuals a child can become attached to. It might be assumed that children do not or cannot form attachments to other children (e.g., siblings) because attachment relies on the presence of an older, wiser, and more capable other (Bowlby, 1984). However, the widespread involvement of siblings in childrearing in many cultures across the globe (e.g., Edwards & Whiting, 1993) suggests that such a cut-and-dried interpretation is likely wrong. We were reminded of a video recording presented by Mesman (2015) from a traditional jungle-dwelling community in which a 1-year-old showed clear attachment behavior toward a remarkably sensitive 3- or 4-year-old sibling. These observations are quite consistent with early data from Stewart and Marvin (1984) in the United States and more recently by Mooya, Sichimba, and Bakermans-Kranenburg (2016) in Zambia. It seemed evident in Mesman's example that the sibling had been socialized to care for younger siblings, and it seems likely the proximate behaviors associated with this led the infant to focus his attachment behavior toward his sibling. We lack good data on what those proximate behaviors are, how infants process and respond to them, and how they adjust their behavior and working models accordingly.

An important question is whether the infant in Mesman's recording had a lasting attachment bond to his sibling. It is tempting to conclude he did, but the presence of attachment behavior may not always imply the presence of a deep affectional bond. These observations point the way to a dynamic conception of children's attachments and underline the fact that children may rely on networks of attachment relationships to meet their needs. These may be fruitful areas of inquiry in future developmental, clinical, and cross-cultural research.

Conclusion

Attachment research has powerfully demonstrated the importance of relationships with caregivers for children's development. Within those relationships, attachment interactions provide children with a vital means of ensuring their protection and comfort. Deep bonds often grow out of such interactions and afford children a sense of security and belonging. As we study populations where opportunities to form new or nonparental attachment relationships exist, it becomes increasingly clear that children can rely on many individuals as lasting or temporary attachment figures, and we are only just beginning to understand how these relationships develop and what their significance might be for child development. It is also a valuable reminder that we know remarkably little about how attachments to even primary caregivers form in the first place.

REFERENCES

Ainsworth, M. D. S. (1989). Attachments beyond infancy. *American Psychologist, 44*(4), 709–716.

Ainsworth, M. D. S. (1991). Attachments and other affectional bonds across the life cycle. In C. M. Parks, J. Stevenson-Hinde, & P. Marris (Eds.), *Attachment across the life cycle* (pp. 33–51). New York: Tavistock/Routledge.

Bifulco, A., Harris, T., & Brown, G. W. (1992). Mourning or early inadequate care?: Reexamining the relationship of maternal loss in childhood with adult depression and anxiety. *Development and Psychopathology, 4,* 433–449.

Bowlby, J. (1984). *Attachment and loss: Vol. 1. Attachment* (2nd ed.). London: Penguin.

De Wolff, M., & van IJzendoorn, M. H. (1997). Sensitivity and attachment: A meta-analysis on parental antecedents of infant attachment. *Child Development, 68*(4), 571–591.

Edwards, C. P., & Whiting, B. B. (1993). Mother, sibling and me: The overlapping roles of caregivers and companions in the social world of two- to three-year-olds in Ngeca, Kenya. In K. MacDonald (Ed.), *Parent–child play: Descriptions and implications* (pp. 305–330). Albany: State University of New York Press.

Granqvist, P., Hesse, E., Fransson, M., Main, M., Hagekull, B., & Bohlin, G. (2016). Prior participation in the strange situation and overstress jointly facilitate disorganized behaviours: Implications for theory, research and practice. *Attachment and Human Development, 18*(3), 235–249.

Hinde, R. A. (1997). *Relationships: A dialectical perspective.* Hove, UK: Psychology Press.

Mesman, J. (2015). *Mothers' and fathers' sensitivity in cultural context.* Keynote lecture, International Attachment Conference, New York, NY.

Mooya, H., Sichimba, F., & Bakermans-Kranenburg, M. (2016). Infant–mother and infant–sibling attachment in Zambia. *Attachment and Human Development, 18*(6), 618–635.

Pinquart, M., Feußner, C., & Ahnert, L. (2013). Meta-analytic evidence for stability in attachments from infancy to early adulthood. *Attachment and Human Development, 15*(2), 189–218.

Rutter, M., Kreppner, J., & Sonuga-Barke, E. (2009). Emanuel Miller lecture: Attachment insecurity, disinhibited attachment, and attachment disorders: Where do research findings leave the concepts? *Journal of Child Psychology and Psychiatry, 50*(5), 529–543.

Seibert, A. C., & Kerns, K. A. (2009). Attachment figures in middle childhood. *International Journal of Behavioral Development, 33*(4), 347–355.

Smyke, A. T., Zeanah, C. H., Gleason, M. M., Drury, S. S., Fox, N. A., Nelson, C. A., & Guthrie, D. (2012). A randomized controlled trial comparing foster care and institutional care for children with signs of reactive attachment disorder. *American Journal of Psychiatry, 169*(5), 508–514.

Spangler, G., Fremmer-Bombik, E., & Grossmann, K. (1996). Social and individual determinants of attachment security and disorganization. *Development and Psychopathology, 7,* 127–139.

Stewart, R. B., & Marvin, R. S. (1984). Sibling relations: The role of conceptual perspective-taking in the ontogeny of sibling caregiving. *Child Development, 55,* 1322–1332.

Stovall-McClough, K. C., & Dozier, M. (2004). Forming attachments in foster care: Infant attachment behaviors during the first 2 months of placement. *Development and Psychopathology, 16*(2), 253–271.

Umemura, T., Jacobvitz, D., Messina, S., & Hazen, N. (2013). Do toddlers prefer the primary caregiver or the parent with whom they feel more secure?: The role of toddler emotion. *Infant Behavior and Development, 36*(1), 102–114.

Zeanah, C. H., & Gleason, M. M. (2015). Annual research review: Attachment disorders in early childhood—clinical presentation, causes, correlates, and treatment. *Journal of Child Psychology and Psychiatry, 56*(3), 207–222.

Zeanah, C. H., Smyke, A. T., Koga, S. F., & Carlson, E. (2005). Bucharest Early Intervention Project Core Group. Attachment in institutionalized and community children in Romania. *Child Development, 76*(5), 1015–1028.

CHAPTER 4

Attachment to Child Care Providers

Lieselotte Ahnert

Children's relationships with care providers are central to the debate on the quality of child care settings and are foremost characterized by child–care provider interactions following guidelines of the educational curriculum. Cognitive and learning theories help to explain the ways in which care providers are involved with the children, passing on knowledge about the world, stimulating language and facilitating learning, and eventually shaping the child–care provider relationship (Hong et al., 2019). Furthermore, some studies have stressed that care providers are also emotionally available and successfully reassure children who seek their proximity when stressful mishaps or peer conflicts occurred throughout the day (more details in Howes & Spieker, 2016). These secure base behaviors of the children and the affective responses of the care providers point to obvious similarities with child–parent attachments, and thus led researchers to examine child–care provider relationships in the framework of attachment theory. In this chapter, we discuss child–care provider attachment or closeness through standardized assessments, reveal their antecedents and peculiarities, report on correlates with child development, and eventually argue that child–care provider attachments differ both functionally and ontogenetically from child–parent attachments.

Description of Child–Care Provider Attachment through Standardized Assessments

Seeking clearer insight into attachment-like phenomena in child care, researchers used the Strange Situation Procedure (SSP; Ainsworth,

Blehar, Waters, & Wall, 1978) or the Attachment Q-set (AQS; Waters, 1995), initially developed to assess mother–child attachment, to further assess child–care provider attachment (Ahnert, 2005). For older children in preschool, researchers captured the connatural construct of closeness using the Student–Teacher Relationship Scale (STRS; Pianta, 2001).

Comparisons of child–parent and child–care provider attachment in young children yielded inconsistent results in terms of the concordance and discordance of these patterns. A meta-analysis (Ahnert, Pinquart, & Lamb, 2006) of nearly 3,000 children from a variety of cultures concluded that secure child–care provider attachments appear less frequently than secure child–parent attachments. Furthermore, the attachments (to mother, father, and care provider) were modestly but significantly inter-correlated, suggesting that children construct intertwined internal working models of significant relationships to adults.

Analyses using the AQS (rated by observers) and SSP revealed similar findings, even though concordance between child–mother and child–care provider attachment was greater in studies using the AQS rather than the SSP. Differences in the behavioral emphases of the two assessments may help explain these discrepancies. The SSP clearly emphasizes security-seeking and proximity-promoting behaviors, which most likely elicit the protective behaviors of mothers. The AQS additionally takes instructional and educational features of the interactions into account, which better characterize care provider behaviors (Ahnert, Rickert, & Lamb, 2000). Overall, the small but significant correlations between child's attachments toward the mother, father, and care provider, as well as distinct discordance between child–parent and child–care provider attachments, suggest that these attachments are functionally adapted to the care environments where they develop.

Peculiarities of Child–Care Provider Attachment

As with parents, attachments with care providers reflect the interactional histories of children, who often spend many hours in child care. However, researchers were puzzled by how the internal working models (IWMs) of these attachments develop and what they mean. For example, Sagi and his colleagues (1995) reported that if more than one care provider cared for a group of children, these care providers were more likely to develop a similar quality of attachment to the children in each group. Howes, Galinsky, and Kontos (1998) found that the security of child–care provider attachment remained the same even when care providers changed. These findings suggest that child–care provider attachments are affected by routine characteristics of the care environment as well as the relationship.

Clearly, child care providers need to divide their attention among several children simultaneously, which makes it difficult to respond promptly to each individual child. Consequently, children in group care may have to wait longer for a response or may even be ignored, which in turn may weaken the security of the child–care provider relationship. If secure attachments, however, derive from sensitivity, the promptness of adult responses to individual children, indicated by short latencies, should be the heart of the relationship formation. Care providers' latencies in response to children's needs and how response latency may predict secure attachment in child care, however, remain almost unknown.

Antecedents of Child–Care Provider Attachment

In a recent study (Zaviska, Mayer, Deichmann, Eckstein-Madry, & Ahnert, 2020), we therefore explored interaction patterns of child–care provider dyads in group care with a special focus on child proximity seeking and the latencies of the care provider's response. Care providers demonstrated promptness to child proximity seeking as a routine part of their care. Promptness was more frequent, with short latencies of 3–7 seconds and was significantly greater for toddlers than for older children, even though children's proximity seeking did not differ across age. Most interestingly, however, care providers' promptness was not associated with the security of all child–care provider attachment relationships, but only with care provider security to toddlers.

To understand the formation of child–care provider attachment beyond toddlerhood, concepts other than promptness must be investigated. First insights came from a meta-analysis (Ahnert et al., 2006), which found that measures of care providers' group-focused sensitivity (i.e., child-oriented involvement while supervising the entire group) were more strongly associated with attachment security (measured with SSP or AQS) than were measures of the same care providers' dyadic sensitivity (i.e., one-on-one positive caregiving). Ereky-Stevens, Funder, Katschnig, Malmberg, and Datler (2018) recently confirmed these findings. Similar to the prediction of child–parent attachment, the care providers' measures of dyadic responsiveness predicted child–care provider attachment in the small groups of the child care centers, which most likely include infants and toddlers (Ahnert et al., 2006). Larger groups typically consist of children beyond toddlerhood, who can process interactional experiences based on expanded social learning while observing others and not only their own involvement in interactions. Observing peers in a group, including how they interact with the care provider with whom the child is also familiar, might thus become a powerful tool in the formation of security of attachment in child care. That is, how a care provider responds, comforts, and helps other children may influence the child's own experience in shaping the security of attachment and the IWMs derived from it (see Waters & Cummings, 2000).

The idea that older children process the complex social experience in group life with their IWMs better than younger children is in line with considerations about the development of IWMs. That is, IWMs become increasingly stable across childhood while their formations also change (Pinquart, Feußner, & Ahnert, 2012). Perhaps IWMs mature into a more generalized type beyond toddlerhood, which includes accumulated experiences of own and observed behaviors of others in attachment-driven contexts as opposed to the simpler IWM during infancy that only encompasses the child's own behaviors.

Gender Bias in Child–Care Provider Attachment

The formation of child–care provider attachments also appear to vary depending on child gender, which is not typically found in studies of attachment. That is, girls tend to develop secure attachments with their child care providers more often than boys (Ahnert et al., 2006; Ereky-Stevens et al., 2018). There are three possible explanations for this:

1. During the formation of gender-based social identity throughout the early years, girls better develop communicative (in contrast to boys' competitive) behaviors and tend to show more positive emotions than boys (Leaper, 2002). This might make interactions and closeness easier with girls.
2. The overwhelming majority of care providers are female, and their engagement and educational goals might be a better match to girls' than boys' social identity.
3. The gender-mixed groups in child care centers tend to segregate into gender-based subgroups where children favor same-sex over cross-sex interactions (Fabes, Hanish, & Martin, 2003). Given the fact that children process their own relationship experiences and those of others with their IWMs, the gender-based subgroup might reinforce the relationship quality of a child with the care provider.

Future research, however, is needed to understand and reflect on these mechanisms in order to avoid gender bias in child–care provider attachment.

Correlates with Child Development

From numerous studies on the associations between child–care provider attachment or child–teacher closeness and children's development, we chose three exemplary studies that go beyond correlational evidence and shed light on the underlying mechanisms of children's (1) cognitive achievement, (2) behavioral adjustment, and (3) stress management.

First, when children's relationships in preschool were characterized as being close, children showed higher levels of classroom participation and pleasure to learn than when they were in more distant relationships (Hamre & Pianta, 2001). The question regarding how child–teacher closeness may predict academic success motivated us to design a study using a priming paradigm (Ahnert, Milatz, Kappler, Schneiderwind, & Fischer, 2013). Preschoolers participated in a laboratory situation in which they worked on computerized tasks thought to govern basic cognitive knowledge. Before each task commenced, however, the image of the child's teacher with whom STRS closeness had previously been measured (i.e., the affective prime stimulus) was displayed for an experimental group of children; a control group was exposed to a neutral prime. Children in the experimental group had shorter solving times than children in the control group the higher the closeness score of the affective prime was. This effect was also evident months later, after children's transition to school. These findings clearly suggest that cognitive processing is much more effective in the psychological presence of close child–teacher relationships, which might eventually lead to higher self-efficacy in the children and more pronounced motivation to learn and achieve.

Second, there is also firm scientific evidence that children who experienced lower attachment security at home are prone to greater externalizing behavior in child care. Greater and more regular exposure to other children in child care centers than is typically experienced at home or in the neighborhood might result in increased amounts of unregulated peer interactions. This could be particularly problematic for children who have limited social competence, which is true for children with lower attachment security at home. Buyse, Verschueren, and Doumen (2011) showed that the insecure children's behavioral maladjustment (specifically, aggressive behavior) was buffered by higher levels of preschool teacher sensitivity. If peers are the cause of behavioral problems, teachers must use group-oriented strategies and respond to adverse peer interactions, not only to the child who misbehaves. For example, Zaviska and colleagues (2020) conducted a longitudinal study following children after child care entry and showed that the earlier and better that children with lower attachment security at home established a child–care provider attachment, the better they were supported during their peer encounters, and the better their behavioral adjustment was. Interestingly, this association was not significant for children with secure child–mother attachment.

Third, current research also provides evidence that child–care provider attachment can influence children's stress management. In a recent study (Eckstein-Madry, Piskernik, & Ahnert, 2020), we hypothesized that care providers in child care might be able to help 3- to 5-year-olds from socioeconomically disadvantaged families with limitations in stress regulation to achieve better regulation. We explored the children's diurnal cortisol rhythm based on 12 saliva samples taken across 3 days a week. These were on Sundays, when the children spend all day at home, and on Mondays and Fridays, when the children spend a substantial amount of time in preschool. Unfortunately, these children had significantly lower AQS scores with their mothers than with their care providers. They also displayed elevated stress in the form of heightened diurnal cortisol release and flatter diurnal cortisol decline (particularly on Sundays), reflecting lower capacities to regulate stress as compared to their peers from families with more socioeconomic resources. Most importantly, greater attachment security to the care providers was associated with greater diurnal cortisol decline, which was particularly obvious on Fridays in children from socioeconomically disadvantaged families.

Conclusion

This chapter provides evidence that child–care provider attachment is both functionally and ontogenetically different than child–parent attachment. In other words, the formation of secure child–care provider attachments emerges differently for children of different ages and gender. Attachment formation in child care seems to be predominantly shaped by care provider behaviors toward the group as a whole. Measures of care providers' dyadic sensitivity (as it is with parents) only predict child–care provider attachment in small groups of infants and toddlers. Measures of care providers' group-focused sensitivity, however, are more strongly associated with secure child–care provider attachment after toddlerhood and reflect the circumstances of the child care setting and the unique role of child care providers. This means that children's social observational learning of how a care provider responds to peers in the group probably adds to the child's own experience in shaping the security of attachment and the IWM that derives from it. In the context of child care, IWMs might be predominantly a more broadly representational type of IWM and less individualized. Furthermore, current research provides detailed evidence on how attachment in child care can affect children's cognitive performance, behavioral adjustment, and stress management. These attachments are less likely to be secure than child–parent attachments, however, despite being influential.

The ontogenetically different process of attachment formation, however, puts greater challenges on the professional practice of child care providers. We thus further need to identify relevant types of care provider behaviors that best promote secure child–care provider relationships and closeness (e.g., van Schaik, Leseman, & de Haan, 2017). As supportive child–care provider relationships are desirable both early and later in the educational process, it is extremely important to assess child–care provider relationships broadly with security of attachment and closeness included.

REFERENCES

Ahnert, L. (2005). Parenting and alloparenting: The impact on attachment in human. In S. Carter, L. Ahnert, K. E. Grossmann, S. B. Hrdy, M. E. Lamb, et al. (Eds.), *Attachment and bonding: A new synthesis* (pp. 229–244). Cambridge, MA: MIT Press.

Ahnert, L., Milatz, A., Kappler, G., Schneiderwind, J., & Fischer, R. (2013). The impact of teacher–child relationships on child cognitive performance as explored by a priming paradigm. *Developmental Psychology, 49,* 554–567.

Ahnert, L., Pinquart, M., & Lamb, M. E. (2006). Security of children's relationships with nonparental care providers: A meta-analysis. *Child Development, 77,* 664–679.

Ahnert, L., Rickert, H., & Lamb, M. E. (2000). Shared caregiving: Comparisons between home and child-care settings. *Developmental Psychology, 36,* 339–351.

Ainsworth, M. D. S., Blehar, M. C., Waters, E., & Wall, S. (1978). *Patterns of attachment: A psychological study of the Strange Situation.* Hillsdale, NJ: Erlbaum.

Buyse, E., Verschueren, K., & Doumen, S. (2011). Preschoolers' attachment to mother and risk for adjustment problems in kindergarten: Can teachers make a difference? *Social Development, 20,* 33–50.

Eckstein-Madry, T., Piskernik, B., & Ahnert, L. (2020). Attachment and stress regulation in socioeconomically disadvantaged children: Can public child-care compensate? *Infant Mental Health Journal.* [Epub ahead of print]

Ereky-Stevens, K., Funder, A., Katschnig, T., Malmberg, L.-E., & Datler, W. (2018). Relationship building between toddlers and new caregivers in out-of-home childcare: Attachment security and caregiver sensitivity. *Early Childhood Research Quarterly, 42,* 270–279.

Fabes, R. A., Hanish, L. D., & Martin, C. L. (2003). Children at play: The role of peers in understanding the effects of child care. *Child Development, 74,* 1039–1043.

Hamre, B. K., & Pianta, R. C. (2001). Early teacher–child relationships and the trajectory of children's school outcomes through eighth grade. *Child Development, 72,* 625–638.

Hong, S. L. S., Sabol, T. J., Burchinal, M. R., Tarullo, L., Zaslow, M., & Peisner-Feinberg, E. S. (2019). ECE quality indicators and child outcomes: Analyses of six large child care studies. *Early Childhood Research Quarterly, 49,* 202–217.

Howes, C., Galinsky, E., & Kontos, S. (1998). Child care caregiver sensitivity and attachment. *Social Development, 7,* 25–36.

Howes, C., & Spieker, S. (2016). Attachment relationships in the context of multiple caregivers. In J. Cassidy & P. R. Shaver (Eds.), *Handbook of attachment:*

Theory, research, and clinical applications (3rd ed., pp. 314–329). New York: Guilford Press.

Leaper, C. (2002). Parenting girls and boys. In M. Bornstein (Ed.), *Handbook of parenting: Vol. 1. Children and parenting* (pp. 189–225). Mahwah, NJ: Erlbaum.

Pianta, R. C. (2001). *STRS. Student-Teacher Relationship Scale.* Lutz, FL: Psychological Assessment Resources.

Pinquart, M., Feußner, C., & Ahnert, L. (2012). Meta-analytic evidence for stability in attachments from infancy to early adulthood. *Attachment and Human Development, 14,* 1–30.

Sagi, A., van IJzendoorn, M. H., Aviezer, O., Donnell, F., Koren-Karie, N., Joels, T., & Harel, Y. (1995). Attachments in multiple-caregiver and multiple-infant environment: The case of the Israeli kibbutzim. *Monographs of the Society for Research in Child Development, 60,* 71–91.

van Schaik, S. D. M., Leseman, P. P. M., & de Haan, M. (2017). Using a group-centered approach to observe interactions in early childhood education. *Child Development, 89,* 897–913.

Waters, E. (1995). The Attachment-Q-Set (Version 3.0). *Monographs of the Society for Research in Child Development, 60,* 71–91.

Waters, E., & Cummings, E. M. (2000). A secure base from which to explore close relationships. *Child Development, 71,* 164–172.

Zaviska, N., Mayer, D., Deichmann, F., Eckstein-Madry, T., & Ahnert, L. (2020). *Care providers' promptness in group care: Relations to children's attachment and behavioral adjustment.* Manuscript submitted for publication.

CHAPTER 5

Defining Attachment Relationships and Attachment Security from a Personality–Social Perspective on Adult Attachment

Phillip R. Shaver
Mario Mikulincer

In this chapter, we deal with two fundamental theoretical issues: (1) the criteria for defining attachment relationships and attachment figures in adulthood and (2) the cognitive–affective aspects of the adult sense of attachment security. Our discussion is based on a personality and social-psychological perspective and informed by the large body of social and personality research on attachment in adulthood (see Mikulincer & Shaver, 2016).

Defining Attachment Relationships and Attachment Figures

Although attachment theory is fairly easy to understand as an account of the formation and maintenance of emotional bonds with relationship partners (i.e., "becoming attached"), it is important to stress the uniqueness of attachment relationships and attachment figures. Attachment figures are not just close, important relationship partners, and not all interactions with attachment figures are attachment-related interactions.

The Uniqueness of Attachment Figures

The term *attachment figure* has a specific meaning in attachment theory. According to the theory (e.g., Ainsworth, 1991; Bowlby, 1988), attachment figures are special individuals who are targets of proximity seeking. People tend to seek and benefit from proximity to their attachment figures in times of need. Moreover, these figures are expected to function as a safe haven in times of need—providing protection, comfort, and relief—and as a secure base, encouraging autonomous pursuit of nonattachment goals while remaining available if needed. When attachment figures accomplish these two functions, they can provide a sense of safety and security, instill feelings of being loved and cared for, and facilitate effective functioning and thriving in nonattachment activities, such as exploration, learning, interpersonal exchanges, and sexual mating. Based on this narrow definition of an attachment figure, a relationship partner becomes such a figure only when he or she is expected to function as a safe haven and secure base and is sought out in times of need with the hope of receiving protection, comfort, and support.

During infancy, primary caregivers (usually one or both parents, but also grandparents, older siblings, or child care providers) are likely to serve attachment functions. In later childhood, adolescence, and adulthood, a wider variety of relationship partners can serve as attachment figures, including siblings, other relatives, familiar coworkers, teachers or coaches, close friends, and romantic partners. There may also be context-specific attachment figures—real or potential sources of comfort and support in specific milieus, such as therapists in therapeutic settings or leaders in organizational settings (e.g., business organizations or the military). Moreover, groups, institutions, pets, and symbolic personages (e.g., God) can become targets of proximity seeking and sources of security (but also see Sroufe, Chapter 2, this volume). There is evidence that many adults believe they can and do obtain protection and comfort from God, leaders, or pets (e.g., Granqvist & Kirkpatrick, 2016; Mayseless & Popper, 2019; Zilcha-Mano, Mikulincer, & Shaver, 2012).

Using cognitive research techniques, Mikulincer, Gillath, and Shaver (2002) provided some of the first experimental evidence for the uniqueness of attachment figures. In their studies, subliminal priming with a threat word (e.g., illness, failure) heightened the cognitive accessibility of mental representations (i.e., names) of people designated as attachment figures. These effects were not found for the names of people other than attachment figures, including family members who were not nominated as attachment security providers. In line with Bowlby's theory, it seems that when threats loom the human mind turns automatically to mental representations of attachment figures, but not to just any relationship partner.

The Uniqueness of Attachment Interactions and Attachment Bonds

Not every interaction with an attachment figure is an attachment-related interaction. A married couple can enjoy making plans for a summer vacation, discuss what to bring to their cabin, and laugh at each other's jokes, but if no partner is frightened or feels threatened by separation, attachment issues are not likely to come to the fore (although such cooperative interactions may help to cement or maintain an emotional bond because they provide evidence of mutual interest, affection, and trustworthiness). Moreover, in relationships between an athlete and his or her coach, many of the interactions may be concerned with teaching, exploring, and learning, without the potential attachment aspects of the relationship being salient. Even in a therapeutic relationship, where one person is formally coming to the other for support and guidance, there are moments of mutual joking and kibitzing that do not necessarily serve attachment functions.

The existence of an attachment relationship may not always be evident. When neither partner is threatened, demoralized, or in need, the two may seem quite autonomous, and their interactions may be more affiliative or exploratory than attachment oriented. But when one person is distressed, and especially if separation is threatened or loss occurs, the attachment bond becomes evident (Bowlby, 1969/1982; Fraley & Shaver, 2016). There are other kinds of emotional bonds, based on familiarity, shared activities, biological relatedness, and respect. When these bonds are threatened or broken, a person may be distressed, but usually not to the same extent or for as long as when attachment bonds are severed.

In adulthood, a long-term romantic or pair-bond relationship is the prototype of adult attachment (Bowlby, 1979; Shaver, Hazan, & Bradshaw, 1988). In fact, attachment researchers have consistently found that romantic partners are often adults' primary attachment figures (Zeifman & Hazan, 2016). Nevertheless, adult pair bonds involve not only the attachment system but also the caregiving and, often, the sexual system (Hazan & Shaver, 1994; Mikulincer & Shaver, 2018). In romantic relationships, partners occupy not only the "person in need" position, expecting to gain security, comfort, and guidance from their mate. They usually also occupy the "caregiver" position, in which they provide empathy, care, and support to their partner in need. In addition, romantic partners are often each other's sole or primary source of sexual gratification and shared reproduction.

The Sense of Attachment Security

When attachment figures successfully provide a safe haven and a secure base in times of need, they instill a sense of attachment security (i.e., confidence that the world is safe, that one is worthy and lovable, and that others will be supportive when needed). This subjective sense is a result of the smooth functioning of the attachment system, including effective support seeking in times of need and the reliable availability of a responsive attachment figure. This sense is renewed every time a person notices that an actual, recalled, or imaginary caring attachment figure is available in times of need. There is evidence that experimentally priming mental representations of a responsive attachment figure (e.g., exposing participants to the name or picture of an attachment figure, consciously or unconsciously) infuses a temporary sense of safety and security, even for chronically insecure people (see Mikulincer & Shaver, 2016).

From our perspective, the sense of attachment security is not just a feeling or the absence of a feeling (e.g., the lack of fear, insecurity, or threat). It is partly "felt" (emotionally), partly assumed and expected (cognitively), and partly unconscious. Moreover, this sense cannot simply be equated with a secure attachment orientation or style. Only when it is the most accessible and dominant representation within a person's network of attachment-related memories and working models does this sense result in a secure style, chronically affecting and reflecting a person's thinking, emotions, and behavior across different relational contexts. For people with a less secure style, the sense of attachment security is also available, but in a less accessible and less dominant position within their attachment-relevant associative network (Mikulincer & Shaver, 2016). At certain times, the sense of security is associated with a specific relationship or relationship partner; at other times, it depends on particular episodic memories or imagined interactions in which a partner was or is responsive in times of need. For the chronically insecure person, these mental processes are neither easily nor frequently engaged. But they can become more accessible in the context of specific security-enhancing relationships, or when an actual, recalled, or imaginary partner is responsive to bids for proximity and support. In other words, even in the most insecure individuals, one can find what we have called "islands of security" (Mikulincer & Shaver, 2016), which can be reached experimentally or naturally, depending on the context.

According to our model of attachment-system functioning in adulthood (Mikulincer & Shaver, 2003), the sense of attachment security includes both declarative and procedural knowledge organized around a relational prototype or "secure base script" (Waters & Waters, 2006; see Waters, Waters, & Waters, Chapter 14, this volume). This script contains something like the following if–then propositions: "If I encounter an obstacle and/or become distressed, I can approach a significant other for help; he or she is likely to be available and supportive; I will experience relief and comfort as a result of proximity to this person; I can then return to other activities." Having many experiences that contribute to the construction of this script within a specific relationship or across different relational contexts helps a person maintain a sense of equanimity, optimism, and hope without necessarily triggering a search for actual support. Indeed, adolescents and adults who score higher on measures of attachment security are more likely to have rich and fully developed secure base scripts in mind when thinking about or narrating threat-related stories or dreams (e.g., Mikulincer, Shaver, Sapir-Lavid, & Avihou-Kanza, 2009).

The sense of attachment security also includes a reservoir of positive beliefs about distress management, other people, and oneself. Interactions with responsive attachment figures make it easy for a person to believe that most of life's problems are solvable and most distress is manageable. These interactions also create positive beliefs about other people and heighten confidence in most relationship partners' benevolence, kindness, and good will. In addition, people learn to perceive themselves as strong and competent, valuable, lovable, and special—thanks to being valued, loved, and viewed as special by caring attachment figures. Of course, people with a secure attachment orientation or style habitually hold positive beliefs about self and others across different relational contexts, whereas people with a less secure style hold these positive beliefs only in contexts in which actual or imagined interactions with a responsive relationship partner arouses feelings of being loved and cared for.

The sense of attachment security also includes a reservoir of useful procedural knowledge concerning emotion regulation and ways to cope with stress. During interactions with a responsive attachment figure, people learn that they can confidently and openly express their vulnerability and neediness and rely on the other's support, and that these actions yield positive outcomes. They also learn that they can often solve important problems themselves, seeking help only when needed, and that turning to others is an effective way to bolster their own considerable coping capacity.

Another aspect of the sense of security concerns attitudes toward one's emotions and other mental states. During security-enhancing interactions with a supportive attachment figure, people learn to expect that awareness of, reflection on, and expression of feelings, desires, and thoughts will result in positive outcomes. These beliefs encourage openness to mental states, nondistorted experience of these states, and accurate expression of feelings to others. This openness is manifested in what Fonagy, Steele, Steele, Moran, and Higgittt (1991) called self-reflective or mentalizing capacity—the ability to notice, think about, and understand mental states, including one's own and those of other people. For individuals whose attachment figures have been available and responsive, the expression of negative mental states usually leads to distress-alleviating support and guidance (Cassidy, 1994).

The sense of security also includes prorelational cognitions—beliefs that closeness is rewarding and that intimate relationships are beneficial. These beliefs make it easier for a person to get psychologically close to a relationship partner, express needs, desires, and hopes, and ask for support when needed. They also predispose a person to feel comfortable with intimacy and interdependence; emphasize the benefits of being together; and offer generous interpretations of a partner's ambiguous or disappointing behavior.

According to our model (Mikulincer & Shaver, 2003), possessing this reservoir of declarative and procedure knowledge makes it less necessary to rely on psychological defenses that distort perception and generate intrapersonal or interpersonal conflict. As a result, the sense of security can lead people to devote mental resources that otherwise would be employed in preventive, defensive maneuvers to more prosocial and growth-oriented activities (e.g., exploration, caregiving). Moreover, by being confident that support is available when needed, people can take calculated risks and accept important challenges that contribute to the broadening of their perspectives and facilitate the pursuit of self-actualization.

Concluding Remarks

One of the most important insights of contemporary psychology and evolutionary biology is that human beings are inherently social—that the human brain is primarily a social device. Attachment theory and research have made important contributions to this realization. By examining the infant–caregiver relationship in detail within a pioneering biosocial-evolutionary framework, Bowlby provided a model for personality and social psychologists who study adult close relationships. In return, their research has provided many insights into adult attachment, the special features of attachment relationships, the crucial role of security in maintaining mental equilibrium, and the various ways in which security can be maintained or undermined.

REFERENCES

Ainsworth, M. D. S. (1991). Attachment and other affectional bonds across the life cycle. In C. M. Parkes, J. Stevenson-Hinde, & P. Marris (Eds.), *Attachment across the life cycle* (pp. 33–51). New York: Routledge.

Bowlby, J. (1979). *The making and breaking of affectional bonds*. London: Tavistock.

Bowlby, J. (1982). *Attachment and loss: Vol. 1. Attachment* (2nd ed.). New York: Basic Books. (Original work published 1969)

Bowlby, J. (1988). *A secure base: Clinical applications of attachment theory*. London: Routledge.

Cassidy, J. (1994). Emotion regulation: Influences of attachment relationships. In N. Fox (Ed.), The development of emotion regulation. *Monographs of the Society for Research in Child Development, 59*(2–3, Serial No. 240), 228–249.

Fonagy, P., Steele, M., Steele, H., Moran, G. S., & Higgitt, P. (1991). The capacity for understanding mental states: The reflective self in parent and child and its significance for security of attachment. *Infant Mental Health Journal, 12,* 201–218.

Fraley, R. C., & Shaver, P. R. (2016). Attachment, loss, and grief: Bowlby's views, new developments, and current controversies. In J. Cassidy & P. R. Shaver (Eds.), *Handbook of attachment: Theory, research, and clinical applications* (3rd ed., pp. 40–62). New York: Guilford Press.

Granqvist, P., & Kirkpatrick, L. A. (2016). Attachment and religious representations and behavior. In J Cassidy & P. R. Shaver (Eds.), *Handbook of attachment: Theory, research, and clinical applications* (3rd ed., pp. 917–940). New York: Guilford Press.

Hazan, C., & Shaver, P. R. (1994). Attachment as an organizational framework for research on close relationships. *Psychological Inquiry, 5,* 1–22.

Mayseless, O., & Popper, M. (2019). Attachment and leadership: Review and new insights. *Current Opinion in Psychology, 25,* 157–161.

Mikulincer, M., Gillath, O., & Shaver, P. R. (2002). Activation of the attachment system in adulthood: Threat-related primes increase the accessibility of mental representations of attachment figures. *Journal of Personality and Social Psychology, 83,* 881–895.

Mikulincer, M., & Shaver, P. R. (2003). The attachment behavioral system in adulthood: Activation, psychodynamics, and interpersonal processes. In M. P. Zanna (Ed.), *Advances in experimental social psychology* (Vol. 35, pp. 53–152). New York: Academic Press.

Mikulincer, M., & Shaver, P. R. (2016). *Attachment in adulthood: Structure, dynamics, and change* (2nd ed.). New York: Guilford Press.

Mikulincer, M., & Shaver, P. R. (2018). A behavioral systems approach to romantic love relationships: Attachment, caregiving, and sex. In R. J. Sternberg & K. Sternberg (Eds.), *The new psychology of love* (2nd ed., pp. 259–279). Cambridge, UK: Cambridge University Press.

Mikulincer, M., Shaver, P. R., Sapir-Lavid, Y., & Avihou-Kanza, N. (2009). What's inside the minds of securely and insecurely attached people?: The secure-base script and its associations with attachment-style dimensions. *Journal of Personality and Social Psychology, 97,* 615–633.

Shaver, P. R., Hazan, C., & Bradshaw, D. (1988). Love as attachment: The integration of three behavioral systems. In R. J. Sternberg & M. Barnes (Eds.), *The psychology of love* (pp. 68–99). New Haven, CT: Yale University Press.

Waters, H. S., & Waters, E. (2006). The attachment working models concept: Among other things, we build script-like representations of secure base experiences. *Attachment and Human Development, 8,* 185–198.

Zeifman, D., & Hazan, C. (2016). Pair bonds as attachments: Mounting evidence in support of Bowlby's hypothesis. In J. Cassidy & P. R. Shaver (Eds.), *Handbook of attachment: Theory, research, and clinical applications* (3rd ed., pp. 416–434). New York: Guilford Press.

Zilcha-Mano, S., Mikulincer, M., & Shaver, P. R. (2012). Pets as safe havens and secure bases: The moderating role of pet attachment orientations. *Journal of Research in Personality, 46,* 571–580.

CHAPTER 6

The Nature and Developmental Origins of Attachment Security in Adulthood

Deborah Jacobvitz
Nancy Hazen

Attachment is a lifelong process influencing humans' capacities to form and maintain our closest relationships. According to Bowlby (1969/1982), attachment behavior evolved to serve the biological function of protecting helpless infants from harm. Attachment security is based on repeated experiences with their primary caregivers during the first years of life. When young children need help or care, their attachment system is activated and they seek their primary caregivers to provide a safe haven. If their caregiver is accessible and responds with comfort and reassurance, infants will form a secure attachment relationship. These early experiences become the basis for trust in the availability of others in times of need. Stronger, wiser, and responsive caregivers can reassure the child, who can then use them as a secure base to explore their environment. But what does it mean to be securely attached as an adult? In this chapter, we discuss the nature and developmental origins of attachment security in adulthood, what kinds of relationships qualify as attachment relationships, and the extent to which early models of attachment can be revised over the lifespan.

Over the lifespan, individuals form multiple attachments, not just with parents or other primary caregivers, but with friends and romantic partners. Ainsworth (1985) defined an affectional bond as a "relatively long-lived tie in which the partner is important as a unique individual, interchangeable with none other, from whom inexplicable, involuntary separation would cause distress, and whose loss would occasion grief" (p. 799). Attachment is a particular type of affectional bond in which the more vulnerable member of the relationship can use their attachment figure as a secure base and safe haven. Because the parent–child relationship is inherently unequal, with parents being the stronger and wiser individuals, children cannot serve as attachment figures to their parents, although this may change when children become adults, and their parents require care. However, adults with secure representations of attachment can take *both* roles in romantic relationships and close friendships. When one person is feeling vulnerable, tired, ill, or fearful, the other can serve as an attachment figure and provide support. As noted by Feeney and Woodhouse (2016), adults' need for emotional support during such times "should not be regarded as childish or immature dependence; instead should be respected as an intrinsic part of human nature that contributes to health and well-being" (p. 827).

Assessment of Attachment Security Using the Adult Attachment Interview

Bowlby (1969/1982) used the term *mental representations of attachment-related experiences* to explain how early experiences shape a person's understanding and expectations of relationships. To operationalize representational models of attachment, Main and colleagues developed the Adult Attachment Interview (AAI; George, Kaplan, & Main, 1985), a semi-structured interview that assesses adults' current state of mind regarding attachment experiences by probing for memories of their relationships with parents during childhood. Adults are faced with the task of producing and reflecting upon attachment-related memories while trying to maintain a collaborative and coherent conversation with the interviewer (Main, Goldwyn, & Hesse, 2003). Attachment classifications assess adults' state of mind with respect to attachment in general, rather than security in specific attachment relationships. The AAI is designed to surprise the unconscious and reveal defensive processes that may impair adults' abilities to provide a secure base and safe haven for their children, and to provide and accept such support in adult attachment relationships.

Main and colleagues developed the AAI categories by examining differences in discourse patterns of mothers according to their mother–infant attachment classification in the Strange Situation Procedure (SSP; Ainsworth, Blehar, Waters, & Wall, 1978). The ability to think openly, flexibly, and coherently about relationships with parents during childhood, including painful early experiences, is a hallmark of security in adulthood (Main et al., 2003). Just as infants classified as secure can flexibly alternate between attachment and exploration in the SSP, adults classified as secure in the AAI can flexibly provide evidence that they value attachment relationships while also providing objective evaluations of their early attachment experiences. Being able to objectively access childhood experiences enables them to mindfully provide sensitive care to their infant, even when those experiences are negative. Indeed, secure AAI classifications have shown robust associations with their infants' attachment security although sensitive caregiving does not fully explain the intergenerational transmission of attachment. van IJzendoorn and Bakermans-Kranenburg (2019) suggest considering the context and infants' differential susceptibility to sensitivity based on temperament, as well as including other aspects of parenting like autonomy support, synchrony, and protective parenting.

Secure attachment also has been linked to the quality of secure base/safe haven support in adult romantic relationships. Similar to children with secure working models, when securely attached adults become emotionally distressed, they are comfortable seeking romantic partners to act as adult "caregivers" by proving safe haven functions (Feeney & Woodhouse, 2016). Secure adults are able also to serve as attachment figures to romantic partners and friends by providing responsive support when they are in need without becoming overinvolved or controlling. For example, adults classified as secure showed greater secure base use, and offered more secure base support, in couple interaction tasks, than those classified as insecure (Crowell et al., 2002). Moreover, female partners classified as secure provided more support to male partners in a stressful situation, but only when the partners sought support, showing sensitivity to the partner (Simpson, Rholes, Oriña, & Grich, 2002).

The three types of insecure attachment classifications—dismissing, preoccupied, and unresolved—are based on the avoidant, ambivalent, and disorganized classifications of infant–caregiver attachment assessed in the SSP. The dismissing pattern is manifested by defensive processes, whereby adults insist they cannot remember early experiences with their parents and often minimize attachment-related distress by speaking glowingly about childhood experiences with parents while simultaneously providing little or no evidence of parental support. Similarly, infants classified as avoidant were observed to minimize expressions of distress so as to not push away a mother who rejects such behavior (Ainsworth et al., 1978). Studies suggest that this minimization of overt distress is based on defensive processes rather than individual traits. When attachment needs are aroused, infants classified as avoidant in the SSP show elevated heart rate, similar to those classified as secure (Spangler & Grossmann, 1993). Similarly, skin conductance measures indicated that adults classified as dismissing in the AAI experience physiological distress when discussing childhood experiences (Dozier & Kobak, 1992).

Adults with dismissing romantic attachment styles (termed *avoidant* in self-report assessments of adult attachment) are theorized to be uncomfortable with close relationships and develop a false sense of self-reliance through defensively excluding painful memories of childhood rejection by their caregivers (see Mikulincer & Shaver, Chapter 26, this volume). Thus, secure base and safe haven needs expressed by their own children or by intimate partners can threaten their defenses, and they lack the trust needed to provide or accept such support from romantic partners (Feeney & Woodhouse, 2016). For example, women higher in attachment avoidance provided less support to their romantic partners in stressful situations than women lower in avoidance, even when their partners sought such support (Simpson et al., 2002). Moreover, avoidant mothers reported feeling more emotionally detached and were less supportive of their preschool children during laboratory tasks (Rholes, Simpson, & Blakely, 1995).

Adults classified as *preoccupied* on the AAI have difficulty providing a coherent overview of experience with parents during childhood; they ramble on and on, angrily recounting their parents' faults, losing track of the discourse context. They have difficulty taking a balanced view of relationships, often blaming parents for relationship difficulties. Similarly, infants classified as ambivalent show dysregulated behavior, alternating between clingy and angry behaviors following separations from their caregiver, and cannot be calmed by the caregiver when distressed (Ainsworth et al., 1978). Main and colleagues (2003) theorized that adults who are preoccupied carry forward patterns of inconsistent care and interfere with their infant's ongoing needs and interests, often leading to an ambivalent attachment relationship with their infant. In adult romantic relationships, individuals showing the preoccupied pattern (termed *anxious* in self-report assessments) also often alternate between clingy, overly dependent behaviors and anger (Feeney & Woodhouse, 2016). For example, in stressful couple interaction tasks, more anxious women displayed strong stress and anxiety and engaged in more negative behavior with partners (Simpson, Rholes, & Phillips, 1996).

Adults are placed in a fourth AAI category, *unresolved with respect to trauma,* based on lapses in the monitoring of reasoning and discourse during discussions of abuse and loss. These lapses involve statements that contradict our understanding of time and causality, for example, "I killed my father by wishing he was dead" or "My mother helps me decide on my career path" (though the mother passed away 10 years prior). Displays of mental disorganization are thought to stem from fear connected with traumatic experiences. Unresolved mothers have been found to engage in frightening/frightened behavior with their infant, which forecasts infant attachment disorganization (Lyons-Ruth & Jacobvitz, 2016). Unresolved adults also tend to be overly controlling with romantic partners and are more likely to experience relationship violence.

Adult Attachment Pairings and Couple Relationship Quality

In infancy, assessment of attachment is relationship-specific, such that infants might have a secure relationship with one caregiver and an insecure relationship with another. In adulthood, however, attachment is assessed at the individual level since it is assumed to have been internalized as a generalized working model and, therefore, to have trait-like characteristics. However, attachment representations have been shown to be modifiable in response to ongoing experiences in relationships, suggesting they are a characteristic of the relationship and not the individual. Adult relationships are interdependent and reciprocal; thus, it is important to examine how partners with different types of attachment representations provide secure base and safe haven support to each other by examining AAI pairings. Few studies have examined this, but findings indicate that secure women's ability to provide and receive such support is hampered if their male partner is insecure. For example, Creasey (2002) found that couple conflict during interactions was greater when the husband was classified as insecure, and a secure wife was unable to buffer the interaction quality. Examining specific insecure classifications, we found that when secure wives interacting with dismissing husbands offer support or seek reassurance, their husbands often use distancing strategies such as derogatory humor and snarky remarks (Jacobvitz et al., 2015). Furthermore, secure parents' caregiving sensitivity is lower when they have an insecure spouse, primarily because mismatches in couples' attachment representations predict marital negativity, which spills over to caregiving quality (Poulsen, Hazen, & Jacobvitz, 2019).

Change and Continuity in Attachment Representations

Infant attachment security predicts security of attachment in adulthood, but considerable discontinuity has also been reported (Sroufe, Egeland, Carlson, & Collins, 2005). Internal working models of attachment evolve and are dynamic rather than static and immutable. Some adults who recount experiences of parental neglect, rejection, and/or abuse can repair past attachment disturbances, break the intergenerational cycle of attachment insecurity, and provide sensitive and responsive care for their children. Main and colleagues (2003) define *earned security* as the ability to have a secure state of mind with respect to attachment despite recounting very unloving relationship experiences with both parents during childhood. Experiencing emotional support from an alternate attachment figure during childhood was associated with adults' capacity to describe early negative experiences coherently, which forecasts developing a secure attachment with their own infant (Saunders, Jacobvitz, Zaccagnino, Beverung, & Hazen, 2011). Therapy can also be effective in helping adults transform insecure working models into secure models. It is unclear, however, whether representational models of attachment are revised based on later attachment-related experiences, or whether adults carry multiple models of different attachment figures, or of the same caregiver, if their relationship with that caregiver changes over time. Evidence that models of attachment with each parent coalesce to some degree come from a study in which AAIs were administered to young adults twice, first with questions that referred to only one parent and later with questions referring to the other parent (Furman & Simon, 2004). While most adults (68%) showed concordant states of mind in both interviews, 38% were relationship specific. However, it is unclear whether adults had similar attachment classifications with each parent during childhood or whether they merged into one working model over time. Understanding whether adults carry multiple models has implications for considering attachment security as an individual or relationship-specific characteristic, and for explaining change and continuity in attachment security over time.

Conclusions and Future Directions

To better understand the meaning of attachment security in adulthood, it is important to investigate the conditions that underlie transformations in attachment security over time. This will be critical for creating effective therapeutic interventions to increase secure attachment. It is also important to study couples' joint attachments to gain more insight into how partners use each other as a secure base and support the sensitive care of their children. Finally, attachment researchers must avoid using attachment to explain every positive or negative developmental outcome. Close relationships serve a variety of functions, and attachment research should focus on secure base and safe haven functions of close relationships. Adults with secure representations of attachment should have an advantage only in relation to behaviors that serve, or relate directly or indirectly to, secure base and safe haven functions.

REFERENCES

Ainsworth, M. D. (1985). Attachments across the life-span. *Bulletin of New York Academy of Medicine, 61*(9), 791–812.

Ainsworth, M. D. S., Blehar, M. C., Waters, E., & Wall, S. (1978). *Patterns of attachment: A psychological study of the Strange Situation*. Mahwah, NJ: Erlbaum.

Bowlby, J. (1982). *Attachment and loss: Vol. 1. Attachment*. New York: Basic Books (Original work published 1969)

Creasey, G. (2002). Associations between working models of attachment and conflict management behavior in romantic couples. *Journal of Counseling Psychology, 49*, 365–375.

Crowell, J. A., Treboux, D., Gao, Y., Fyffe, C., Pan, H., & Waters, E. (2002). Assessing secure base behavior in adulthood: Development of a measure, links to adult attachment representations and relations to couples' communication and reports of relationships. *Developmental Psychology, 38*(5), 679–693.

Dozier, M., & Kobak, R. R. (1992). Psychophysiology in attachment interviews: Converging evidence for deactivating strategies. *Child Development, 63,* 1473–1480.

Feeney, B. C., & Woodhouse, S. S. (2016). Caregiving. In J. Cassidy & P. R. Shaver (Eds.), *Handbook of attachment: Theory, research, and clinical applications* (3rd ed., pp. 827–851). New York: Guilford Press.

Furman, W., & Simon, V. A. (2004). Concordance in states of mind and styles with respect to mothers and father. *Developmental Psychology, 6,* 1239–1247.

George, C., Kaplan, N., & Main, M. (1985). *Adult Attachment Interview.* Unpublished manuscript, University of California, Berkeley.

Jacobvitz, D., Messina, S., Reisz, S., Pettit, K., Poulsen, H., & Hazen, N. (2015, March). *Family dynamics from an attachment perspective: Parents' attachment pairings predict couple and parent–infant interactions.* Paper presented at the biannual meeting of the Society for Research in Child Development, Philadelphia, PA.

Lyons-Ruth, K., & Jacobvitz, D. (2016). Attachment disorganization from infancy to adulthood: Neurobiological correlates, parenting contexts, and pathways to disorder. In J. Cassidy & P. R. Shaver (Eds.), *Handbook of attachment: Theory, research, and clinical applications* (3rd ed., pp. 667–695) New York: Guilford Press.

Main, M., Goldwyn, R., & Hesse, E. (2003). *Adult attachment scoring and classification system. Version 7.2.* Unpublished manuscript, University of California, Berkeley, CA.

Poulsen, H. B., Hazen, N., & Jacobvitz, D. (2019). Parents' joint attachment representations and caregiving: The moderating role of marital quality. *Attachment and Human Development, 21,* 597–615.

Rholes, W. S., Simpson, J. A., & Blakely, B. S. (1995). Adult attachment styles and mothers' relationships with their young children. *Personal Relationships, 2,* 35–54.

Saunders, R. S., Jacobvitz, D., Zaccagnino, M., Beverung, L. M., & Hazen, N. (2011). Pathways to earned-security: The role of alternative support figures. *Attachment and Human Development, 13,* 403–420.

Simpson, J. A., Rholes, W. S., Oriña, M. M., & Grich, J. (2002). Working models of attachment, support giving, and support seeking in a stressful situation. *Personality and Social Psychology Bulletin, 28,* 598–608.

Simpson, J. A., Rholes, W. S., & Phillips, D. (1996). Conflict in close relationships: An attachment perspective. *Journal of Personality and Social Psychology, 71,* 889–914.

Spangler, G., & Grossmann, K. E. (1993). Biobehavioral organization in securely and insecurely attached infants. *Child Development, 64,* 1439–1450.

Sroufe, L. A., Egeland, B., Carlson, E. A., & Collins, W. A. (2005). *The development of the person: The Minnesota Study of Risk and Adaptation from Birth to Adulthood.* New York: Guilford Press.

van IJzendoorn, M. H., & Bakermans-Kranenberg, M. J. (2019). Bridges across the intergenerational transmission of attachment gap. *Current Opinion in Psychology, 25,* 31–36.

CHAPTER 7

Casting a Wider Net

Parents, Pair Bonds, and Other Attachment Partners in Adulthood

Ashleigh I. Aviles
Debra M. Zeifman

> All of us, from the cradle to the grave, are happiest when
> life is organized as a series of excursions, long or short,
> from the secure base provided by our attachment figures.
> —JOHN BOWLBY (1988)

When the 2020 coronavirus pandemic required individuals to physically distance themselves from others, a common ritual emerged across the world: porch visits in which grown children of elderly parents visited while standing at a safe distance apart. The universal need to "touch base" with loved ones in order to feel whole reflects the important role attachment relationships play in supporting health and well-being throughout life. Adults, like children, seek contact with attachment figures who provide a sense of emotional security. Building upon Bowlby's theory, adult attachment researchers have argued that attachment needs in adults are typically met within the context of sexual pair bonds—partnerships between sexual mates that also involve intense emotional bonds (Hazan & Shaver, 1987; Zeifman & Hazan, 2016). Many of the same features that characterize infant–caregiver attachments also distinguish adult pair bonds, including a desire to protect and maintain the relationship, and a strong resistance to separation. In addition to having similar psychological and behavioral dynamics, adult romantic relationships and childhood attachments also share similar neurochemical underpinnings (Feldman, 2017).

While adult pair bonds are the most common manifestation of adult attachment, shifting cultural norms and demographic patterns in recent decades suggest that, for a growing segment of society, attachment figures may include other types of close relationship partners. DePaulo and others have argued that friends and family members, such as siblings, often provide the same support that spouses do in marriage (DePaulo & Morris, 2005). One profound difference between attachment in childhood versus in adulthood is that adults have the ability to choose, replace, or forgo attachment partners. In this chapter, we argue that future attachment research should explore the full range and diversity of adult relationships. As increasing numbers of adults delay or abstain from long-term sexual partnerships, researchers need to consider whether and how various types of nonsexual relationships function to satisfy attachment needs.

Because sexual partnerships are the most common context in which children are reared and long-term emotional bonds usually accompany sexual interactions, evolutionary psychologists have argued that pair bonds evolved because they confer unique advantages to individuals and their offspring. Having strong ties to sexual partners is associated with higher levels of life satisfaction and improved health outcomes for adult pairs, as well as for their children. A common view is that sexual attraction brings sexual partners together initially, and rewarding sexual interactions then promote the formation and persistence of emotional bonds (Zeifman, 2019). A logical question might therefore be: In the absence of sex, what serves to unite partners and keep them attached? Are close friendships characterized by the same features as attachment relationships? Are bonds between nonsexual partners as intense and enduring as sexual pair bonds? These are significant empirical questions that require further research.

In efforts to distinguish attachment relationships from other social relationships, attachment researchers have argued that four features characterize attachment relationships: a drive to maintain proximity to the attachment figure, the use of the attachment figure both as a safe haven and as a secure base in times of stress, and strong distress at separation (Zeifman & Hazan, 2016). Infant–caregiver relationships and adult sexual pair bonds typify these features, but do other relationships encompass these features as well? A central tenet of Bowlby's observations of children and Harlow's seminal work with monkeys is that close physical contact fosters the development of emotional bonds. In most cultures, intimate physical contact in adults is restricted to parents with their own children and sexual partners (Zeifman, 2019). Presumably, the psychological security derived from touch is at least in part mediated by the physiological changes induced by close physical contact. A recent study in which romantic couples were randomly assigned to touching or nontouching conditions demonstrated the positive effect of touch for producing feelings of emotional security (Jakubiak & Feeney, 2016). Repeated intimate contact surrounding caregiving in infancy and sexual encounters in adulthood is rewarding, and at least partly responsible for the development of emotional interdependence (Zeifman & Hazan, 2016).

As a result of repeated, soothing physical contact, one hallmark feature of attachment relationships is that they are mutually physiologically regulating (Zeifman, 2019). Infants use their caregivers as a source of comfort, the person to retreat to in times of distress. Similarly, adults seek partners to reduce aversive arousal. For example, holding the hand of a spouse attenuates neural responses associated with threat of electrical shock in married women (Coan, Schaefer, & Davidson, 2006). Although holding the hand of a male stranger attenuates threat response as well, a spouse is more effective, and the magnitude of threat attenuation is associated with marital quality. Thus, the stress-modulating impact of adult relationships is similar to the caregiver's ability to buffer an infant's distress, an effect that is partially modulated by the quality of the attachment (Gunnar & Donzella, 2002). Both infants and their caregivers as well as pair-bonded couples experience distress at separation, and remain alert to perceived threats to themselves, their attachment figure, and the relationship. Although most adults are capable of tolerating longer separations from attachment partners than children are, even adults become dysregulated when they experience unanticipated or permanent separations from attachment figures (Weiss, 1976).

Neurochemical evidence points to distinct characteristics of pair-bonded couples' interactions that may not generalize to platonic friends. Cortisol levels are linked between romantic partners but not friends (Feldman, 2017). Oxytocin, a neuropeptide produced during labor and breastfeeding that is associated with feelings of closeness and well-being, is also released in a pulsatile fashion during sexual intercourse (Feldman, 2017). Although oxytocin is also released during interactions with friends, there is no evidence of a coupling of oxytocin response as there is with parent–child and romantic partners (Feldman, 2017). Like infant attachments, adult attachment relationships develop over time. This suggests that, at any age, attachments require experience with a particular significant other, learning, and repeated neurohormonal transformations.

The case for pair bonds as attachments has been made elsewhere and often, but shifting demographics suggest that additional relationships might also qualify as attachment relationships. Increasing numbers of adults are delaying marriage into middle age or are choosing to remain single (DePaulo & Morris, 2005). Slightly over 50% of adults aged 18–34 did not have a steady partner in 2018 (Bonos & Guskin, 2019). These changing demographics raise important questions for attachment researchers. As more adults remain single for longer periods of time (Pepping & MacDonald, 2019), how are uncoupled adults getting their attachment needs met? Attachment researchers are only beginning to explore these questions and employ comparison groups that could shed light on what types of relationships serve key attachment functions. A recent follow-up to the original Coan and colleagues (2006) study demonstrated that holding the hand of a close relative or friend was as effective as holding the hand of a spouse for attenuating neural threat response (Coan et al., 2017). Another study in which individuals envisioned being touched by a close friend or romantic partner demonstrated that the two were equally effective in producing feelings of security (Jakubiak & Feeney, 2016). In a second experiment in the same study, adults receiving touch from a romantic partner increased feelings of security to an even greater degree than just imagining touch, but this study did not examine the *actual* touch of a close friend. Further research should include various categories of relational partners and compare their effectiveness for promoting feelings of emotional security.

Adult attachment researchers have sometimes been criticized for implying that many adults who remain single do so because of personal deficiencies (DePaulo & Morris, 2005). Some recent studies have examined the trajectories of singles who are single by choice versus those who are single due to relationship difficulties, highlighting differences in outcomes between these groups. Individuals who are happily single cite their relationships with close friends and family as a key factor underlying satisfaction (Pepping & MacDonald, 2019). There is a dearth of research about close familial relationships and friendships in adulthood; studies often focus on these bonds only in adolescence. Future research ought to examine the range of single adults' attachments more fully and distinguish among types of friendships. In the same way that not all romantic relationships are full-blown attachments, not all friendships are attachments. It is also possible that close friendships function as attachments only when one or both friends are not in serious romantic or pair-bonded relationships with others, or when sexual relationships are insecure. Some studies suggest that adults high in attachment anxiety are more likely to develop nonsexual close relationships that satisfy some attachment needs (e.g., Pepping & MacDonald, 2019). Prospective studies would be helpful for understanding the developmental roots of choosing sexual partners versus friends as a primary means of satisfying attachment needs.

Another presumption of attachment theory challenged by modern trends is the assumption that attachment relationships are exclusive. An infant's preference for one caregiver over any other and explicit rejection of strangers is a tell-tale sign that a bond has been formed. Similarly, most conceptualizations of romantic sexual love assume or idealize exclusivity. There is, however, a growing trend for individuals to identify as polyamorous and choose to be in consensual, nonmonogamous relationships. Almost no empirical data has addressed the attachment dynamics of polyamorous relationships; what few data exist suggest that the majority of individuals in consensually nonmonogamous relationships have secure romantic attachment orientations (Moors, Ryan, & Chopik, 2019). The fact that polyamorous individuals can be secure with their primary attachment partners suggests that sexual exclusivity is neither necessary nor sufficient for becoming attached. It would be valuable to understand the conditions, other than gratification of sexual needs, which promote the development of lasting emotional bonds. If sexual encounters are rewarding and promote bonding, why do some sexual relationships become attachments whereas others do not? In the context of multiple attachment targets, are all targets equal?

One possibility proposed by Fraley (2019) and others is that adults have attachment networks rather than hierarchies in which one attachment figure occupies a privileged position at the pinnacle (see also Fearon & Schuengel, Chapter 3, this volume). Although Bowlby (1969/1982) emphasized the primacy of the *primary* caregiver as the preferred source of comfort and security, adults may rely on multiple attachment figures to meet their needs, and this tendency may be functionally adaptive. The idea that having an attachment network might be an adaptive strategy for supporting adult mental health is also consistent with other recent conceptualizations of adult attachment. Finkel and his colleagues have argued that the expectation that a single marital partner can satisfy all of an individual's needs from physiological, to emotional, to higher-order needs such as self-actualization, is unrealistic, and is creating a crisis in marital satisfaction and personal well-being (Finkel, Hui, Carswell, & Larson, 2014).

Despite these controversies, throughout life, it is clear that individuals thrive when they have close relationships that confer feelings of security. Pair bonds remain a common source of attachment security in adulthood, but there is growing evidence that adults derive security from other social bonds as well. Given that many adults are increasingly postponing or forgoing marriage, future research should explore how attachment needs are being met during protracted periods of singlehood, and whether, and to what extent, friendships serve as attachments. If close friendships do serve as attachments and are equally effective in providing security, one important question is: How are attachment bonds among platonic friends formed and what neurohormonal processes underlie closeness? It is noteworthy that friendships forged during times of extreme stress, such as in the armed service, are notoriously intense, and that friendship bonding rituals, such as fraternity hazing practices, often involve artificially heightening arousal by placing individuals in physically or emotionally dangerous or distressing situations. Attempts to engage or coopt the distress–relief sequence that is at the heart of attachment processes may also explain why self-disclosure, which heightens personal vulnerability, is a common means of enhancing closeness as friendships are forming. Researchers are beginning to investigate the hormonal underpinnings and dynamics of friendship development (Ketay, Welker, & Slatcher, 2017), but this research is still in its infancy, and more comparative research is needed.

Adult attachment researchers have always acknowledged important differences between attachment in infancy and later in life. Older children and adults are capable of mentally representing an attachment figure who is not physically present, and this capacity leads to a tolerance for longer periods of separation. Yet, despite this capacity, even adults find physical contact comforting and ultimately necessary. The proliferation of popular articles with titles such as "Why Zoom Is Terrible," and "The Stark Loneliness of Digital Interaction" during the 2020 pandemic drives home the inadequacy of mental imagery or physically restrained porch visits. Digital communications and porch visits are meager substitutes for the rich, physical closeness humans crave and need from friends and loved ones. One reason might be that close physical contact is, as many attachment researchers have surmised, the bedrock of attachment.

REFERENCES

Bonos, L., & Guskin, E. (2019, March 21). It's not just you: New data shows more than half of young people in America don't have a romantic partner. Retrieved from *www.washingtonpost.com/lifestyle/2019/03/21/its-not-just-you-new-data-shows-more-than-half-young-people-america-dont-have-romantic-partner*.

Bowlby, J. (1982). *Attachment and loss: Vol. 1. Attachment* (2nd ed.). New York: Basic Books. (Original work published 1969)

Bowlby, J. (1988). *A secure base: Parent–child attachment and healthy human development*. New York: Basic Books.

Coan, J. A., Beckes, L., Gonzalez, M. Z., Maresh, E. L., Brown, C. L., & Hasselmo, K. (2017). Relationship status and perceived support in the social regulation of neural responses to threat. *Social Cognitive and Affective Neuroscience, 12*(10), 1574–1583.

Coan, J. A., Schaefer, H. S., & Davidson, R. J. (2006). Lending a hand: Social regulation of the neural response to threat. *Psychological Science, 17,* 1032–1039.

DePaulo, B. M., & Morris, W. L. (2005). Singles in society and in science. *Psychological Inquiry, 1*(6), 57–83.

Entis, L. (2020, May 26). The stark loneliness of digital interactions. Retrieved from *www.vox.com/the-highlight/2020/5/26/21256190/zoom-facetime-skype-coronavirus-loneliness*.

Feldman, R. (2017). The neurobiology of human attachments. *Trends in Cognitive Sciences, 21,* 80–99.

Finkel, E. J., Hui, C. M., Carswell, K. L., & Larson, G. M. (2014). The suffocation of marriage: Climbing Mount Maslow without enough oxygen. *Psychological Inquiry, 25,* 1–41.

Fraley, R. C. (2019). Attachment in adulthood: Recent developments, emerging debates, and future directions. *Annual Review of Psychology, 70,* 401–422.

Gunnar, M. R., & Donzella, B. (2002). Social regulation of the cortisol levels in early human development. *Psychoneuroendocrinology, 27*(1–2), 199–220.

Hazan, C., & Shaver, P. (1987). Romantic love conceptualized as an attachment process. *Journal of Personality and Social Psychology, 52,* 511–524.

Jakubiak, B. K., & Feeney, B. C. (2016). A sense of security: Touch promotes state attachment security. *Social Psychological and Personality Science, 7*(7), 745–753.

Ketay, S., Welker, K. M., & Slatcher, R. B. (2017). The roles of testosterone and cortisol in friendship formation. *Psychoneuroendocrinology, 76,* 88–96.

Moors, A. C., Ryan, W., & Chopik, W. J. (2019). Multiple loves: The effects of attachment with multiple concurrent romantic partners on relational functioning. *Personality and Individual Differences, 147,* 102–110.

Murphy, K. (2020, April 29). Why Zoom is terrible. Retrieved from *https://nyti. ms/35hnfN7.*

Pepping, C. A., & MacDonald, G. (2019). Adult attachment and long-term singlehood. *Current Opinion in Psychology, 25,* 105–109.

Weiss, R. S. (1976). The emotional impact of marital separation. *Journal of Social Issues, 32*(1), 135–145.

Zeifman, D. M. (2019). Attachment theory grows up: A developmental approach to pair bonds. *Attachment in Adulthood, 25,* 139–143.

Zeifman, D. M., & Hazan, C. (2016). Pair bonds as attachments: Mounting evidence in support of Bowlby's hypothesis. In J. Cassidy & P. R. Shaver (Eds.), *Handbook of attachment: Theory, research, and clinical applications* (3rd ed., pp. 416–434). New York: Guilford Press.

TOPIC 2

MEASURING THE SECURITY OF ATTACHMENT

- How should attachment security be assessed?

- What are the advantages and challenges of alternative measurement approaches?

CHAPTER 8

Categorical Assessments of Attachment
On the Ontological Relevance of Group Membership

Howard Steele
Miriam Steele

Measures of attachment, in their origins, have consistently relied on categories or patterns of assessment, and none have been more fundamental than insecure versus secure (Ainsworth, Blehar, Waters, & Wall, 1978) and disorganized versus organized (Main & Hesse, 1990a, 1990b). This chapter will focus on the ongoing utility of these categorical group membership approaches, despite much evidence that dimensional approaches may be more valuable than categorical approaches when it comes to making statistical predictions to outcome variables (see Raby, Fraley, & Roisman, Chapter 9, this volume). Dimensional approaches may also prove more relevant for identifying clinical subtypes of personality disorder (e.g., Chiesa, Williams, Nassisi, & Fonagy, 2017).

While the distinction, for example, between the insecure-avoidant and insecure-resistant categories from the Strange Situation is well established, as is the overall distinction between insecure and secure infant–parent attachment, these categorical assignments may be best rendered as scores along avoidance, resistance, and secure dimensions so that low, moderate, and high scores all contribute to predicting outcomes. As Raby and colleagues (Chapter 9, this volume) demonstrate, dimensional approaches maximize variance in attachment measures, while categorical approaches lessen variance by assigning individuals with varying scores to one group, nominally defined. Yet among the chief benefits delivered by categorical approaches is that they conform, especially in their binary formulation, with the way human (and other animal) brains work (Anderson, Silverstein, Ritz, & Jones, 1977).

Thus, as we argue below, categorical approaches are here to stay because communication about attachment would be radically limited without them. By the same token, dimensions or scores are vital to the formation of categories, as for every category there is a cutoff value along a dimension where, once reached, the category applies. Short of reaching that value, category membership does not apply. This chapter discusses (1) the ontological and epistemological basis for categorical judgments, and then provides an overview of the utility of (2) infant and child categories of attachment, (3) adult categories of attachment, and (4) special considerations regarding loss and trauma, before concluding with (5) some final arguments regarding the ongoing requirement for, and relevance of, categorical assessments of attachment.

The Ontological Basis and Epistemological Foundation of Categorical Judgments

Categorical judgments are embedded in the way human and other animal brains work. Our survival depends on it. We need to know quickly when and where danger looms, so the judgment regarding what is "safe" and what is "dangerous" is essentially a necessary categorical judgment. We make such decisions in microseconds, often below the threshold of awareness. Haidt (2012) shows that this process of quick categorical emotional decisions underpins our sense of morality, with nonconscious intuitive binary judgments (e.g., care/harm, loyalty/betrayal, sanctity/degradation) underlying our sophisticated multidimensional moral judgments. This mental, emotional, and cognitive process is hard-wired in our brains, a reflection of our shared evolutionary heritage. This is also reflected in our language, rife with binary terms for dividing up the world of experience into clearly demarcated categorical groups, for example, safe/dangerous, in/out, on/off, mine/yours, raw/cooked, good/bad, right/wrong, north/south, and so on. Our language seems to possess an infinite number of categorical contrasts that are immediately recognized and frequently used in language linked to actions in the world. Harnad (2003) summarized how language itself is based on categorical speech perception—that is, the capacity to hear meaningful words and to parse them into sentences when listening to the continuous stream of sounds coming from a speaker. So even if we tried to rely on dimensional measurements alone, categorical assessments would insist on being part of the appraisal process as we are drawn to think of attachment, like so many other domains of knowledge, in binary or nominal terms: insecure versus secure; disorganized versus organized, avoidant versus resistant, dismissing versus preoccupied.

Infant and Child Attachment Categories

With the publication of *Patterns of Attachment* (Ainsworth et al., 1978), the categorical assessment of attachment was launched. Notably, when researchers are trained in categorizing infant–parent patterns of attachment, the first lesson is that one first rates, on 7-point scales, the infant's interactive behavior, and only after ratings are completed and examined is a pattern or category of attachment assigned. There is an appendix to the 1978 book that shows typical interactive behavior scores for (1) proximity seeking, (2) contact maintaining, (3) avoidance, and (4) resistance that are typically assigned to categories (A, B, C) and subcategories (A1, A2, B1, B2, B3, B4, C1, or C2) of infant–caregiver attachment. Interobserver agreement is mostly easily obtained on the principal three-way (A, B, or C) category assignments. Correspondingly the literature on infant–parent attachment was for two decades or more governed by reports of principal categorical assessments, their stability over time (Waters, 1978), and their antecedents and links to later developmental outcomes, all of which were neatly summarized by Ainsworth (1985). The one secure pattern in contrast to the two insecure patterns was reified. And this categorical distinction has been further reified in multiple independent longitudinal studies and many meta-analytic reports (e.g., Groh et al., 2014).

But the avoidant versus resistant reification was altered after the "discovery" of the disorganized-disoriented infant response to the Strange Situation (Main & Solomon, 1990), the concordance between infants' disorganized-disoriented patterns of response to the Strange Situation with their caregivers' unresolved loss or unresolved trauma responses to the Adult Attachment Interview (Main & Hesse, 1990a), and the link to frightening or frightened maternal behavior (Main & Hesse, 1990b). Suddenly, in 1990, the organized insecure patterns of attachment (A and C) were seen to have more in common with the organized secure pattern (B), in contrast to the disorganized-disoriented (D) response. As a consequence, research papers, especially clinical outcome papers gathering data from high-risk samples where disorganization is often the predominant category, reported on organized (A, B, and C) versus disorganized (D) patterns of infant–caregiver attachment. Clinical interventions with parents and young children are often focused on the movement observed from disorganized to organized groups as a result (Facompré, Bernard, & Waters, 2018).

Adult Attachment Patterns or Categories

With the publication of Main, Kaplan, and Cassidy (1985), showing how parents' patterns of attachment mapped on to their children's attachment patterns, the Adult Attachment Interview (AAI; George, Kaplan, & Main,

1985) and a corresponding AAI rating and classification manual (Main, Goldwyn, & Hesse, 2003) entered the scientific literature, for circulation to participants of AAI institutes, and summarized in a 2008 chapter (Main, Hesse, & Goldwyn, 2008). The AAI manual evolved in subtle ways from its beginnings in the late 1980s through the present, yet both ratings (bottom-up appraisal processes) and classifications (top-down appraisal processes) inform the measurement of attachment in response to the AAI (Main et al., 2003, 2008). Literally tens of thousands of AAIs have been collected, transcribed, rated, and classified. These AAIs have come increasingly from clinical samples as attachment research has become deeply relevant to clinical psychological research and practice. This was made clear by the meta-analytic report from Bakermans-Kranenburg and van IJzendoorn (2009) on the "first 10,000 AAIs," the bulk of which came from clinical samples, revealing the standardization of the categorical approach and its reliability and validity in the domains of developmental and clinical psychology.

Unresolved Loss and Unresolved Trauma

The term *disorganized-disoriented* was used by Bowlby (1980) to describe the typical human response to loss. Bowlby described being *disorganized* as the state of being deeply unsure of one's surroundings, physically, emotionally, and cognitively, and *disoriented* in terms of temporal judgments, being deeply uncertain of the direction to follow given the grievously unsetting experience one is overcome by. For Bowlby, loss, especially sudden and unexpected loss, places one in a categorically distinct state of mind—different from the state of mind that would have held had the traumatic event or loss not occurred. For this reason, AAIs are scored for evidence of unresolved loss or unresolved trauma on 9-point scales, with specified speech markers indicating when to give high scores. A final judgment is then made as to whether the AAI is deemed one that carries the categorical assignment of Unresolved Loss (U-Loss) and/or Unresolved Trauma (U-Trauma). Scores of 6 or higher on the 9-point scale are so assigned. A score of 5 leaves the matter of assignment of U-Loss to the discretion of the AAI rater, who must weigh the extent of slips of the tongue and lapses in the monitoring of speech and reason, the salience of absorption and guilt, that when firmly in view mandate assigning the interview to the U-Loss or U-Trauma category, alongside the best-fitting alternative assignment to Dismissive, Preoccupied, or Autonomous (secure) categories. Given the robust and extensive evidence that such U-status in the AAI is linked to disorganized child attachments, and all range of adult psychopathological outcomes, it is vital to make the categorical assignment correctly (Bakermans-Kranenburg & van IJzendoorn, 2009).

With regard to both infant disorganization evident on reunion in the Strange Situation and unresolved loss or trauma in adulthood, Bowlby's (1980) view reflects these reliably identified behavioral and psychological phenomena to indicate a categorically different "state of mind"—not simply a high or extreme score on a dimension. And despite dimensional approaches to both anxious and resistant Strange Situation behavior (Fraley & Spieker, 2003) and dismissing and preoccupied attachment in response to the AAI (Haydon, Roisman, Marks, & Fraley, 2011), no dimension has yet been proposed to represent either disorganized attachment in infancy, or unresolved loss or trauma in adulthood. In other words, there are extremes of human experience involving fear and loss that place one in a categorically distinctive psychological state.

Conclusion

The arguments advanced in this chapter in favor of a categorical approach to attachment can be summed up as follows: (1) Humans think categorically about matters basic to survival and well-being, and security (vs. insecurity) is likely to be one of these because it is associated with safety (vs. danger); (2) dimensions of variability related to anxiety or avoidance capture some of the important variability in infant attachment classifications, but do not begin to capture the significance of disorganization that has proven to be of clinical value; (3) adult attachment can likewise be represented by dimensions related to dismissal or preoccupation, but AAI classifications are multidimensional and important variance related to the "states of mind" captured in AAI categories is missed in these dimensional assessments; like clinical diagnostic categories (with which they are associated), these differences are of *kind* and not of *degree*; and (4) the unique "state of mind" associated with unresolved loss and trauma is likewise a matter of *quality* and not *quantity*. Dimensional approaches, while valuable, are unlikely to accomplish what current categorical approaches do for the study of attachment. As Bowlby (1969) articulated, the propensity to seek out, hold on to, and prefer attachment figures deemed wiser and stronger is embedded in the makeup of our and other animals' brains and inborn behavior.

We finish with an anecdote regarding the enduring scientific value of attachment categories. We recall seeing and hearing John Bowlby at the Regent's Park Zoo in 1987 on the occasion of his 80th birthday. It was a festive meeting with multiple plenary presentations, many reporting on attachment categories, followed by questions at the end of the day. One questioner asked about the "idiosyncratic" categorical language in use throughout the day to speak of groups of children A, B, C, D and adults D, E, F, U, saying with some irritation, "This sounds like a language all its own?!" There was silence, and then after some seconds, John Bowlby leaned forward into his microphone and replied firmly, "The discussion of attachment categories comprises a unique scientific language indeed, and that language is one that is well worth learning!"

REFERENCES

Ainsworth, M. D. (1985). Patterns of infant–mother attachments: Antecedents and effects on development. *Bulletin of the New York Academy of Medicine, 61*(9), 771–791.

Ainsworth, M. D. S., Blehar, M. C., Waters, E., & Wall, S. (1978). *Patterns of attachment: A psychological study of the Strange Situation.* Hillsdale, NJ: Erlbaum.

Anderson, J. A., Silverstein, J. W., Ritz, S. A., & Jones, R. S. (1977). Distinctive features, categorical perception, and probability learning: Some applications of a neural model. *Psychological Review, 84*(5), 413–451.

Bakermans-Kranenburg, M. J., & van IJzendoorn, M. H. (2009). The first 10,000 Adult Attachment Interviews: Distributions of adult attachment representations in clinical and non-clinical groups. *Attachment and Human Development, 11*(3), 223–263.

Bowlby, J. (1969). *Attachment and loss: Vol. 1. Attachment.* New York: Basic Books.

Bowlby, J. (1980). *Attachment and loss: Vol. 3. Loss, sadness and depression.* New York: Basic Books.

Chiesa, A. C., Williams, R., Nassisi, V., & Fonagy, P. (2017). Categorical and dimensional approaches in the evaluation of the relationship between attachment and personality disorders: An empirical study. *Attachment and Human Development, 19,* 151–169.

Facompré, C., Bernard, K., & Waters, T. (2018). Effectiveness of interventions in preventing disorganized attachment: A meta-analysis. *Development and Psychopathology, 30*(1), 1–11.

Fraley, R. C., & Spieker, S. J. (2003). Are infant attachment patterns continuously or categorically distributed?: A taxometric analysis of Strange Situation behavior. *Developmental Psychology, 39,* 387–404.

George, C., Kaplan, N., & Main, M. (1985). *The Adult Attachment Interview protocol.* Unpublished manuscript, University of California, Berkeley.

Groh, A. M., Fearon, R. P., Bakermans-Kranenburg, M. J., van IJzendoorn, M. H., Steele, R. D., & Roisman, G. R. (2014). The significance of attachment security for children's social competence with peers: A meta-analytic study. *Attachment and Human Development, 16*(2), 103–136.

Haidt, J. (2012). *The righteous mind.* New York: Pantheon Books.

Harnad, S. (2003). Categorical perception. In L. Nadel (Ed.), *Encyclopedia of cognitive science.* New York: Nature Publishing Group/Macmillan.

Haydon, K. C., Roisman, G. I., Marks, M. J., & Fraley, R. C. (2011). An empirically derived approach to the latent structure of the Adult Attachment Interview: Additional convergent and discriminant validity evidence. *Attachment and Human Development, 13,* 503–524.

Main, M., Goldwyn, R., & Hesse, E. (2003). *Adult Attachment Classification system Version 7.2.* Unpublished manuscript, University of California, Berkeley.

Main, M., & Hesse, E. (1990a). Parent's unresolved traumatic experiences are related to infant disorganized/disoriented attachment status: Is frightened and/or frightening parental behavior the linking mechanism? In M. T. Greenberg, D. Cicchetti, & E. M. Cummings (Eds.), *Attachment in the preschool years: Theory, research, and intervention* (pp. 161–182). Chicago: University of Chicago Press.

Main, M., & Hesse, E. (1990b). Adult lack of resolution of attachment-related trauma related to infant disorganized/disoriented behavior in the Ainsworth Strange Situation: Linking parental states of mind to infant behavior in a stressful situation. In M. T. Greenberg, D. Cicchetti, & E. M. Cummings (Eds.), *Attachment in the preschool years: Theory, research and intervention* (pp. 339–426). Chicago: University of Chicago Press.

Main, M., Hesse, E., & Goldwyn, R. (2008). Studying differences in language use in recounting attachment history. In H. Steele & M. Steele (Eds.), *Clinical applications of the Adult Attachment Interview* (pp. 31–68). New York: Guilford Press.

Main, M., Kaplan, N., & Cassidy, J. (1985). Security in infancy, childhood and adulthood: A move to the level of representation. *Monographs of the Society for Research in Child Development, 50*(1–2, Serial No. 209), 66–104.

Main, M., & Solomon, J. (1990). Procedures for identifying infants as disorganized/disoriented during the Ainsworth Strange Situation. In M. T. Greenberg, D. Cicchetti, & E. M. Cummings (Eds.), *Attachment in the preschool years: Theory, research, and intervention* (pp. 121–160). Chicago: University of Chicago Press.

Waters, E. (1978). The reliability and stability of individual differences in infant–mother attachment. *Child Development, 49,* 483–494.

CHAPTER 9

Categorical or Dimensional Measures of Attachment?
Insights from Factor-Analytic and Taxometric Research

K. Lee Raby
R. Chris Fraley
Glenn I. Roisman

A long-standing debate among attachment researchers is whether individual differences in attachment are more accurately captured with categorical or dimensional measures. The practice of operationalizing individual differences in attachment using categorical measures can be traced to Mary Ainsworth's landmark research on the quality of infants' attachment to their parents. Ainsworth and colleagues (Ainsworth, Blehar, Waters, & Wall, 1978/2015) assigned dimensional ratings for infants' attachment behaviors during the Strange Situation Procedure, but these ratings were ultimately used to inductively sort the children into one of three mutually exclusive attachment categories. Young children were classified as securely attached if they sought interaction and/or proximity with their parents during the reunions and were effectively comforted by their parents. In contrast, children were classified as having formed an avoidant attachment if they ignored the parent during the reunion episodes, whereas children were classified as having a resistant attachment if they both sought and resisted contact with the parent (i.e., became angry and/or passive) while interacting with their parents. Main and Solomon (1990) later introduced a fourth category for infants who exhibited disorganized or disoriented attachment behaviors.

Ainsworth and colleagues' categorical system served as a blueprint for assessments of adult attachment that were developed in the 1980s.

For example, the traditional system for coding the Adult Attachment Interview—the most commonly used measure in developmental science for assessing adults' attachment representations—recommends classifying individuals into one of four categories that are conceptual analogues to the infant attachment classifications (Main, Kaplan, & Cassidy, 1985). Similarly, early measures of adults' self-reported attachment style involved placing adults into the best-fitting category, and the category descriptions were based on the infant attachment typology (e.g., Hazan & Shaver, 1987).

Each of these categorical measurement systems includes two tacit assumptions about the latent structure of individual differences in attachment quality. One assumption is that variability in attachment reflects categorical, rather than dimensional, distinctions. Although these systems recognize that not all individuals assigned the same classification exhibit the exact same behaviors, the implicit assumption in these categorical systems is that the variation within each of the categories is less meaningful than the variation between categories. The second assumption pertains to the nature and number of distinct phenomena that purportedly are being measured. Specifically, the traditional coding systems imply that four relatively independent latent constructs underlie the variation in young children's and adults' attachment-related thoughts, feelings, and behaviors.

When the systems for measuring attachment during infancy and adulthood were initially developed, it was necessary to make formal assumptions about the number of constructs being assessed and whether the variation within the constructs was categorical or dimensional. Moreover, these assumptions were reasonable. Ainsworth and colleagues (1978/2015) offered several explanations why they favored categorical measures of infant attachment over dimensional ones. First, they felt that the "classificatory groups [help] retain the picture of patterns of behavior, which tend to become lost in—or at least difficult to retrieve from—the quantification process" (p. 57). Second, they suggested that it "would be foolish to believe that the dimensions that we have so far subjected to quantification take into account all of the behaviors that are important components to the patterning of individual differences. . . . To abandon the classificatory system in favor of our present set of component behavioral scales . . . would freeze our knowledge in its present state" (p. 57). Third, they felt that "the patternings described and differentiated within a classificatory system keep . . . [the issue of developmental origins] to the forefront rather than burying it in a welter of refined statistics" (p. 57). Over time, assumptions about the categorical structure of attachment have been accepted as facts, and the traditional categorical measurement systems have dominated attachment research.

It is important to recognize that claims about the latent structure of a psychological phenomenon (including attachment) can be empirically

evaluated. Specifically, factor-analytic methods can help identify the number of distinct constructs that underlie a set of observations, and taxometric procedures can help determine whether variability in a latent construct reflects categorical or dimensional differences (Ruscio, Haslam,
& Ruscio, 2006). These statistical techniques were fully developed after
the traditional attachment measurement systems were created. However,
these tools allow us to evaluate the early assumptions about latent structure and therefore improve the measurement systems used to assess individual differences in attachment.

Fraley and Spieker (2003) conducted the first study of the latent structure of infant attachment quality. They began by conducting exploratory
factor analyses of the ratings of infants' behaviors during the Strange Situation collected from over 1,000 15-month-old children from the NICHD
Study of Early Child Care and Youth Development. In so doing, Fraley
and Spieker (2003) identified two latent factors as the most parsimonious
fit to the data. The first included the ratings traditionally used to classify
infants as having developed an avoidant versus a secure attachment. Specifically, this factor reflected the extent to which infants avoided their parents during the reunion episodes or sought proximity and actively maintained physical contact with their parents. The second factor included
ratings traditionally used to classify infants as having developed a resistant or a disorganized attachment. In this way, this second factor reflected
the extent to which infants became emotionally overwhelmed, conflicted,
and/or disoriented. This two-factor structure was replicated in a separate
sample (Groh et al., 2019). Fraley and Spieker (2003) also conducted a
set of taxometric analyses of the infants' attachment behaviors, and the
results indicated that the variation within each of the two latent factors
was more consistent with a dimensional rather than categorical model.

A substantial amount of research has examined the latent structure
of the Adult Attachment Interview (for reviews, see Booth-LaForce & Roisman, 2014; Roisman & Cicchetti, 2017). Perhaps most notably, these issues
were recently examined using data from over 3,000 individuals compiled
by the Collaboration on Attachment Transmission Synthesis (Raby et
al., 2020). The results of the factor analyses were consistent with prior
evidence indicating that variation in adults' attachment states of mind
can be captured by two factors. The first factor represents the extent to
which adults idealize their childhood relationships with their parents and
claim to not remember past attachment experiences (dismissing states
of mind). The second factor captures the extent to which adults become
emotionally distressed when discussing childhood experiences with parents or become confused when discussing the loss of a loved one or experiences of trauma (preoccupied states of mind). Although a three-factor
model that separated the traditional indicators of a preoccupied state
of mind from the traditional indicators of an unresolved state of mind

also provided a satisfactory fit to the data, the empirical overlap between the preoccupied and unresolved latent factors was substantial ($r = .87$). Thus, the two-factor model appears to be the most parsimonious solution. Moreover, the results of the taxometric analyses reported by Raby and colleagues (2020) were more consistent with a dimensional model for all latent factors, including unresolved states of mind when treated as distinct from preoccupied states of mind.

Factor analyses of adults' self-report attachment styles have also identified two latent factors underlying the various questionnaire items (for a review, see Brennan, Clark, & Shaver, 1998). The avoidance factor represents the extent to which adults value intimacy and easily rely on others in times of need versus being uncomfortable with closeness and dependency in close relationships. The anxiety factor represents the extent to which people experience emotional distress within close relationships. Moreover, taxometric analyses have consistently revealed that variation in both avoidance and anxiety is dimensional rather than categorical (Fraley, Hudson, Heffernan, & Segal, 2015; Fraley & Waller, 1998).

To summarize, factor and taxometric analyses of the three most commonly used measures of attachment indicate individual differences during infancy and adulthood can be parsimoniously characterized using two dimensions. The consistency of the results across measures of observed behavior, narrative-based assessments of attachment representations, and self-reported thoughts, feelings, and behaviors increases confidence in the validity of the findings. In general, the first dimension involves the degree to which individuals are comfortable engaging with versus defensively avoid attachment-related thoughts, feelings, and relationship partners, whereas the second dimension involves the degree to which individuals exhibit emotional distress versus are emotionally composed in attachment situations (Roisman, 2009). The traditional attachment classifications can be reconceptualized as combinations of these two dimensions (see Figure 9.1). Specifically, classifications of attachment security or autonomous states of mind involve the co-occurrence of relational engagement and emotional composure in attachment situations. Classifications of avoidance or dismissing states of mind are a mixture of relational avoidance and emotional composure, whereas classifications of resistance or preoccupied states mind are a blend of relational engagement and emotional distress. Finally, individuals classified as having a fearful attachment style or are assigned a cannot-classify label exhibit both relational avoidance and emotional distress in attachment situations.

This empirically based, two-dimensional model departs from the traditional view of individual differences in attachment in two key ways. First, this model suggests that variation in attachment exists on a graded continuum rather than being categorical. In other words, individual differences in attachment quality appear to be a matter of degree rather

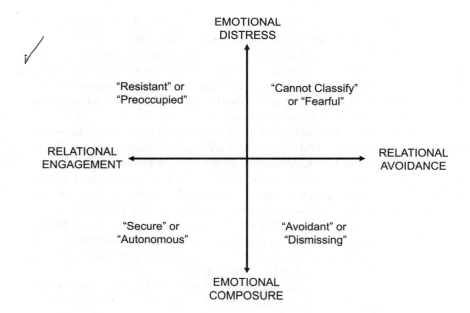

FIGURE 9.1. The two-dimensional model of individual differences in attachment quality. The horizontal and vertical axes represent the two dimensions identified in factor and taxometric analyses of infants' attachment behavior during the Strange Situation, adults' attachment states of mind as assessed by the Adult Attachment Interview, and adults' self-reported attachment styles. The traditional attachment classifications are listed in each of the quadrants to illustrate how the classifications can be represented as combinations of the two dimensions.

than kind. The second key difference from the traditional perspective is that individual differences in attachment are due to two (rather than four) latent constructs. Attachment disorganization and unresolved states of mind do not appear to be unique constructs but may instead be additional manifestations of attachment-related distress. In addition, this model suggests that attachment security is not a unitary construct but rather is a mixture of two attachment-related processes. To be clear, the factor and taxometric findings do not challenge the validity of the Strange Situation Procedure, the Adult Attachment Interview, or self-report questionnaires as instruments for collecting information about variation in attachment. Rather, the latent structure evidence supports an alternative approach to operationalizing individual differences in attachment using the information these instruments generate.

The traditional, categorical systems have been heuristically valuable for the field of attachment research. Over the past several decades, a sizable number of studies have used the classifications to test theoretical claims about individual differences in attachment, including the hypothesis that they are rooted in early experiences in parent–child relationships, are relatively stable over time, are associated with social and emotional functioning across the lifespan, and are transmitted across generations (e.g., Verhage et al., 2018). That said, the use of these empirically based, dimensional indices in research can deepen our understanding of the origins, stabilities, and consequences of variation in attachment quality. One reason for this is that dichotomizing dimensional constructs (as the traditional classifications do) can reduce statistical power, produce biased parameter estimates, and increase the risk of both type I (false-positive) and type II (false-negative) errors (MacCallum, Zhang, Preacher, & Rucker, 2002). Thus, research that uses the dimensional indices of attachment identified by the factor-analytic and taxometric studies will often have more statistical power and will yield more accurate estimates of the associations between individual differences in attachment and other theoretically relevant variables than research that uses the traditional categorical measures.

Operationalizing individual differences in attachment as two dimensions also can advance our understanding of the unique correlates of the resistant/preoccupied and avoidant/dismissing attachment patterns. Studies that have used the traditional classifications often report relatively low base rates for the various subtypes of attachment insecurity. As a result, a common practice has been to combine these subtypes into a general insecurity classification. This is despite the theoretical ideas that the avoidant/dismissing and resistant/preoccupied attachment patterns represent distinct strategies that have unique origins and sequelae. Research that uses the two attachment dimensions is well positioned to test these theoretical hypotheses. For example, a growing number of studies have used the dimensional indices of adults' attachment states of mind and adults' self-reported attachment styles to document that the dismissing/avoidance and preoccupied/anxiety dimensions are predicted by distinct sets of childhood caregiving experiences and are associated with distinct social-emotional outcomes (e.g., Booth-LaForce & Roisman, 2014; Fraley, Roisman, Booth-LaForce, Owen, & Holland, 2013). A critical task for future research will be to leverage the dimensional measures of infants' attachment strategies to better understand whether attachment avoidance and resistance during these early years have unique antecedents and/or unique consequences for later adaptation.

To date, nearly all of the factor-analytic and taxometric studies of attachment have focused on measures designed for infants or adults. As a result, there is a general lack of information about the latent structure of the measures of attachment that have been developed for children and adolescents (cf. Waters et al., 2019). In order to address this gap in our knowledge, it is essential that the coding systems developed for these ages undergo empirical tests of the factor structure by including a sufficient number of rating scales that thoroughly capture the various indicators of attachment quality. It is also important that data are collected from several hundred individuals or more to allow for appropriately powered tests of whether the variation is categorical or dimensional. Aggregating data collected from several research labs is one possible solution to this logistical obstacle (e.g., Verhage et al., 2018). Altogether, these efforts to continue to refine the measures that undergird attachment research will help the field answer both the long-lasting and novel questions regarding the significance of attachment for human health and development.

REFERENCES

Ainsworth, M. D. S., Blehar, M. C., Waters, E., & Wall, S. N. (2015). *Patterns of attachment: A psychological study of the Strange Situation.* New York: Psychology Press. (Original work published 1978)

Booth-LaForce, C., & Roisman, G. I. (Eds). (2014). The Adult Attachment Interview: Psychometrics, stability and change from infancy, and developmental origins. *Monographs of the Society for Research in Child Development, 79,* 1–185.

Brennan, K. A., Clark, C. L., & Shaver, P. R. (1998). Self-report measurement of adult attachment: An integrative overview. In J. A. Simpson & W. S. Rholes (Eds.), *Attachment theory and close relationships* (pp. 46–76). New York: Guilford Press.

Fraley, R. C., Hudson, N. W., Heffernan, M. E., & Segal, N. (2015). Are adult attachment styles categorical or dimensional?: A taxometric analysis of general and relationship-specific attachment orientations. *Journal of Personality and Social Psychology, 109,* 354–368.

Fraley, R. C., Roisman, G. I., Booth-LaForce, C., Owen, M. T., & Holland, A. S. (2013). Interpersonal and genetic origins of adult attachment styles: A longitudinal study from infancy to early adulthood. *Journal of Personality and Social Psychology, 104,* 817–838.

Fraley, R. C., & Spieker, S. J. (2003). Are infant attachment patterns continuously or categorically distributed?: A taxometric analysis of strange situation behavior. *Developmental Psychology, 39,* 387–404.

Fraley, R. C., & Waller, N. G. (1998). Adult attachment patterns: A test of the typological model. In J. A. Simpson & W. S. Rholes (Eds.), *Attachment theory and close relationships* (pp. 77–114). New York: Guilford Press.

Groh, A. M., Propper, C., Mills-Koonce, R., Moore, G. A., Calkins, S., & Cox, M. (2019). Mothers' physiological and affective responding to infant distress: Unique antecedents of avoidant and resistant attachments. *Child Development, 90,* 489–505.

Hazan, C., & Shaver, P. (1987). Romantic love conceptualized as an attachment process. *Journal of Personality and Social Psychology, 52,* 511–524.

MacCallum, R. C., Zhang, S., Preacher, K. J., & Rucker, D. D. (2002). On the practice of dichotomization of quantitative variables. *Psychological Methods, 7,* 19–40.

Main, M., Kaplan, N., & Cassidy, J. (1985). Security in infancy, childhood, and adulthood: A move to the level of representation. In I. Bretherton & E. Waters (Eds.), Growing points of attachment theory and research. *Monographs of the Society for Research in Child Development, 50*(1–2, Serial No. 209), 66–104.

Main, M., & Solomon, J. (1990). Procedures for identifying infants as disorganized/disoriented during the Ainsworth Strange Situation. In M. T. Greenberg, D. Cicchetti, & E. M. Cummings (Eds.), *Attachment in the preschool years: Theory, research, and intervention* (pp. 121–160). Chicago: University of Chicago Press.

Raby, K. L., Verhage, M. L., Fearon, R. M. P., Fraley, R. C., Roisman, G. I., van IJzendoorn, M. H., . . . The Collaboration on Attachment Transmission Synthesis. (2020). The latent structure of the Adult Attachment Interview: Large sample evidence from the Collaboration on Attachment Transmission Synthesis. *Development and Psychopathology.* [Epub ahead of print]

Roisman, G. I. (2009). Adult attachment: Toward a rapprochement of methodological cultures. *Current Directions in Psychological Science, 18,* 122–126.

Roisman, G. I., & Cicchetti, D. (2017). Editorial: Attachment in the context of atypical caregiving. *Development and Psychopathology, 29,* 331–335.

Ruscio, J., Haslam, N., & Ruscio, A. M. (2006). *Introduction to the taxometric method: A practical guide.* Mahwah, NJ: Erlbaum.

Verhage, M. L., Fearon, R. M. P., Schuengel, C., van IJzendoorn, M. H., Bakermans-Kranenburg, M. J., Madigan, S., . . . The Collaboration on Attachment Transmission Synthesis. (2018). Examining ecological constraints on the intergenerational transmission of attachment via individual participant data meta-analysis. *Child Development, 89,* 2023–2037.

Waters, T. E. A., Facompré, C. R., Dujardin, A., Van De Walle, M., Verhees, M., Bodner, N., . . . Bosmans, G. (2019). Taxometric analysis of secure base script knowledge in middle childhood reveals categorical latent structure. *Child Development, 90,* 694–707.

CHAPTER 10

Representational Measures of Attachment
A Secure Base Script Perspective

Theodore E. A. Waters

The "move to the level of representation" in attachment research (e.g., Main, Kaplan, & Cassidy, 1985) ushered in a much-needed new era of theoretical and methodological advances. Prior to Main and colleagues' work, attachment research was largely confined to observations of infant–parent dynamics during distress and exploration. With no way to easily evaluate the primary caregiver's attachment history, developmental psychologists were unable to examine Bowlby's (e.g., 1969) most ambitious theoretical predictions. Most critical among them was the idea that early caregiving experiences are organized and carried forward by the cognitive system and brought to bear in attachment-relevant relationship contexts across the lifespan. Without a window into what Bowlby (e.g., 1969) termed the *internal working model (IWM)*, or an individual's attachment representations, studying the formation, stability, change, and impact of the IWM was limited.

However, once assessments targeting attachment representations were validated, more rigorous (and dangerous) tests leveraging longitudinal data and examining the intergenerational transmission of attachment representations became possible. Long-term longitudinal studies focused on the antecedents and consequences of individual differences in adult attachment representations went a long way toward informing Bowlby's predictions and answering thoughtful critiques of attachment theory (e.g., Grossmann, Grossmann, & Waters, 2006). However, even with those advances, the contents of an individual's attachment representations and how those contents may develop and change over time *remain* fundamental questions in attachment research.

Attachment Representations:
Adult Attachment Interview Coherence and Beyond

The introduction of the Adult Attachment Interview (AAI) allowed researchers to study attachment representations for the first time. Attachment theory was clearly strengthened by the tremendous success of the measure. But when asked "What is in an IWM?," attachment researchers had to be satisfied with the answer "Whatever the AAI is measuring." However, this answer is unsatisfactory for three reasons: (1) There is substantial conceptual distance between the AAI's traditional coding system and the behaviors it is meant to explain (Waters & Facompré, in press); (2) the AAI has produced smaller than expected associations in several domains of attachment research (i.e., an individual's attachment classification in infancy and the classification of infants in the next generation; see Groh et al., 2014; Verhage et al., 2018); and (3) mental representations of attachment are likely more multifarious than the AAI and its traditional coding system are designed to capture (Waters & Waters, 2006).

The AAI scoring emphasizes the coherence of autobiographical recollections of early attachment experience during a retrospective interview (e.g., Hesse, 2008). But narrative coherence, the extent to which narratives are detailed, direct, and not emotionally overwrought, is a far cry from the secure base interactions thought to give rise to attachment representations and the secure base behaviors attachment representations are thought to inform. In fact, coherence coding largely overlooks secure base content provided during the AAI in favor of more stylistic elements related to Gricean maxims of conversational implicature (Grice, 1975). Furthermore, it is not well described *how* coherence or incoherence leads to any given behavior in a particular attachment context. Waters, Brockmeyer, and Crowell (2013) termed this conceptual distance between coherence coding and the secure base behaviors so central to Bowlby–Ainsworth attachment theory the *explanation gap*.

In addition to the conceptual problems associated with an emphasis on AAI coherence, the AAI has produced modest association with central attachment outcomes (e.g., infant attachment; Verhage et al., 2018). These modest results indicate that attachment researchers are leaving substantial variance unaccounted for and that attention needs to be paid not only to explaining the variance we can account for but also to explaining *more* of the individual differences in our assessments. This, along with the existence of an extensive cognitive literature on mental representations, necessitates a broader view of what we mean by attachment representations.

Along these lines, Waters and Waters (2006) argued that mental representations of attachment are multifaceted and include more than just autobiographical memories of attachment experiences (i.e., the emphasis of the AAI). They also include a cognitive script summarizing the basic elements of an individual's experiences with secure base use and support in times of need (i.e., the secure base script). Several studies find that the secure base script construct complements and adds incrementally to the ability of AAI coherence to account for attachment outcomes (e.g., Waters et al., 2013; Waters, Raby, Ruiz, Martin, & Roisman, 2018).

Assessing the Secure Base Script

Two primary measures for assessing secure base script knowledge have emerged: the Attachment Script Assessment (ASA; Waters & Rodrigues-Doolabh, 2001, 2004) and a secure base script scale for use with the AAI (AAI$_{sbs}$; Waters & Facompré, in press; see Vaughn, Posada, Veríssimo, Lu, & Nichols, 2019, for additional approaches used for toddlerhood). Both measures attempt to quantify individual differences in secure base script knowledge reflected in attachment narratives. The ASA uses a word-prompt methodology and asks participants to construct fictional narratives using a series of word lists outlining various attachment scenarios (e.g., a child falling off a bike and needing to go to the doctor), with different story sets adapted for typical child, adolescent, or adult attachment needs. In contrast, the AAI$_{sbs}$ assesses secure base script knowledge from autobiographical narratives produced during the semistructured AAI (Main et al., 1985) used with adolescence and adult samples.

Despite notable methodological differences, the ASA and AAI both produce comparable secure base script content that can be coded using parallel scoring criteria emphasizing the extent to which an attachment narrative reflects and elaborates on the secure base script. They are also well validated in terms of test–retest reliability and share similar theory-consistent correlations (e.g., predicted by early caregiving; Waters & Roisman, 2019). Strengths of the ASA include ease of use, adaptability to a broad range of ages and cultures, and consistency of administration across participants (all participants are given the same outlines and the same instructions). Strengths of the AAI$_{sbs}$ include the ability to collect and code shortened AAI interviews and to code and reanalyze existing AAI data from a secure base script perspective. Given these strengths, the last 15 years has seen the secure base script approach to assessing attachment representations progress relatively quickly with studies focused on childhood up to midlife and coming from a variety of cultural contexts.

Attachment Representations: Development and Change

With the emergence of the secure base script perspective (see Waters & Roisman, 2019, for a recent review) and the already extensive literature on attachment representations focused on the AAI, researchers were confronted with how to reconcile the existence of two forms of mental representations, one rooted in autobiographical memory (AAI coherence) and one in semantic memory (secure base script knowledge). Both constructs have similar antecedents and predict theoretically consistent outcomes in a similar way (e.g., Steele et al., 2014; Waters et al., 2018). Furthermore, they are only moderately correlated with each other, which suggests that each method reflects distinct aspect of the IWM. Given this, the question becomes "do autobiographical and schematic attachment representations develop in parallel or in series?"

Using data from the Minnesota Longitudinal Study of Risk and Adaptation (MLSRA; Sroufe, Egeland, Carlson, & Collins, 2005), Waters, Ruiz, and Roisman (2017) tested the hypothesis that attachment representations develop sequentially with secure base script knowledge emerging first and helping to structure and organize the later emerging autobiographical representations tapped by the AAI. They based their hypothesis on the memory development literature, which suggests that scripts serve as an early form of event memory and that the ability to connect autobiographical memories together and abstract larger meaning emerges later in development (during late adolescence) and relies in part on schemas (e.g., Habermas & de Silveira, 2008; Nelson & Fivush, 2004). In support of this prediction, they found that secure base script knowledge mediated the link between early caregiving experiences and AAI coherence in young adulthood. This suggested that the secure base script is organized prior to aspects of the IWM tapped by the coherence coding system of the AAI and helps to facilitate the organization and coherence of autobiographical memories of early attachment experiences later in development.

These results suggested that the reason early secure base experience informs the coherence of our autobiographical narratives in adulthood is because they first give rise to the secure base script. Once established, the script provides a guide for what information is most central to caregiving interactions and how to organize those interactions with a beginning–middle–end structure (see Waters et al., 2013).

The development of attachment representations is, of course, more complicated than simply scripts preceding autobiographical representations. Each form of attachment representation likely develops along with, or is impacted by, the development of the cognitive system within which it is housed. Scripts are thought to undergo change or develop via two distinct processes: generalization and elaboration. Within the context of attachment, generalization refers to the extent to which attachment security is relationship specific or generalized across attachment relationships, reflecting a characteristic of the individual rather than a given relationship (e.g., security to mother and father are independent rather than overlapping).

Waters and colleagues (2015) examined the generalization of secure base script knowledge across multiple relationships in two large samples of normative risk adolescents and adults, respectively. The convergence of secure base script knowledge indicators for mother and father (adolescent sample) and for parents and romantic partners (adult sample) were examined. Results indicated that secure base script knowledge on mother–child and father–child items were highly correlated and reflected a common underlying factor in the adolescent sample. Similar results were obtained for parent–child and romantic-partnership items in the adult sample. Given that attachment security to mother and to father is generally uncorrelated during infancy (van IJzendoorn & De Wolff, 1997), these results suggest that attachment representations undergo a process of generalization, at least in normative risk contexts.

Aside from generalization, scripts also undergo a process of elaboration. Scripts become increasingly detailed and nuanced as more script-relevant contexts are encountered. Just as a script for going to a restaurant becomes more nuanced as one dines at different restaurants, the secure base script may become more elaborated as individuals encounter novel attachment contexts (e.g., forming romantic relationships for the first time). To examine this process, Waters and colleagues conducted a pair of studies on the latent structure of secure base script knowledge (Waters et al., 2015; Waters, Facompré, Dujardin, et al., 2019). Using taxometric analysis to examine whether or not individual differences in secure base script knowledge were categorical in nature (secure or insecure) or continuous (differing degrees of security), they found that during middle childhood, it was categorical, but it was continuous in adolescence and adulthood. This change maps onto a pattern of elaboration: As more diverse attachment contexts are encountered, individual differences become more nuanced as reflected in a continuous latent structure.

Waters, Facompré, Van de Walle, and colleagues (2019) also found that increases in secure base script knowledge across middle childhood and early adolescence were associated with higher levels of minor everyday stressors. They argued that more frequent opportunities and diverse contexts in which to practice secure base use facilitates its development and elaboration. Taken together, this work suggests that attachment representations are subject to substantial development and change. Bowlby's IWM seems to contain multiple constructs that unfold in a particular developmental sequence, change in latent structure, and undergo extensive generalization and elaboration across development.

Challenges

The emergence of the secure base script perspective allows for a more nuanced and dynamic picture of attachment representations to emerge. When developing a new assessment tool in any field, researchers must articulate the theoretical and practical utility of the new construct/ measure in the service of demonstrating added value rather than added complexity and addressing "old wine in new bottles" critiques. An argument can be made that AAI coherence is only part of a larger IWM and researchers do themselves a disservice in terms of variance accounted for and theoretical clarity by emphasizing only one aspect of attachment representations. Furthermore, for many, the traditional use of the AAI is prohibitively resource intensive. In contrast, the current assessments of the secure base script are relatively economical (Table 10.1).

That said, measurement selection should not be based on convenience. As attachment research moves forward, articulating when scripts and/or autobiographical attachment representations are at play is an important challenge. The secure base script is probably best thought of as a heuristic, a cognitive representation in which detail is sacrificed in the service of speed and efficiency. It can guide behavior in high arousal/ stress situations in which more implicit and automatic processing is advantageous. What autobiographical memories lack in speed and efficiency, they make up for with detail, nuance, and meaning. Autobiographical representations are more likely to facilitate attachment behaviors in more

TABLE 10.1. Comparison of Approaches to Assessing Adult Attachment Representations in the Developmental Psychology Tradition

	$AAI_{traditional}$	AAI_{sbs}	ASA
Data collection	1–2 hours	30–60 minutes (first six questions only)	15–30 minutes
Transcription	10 hours/AAI	4–5 hours/AAI	1–2 hours
Coder training[a]	2 weeks	2–3 days	2–3 days
Reliability test	1–1.5 years	1 month	2–4 weeks
Coding time	2–3 hours/AAI	30–45 minutes/AAI	15–20 minutes/ASA (four stories total)

Note. All information presented in the above table are informed estimates meant to illustrate differences in coding training and implementation of each coding system.

[a]Costs associated with training and reliability are not presented. $AAI_{traditional}$ coder training typically includes tuition plus travel expenses. Both the AAI_{sbs} and ASA trainings are tuition-free but may include travel expenses.

deliberate and planful interactions. Although the secure base script may lead us to offer comfort when our child or romantic partner is distressed, it offers little in the way of what that comfort should look like or what should be said or done. In addition, recalling moments of comfort and support from the past may serve to buoy our confidence to explore in the face of distress and adversity in the future. With more than one possibility for how to measure attachment representations, understanding the costs, benefits, and implications associated with each approach must always be a priority.

REFERENCES

Bowlby, J. (1969). *Attachment and loss: Vol. 1. Attachment*. New York: Basic Books.

Grice, H. P. (1975). Logic and conversation. In P. Cole & J. Morgan (Eds.), *Syntax and semantics: Vol. 3. Speech acts* (pp. 43–58). New York: Academic Press.

Groh, A. M., Roisman, G. I., Booth-LaForce, C., Fraley, R. C., Owen, M. T., Cox, M. J., & Burchinal, M. R. (2014). The Adult Attachment Interview: Psychometrics, stability and change from infancy, and developmental origins: IV. Stability of attachment security from infancy to late adolescence. *Monographs of the Society for Research in Child Development, 79*(3), 51–66.

Grossmann, K. E., Grossmann, K., & Waters, E. (Eds.). (2006). *Attachment from infancy to adulthood: The major longitudinal studies*. New York: Guilford Press.

Habermas, T., & de Silveira, C. D. (2008). The development of global coherence in life narratives across adolescence. *Developmental Psychology, 44*, 707–721.

Hesse, E. (2008). The Adult Attachment Interview: Protocol, method of analysis, and empirical studies. In J. Cassidy & P. R. Shaver (Eds.), *Handbook of attachment: Theory, research, and clinical applications* (2nd ed., pp. 552–598). New York: Guilford Press.

Main, M., Kaplan, N., & Cassidy, J. (1985). Security in infancy, childhood, and adulthood: A move to the level of representation. In I. Bretherton & E. Waters (Eds.), *Growing points of attachment theory and research. Monographs of the Society for Research in Child Development, 50*(1–2, Serial No. 209), 66–104.

Nelson, K., & Fivush, R. (2004). The emergence of autobiographical memory: A social cultural developmental theory. *Psychological Review, 111*(2), 486–511.

Sroufe, L. A., Egeland, B., Carlson, E. A., & Collins, W. A. (2005). *The development of the person: The Minnesota Study of Risk and Adaptation from Birth to Adulthood*. New York: Guilford Press.

Steele, R. D., Waters, T. E. A., Bost, K. K., Vaughn, B. E., Truitt, W., Waters, H. S., . . . Roisman, G. I. (2014). Caregiving antecedents of secure base script knowledge: A comparative analysis of young adult attachment representations. *Developmental Psychology, 50*(11), 2526–2538.

van IJzendoorn, M. H., & De Wolff, M. S. (1997). In search of the absent father— Meta-analysis of infant–father attachment: A rejoinder to our discussants. *Child Development, 68*, 604–609.

Vaughn, B. E., Posada, G., Veríssimo, M., Lu, T., & Nichols, O. I. (2019). Assessing and quantifying the secure base script from narratives produced by preschool age children: Justification and validation tests. *Attachment and Human Development, 21*(3), 225–237.

Verhage, M. L., Fearon, P., Schuengel, C., van IJzendoorn, M. H., Bakermans-Kranenburg, M. J., Madigan, S., . . . Collaboration on Attachment Transmission Synthesis. (2018). Examining ecological constraints on the intergenerational transmission of attachment via individual participant data meta-analysis. *Child Development, 89*(6), 2023–2037.

Waters, H. S., & Rodrigues-Doolabh, L. M. (2001, April). *Are attachment scripts the building blocks of attachment representations?* Paper presented at the biennial meeting of the Society for Research in Child Development, Washington, DC.

Waters, H. S., & Rodrigues-Doolabh, L. M. (2004). *Manual for scoring secure base narratives.* Unpublished manuscript, State University of New York at Stony Brook.

Waters, H. S., & Waters, E. (2006). The attachment working models concept: Among other things, we build script-like representations of secure base experiences. *Attachment and Human Development, 8,* 185–197.

Waters, T. E. A., Brockmeyer, S., & Crowell, J. A. (2013). AAI coherence predicts caregiving and care seeking behavior in couple problem solving interactions: Secure base script knowledge helps explain why. *Attachment and Human Development, 15*(3), 316–331.

Waters, T. E. A., & Facompré, C. R. (in press). Measuring secure base content in the Adult Attachment Interview. In E. Waters, B. E. Vaughn, & H. S. Waters (Eds.), *Measuring attachment.* New York: Guilford Press.

Waters, T. E. A., Facompré, C. R., Dujardin, A., Van de Walle, M., Verhees, M., Bodner, N., . . . Bosmans, G. (2019). Discontinuity in the latent structure of the secure base script: Taxometrics reveal a representational shift in middle childhood. *Child Development, 90*(3), 694–707.

Waters, T. E. A., Facompré, C. R., Van de Walle, M., Dujardin, A., De Winter, S., Heylen, J., . . . Bosmans, G. (2019). Stability and change in secure base script development during middle childhood and early adolescence: A three-year longitudinal study. *Developmental Psychology, 55*(11), 2379–2388.

Waters, T. E. A., Fraley, R. C., Groh, A. M., Steele, R. D., Vaughn, B. E., Bost, K. K., . . . Roisman, G. I. (2015). The latent structure of secure base script knowledge. *Developmental Psychology, 51,* 823–830.

Waters, T. E. A., Raby, K. L., Ruiz, S. K., Martin, J., & Roisman, G. I. (2018). Adult attachment representations and the quality of romantic and parent–child relationships: An examination of the contributions of coherence of discourse and secure base script knowledge. *Developmental Psychology, 54*(12), 2371–2381.

Waters, T. E. A., & Roisman, G. I. (2019). The secure base script concept: An overview. *Current Opinion in Psychology, 25,* 162–166.

Waters, T. E. A., Ruiz, S. K., & Roisman, G. I. (2017). Origins of secure base script knowledge and the developmental construction of attachment representations. *Child Development, 88,* 198–209.

CHAPTER 11

Measuring the Security of Attachment in Adults
Narrative Assessments and Self-Report Questionnaires

Judith A. Crowell

Research in adult attachment emerged in the mid-1980s with two types of measures. In the developmental domain, George, Kaplan, and Main created the Adult Attachment Interview (AAI) to capture a narrative "to assess the security of the adult's overall working model of attachment, . . . the security of the self in relation to attachment in its generality rather than in relation to any particular . . . relationship" (Main, Kaplan, & Cassidy, 1985, p. 78). Social psychologists Hazan and Shaver (1987) hypothesized that attachment theory could illuminate the study of romantic relationships and developed the first questionnaire based on the infant attachment classification patterns. The two lines of research developed very differently and not without controversy. These assessments of attachment do not converge empirically, despite their foundations in theory and some similar relations to outcomes (Crowell, Fraley, & Roisman, 2016).

The AAI inquires about autobiographical childhood attachment memories. It does not ask a person about security or even mention attachment, nor does it probe for specific types of feelings or behaviors. Rather, it asks for general and specific memories of attachment experiences and the meaning of those experiences for the adult's development. It is scored with respect to language, organization, believability, and flexible transitioning between generalized and specific memories. In contrast, the questionnaire measures inquire directly into specific types of feelings and behaviors in relationships. As such, they are very much a self-report about attachment. In this chapter, we focus on these two domains of assessment: the AAI and self-report questionnaires of attachment style, focusing on the Experiences in Close Relationships Scale (Brennan, Clarke, & Shaver, 1998).

Background

The attachment system is an evolutionarily adaptive motivational–behavioral control system. Attachment behavior is activated in times of danger, stress, or novelty, with the goal of gaining and maintaining proximity and contact with the caregiver for protection and reassurance. Under ordinary circumstances, the child confidently explores the environment with the active support of the caregiver, secure in the knowledge that this person is available if need should arise (i.e., the secure base phenomenon). Thus, the behaviors are most apparent at times of stress, although aspects of the system are active at all times (Bretherton, 1985). Bowlby hypothesized that infants develop representations of the functioning and significance of close relationships that make early experiences "portable" to other interpersonal contexts across the lifespan (Bowlby, 1988).

Measurement of attachment in adults draws heavily on this concept of internal working models (IWMs). IWMs consist of beliefs and expectations about how attachment relationships operate. They are hypothesized to be relatively stable and to operate without the need for conscious appraisal; they guide behavior in relationships, influencing expectations and strategies (Bretherton, 1985; Main et al., 1985). They are open to revision as a function of attachment-related experiences and formal operational thought (Crowell, Treboux, & Waters, 2002). Both narrative and self-report questionnaires aim to assess the IWM and are based on the assumption that adult patterns of attachment parallel the individual differences in infancy (Hazan & Shaver, 1987; Main et al., 1985).

Narrative Assessments

The use of narratives to assess attachment started with the premise that "mental processes vary as distinctively as do behavioral processes" (Main et al., 1985, p. 78), and organized behavioral, cognitive, and affective processes are reflected in coherent, organized language. The AAI is the most widely used of the narrative assessments, but we also provide some discussion of the Current Relationship Interview (CRI), a related but distinct form of narrative assessment.

The AAI is based on the core hypotheses about IWMs noted above. It probes for an attachment "script" that develops and elaborates with experience, and guides attachment-relevant behavior and thoughts (Waters, Brockmeyer, & Crowell, 2013; see also Waters, Waters, & Waters, Chapter 14, this volume).

Scoring of the interview transcript includes (1) the coder's assessment of childhood experiences with parents, (2) language used, and

(3) coherence—the ability to give an integrated, believable account of experiences and their meaning (Main, Goldwyn, & Hesse, 2003). Scale scores are used to assign the adult to one of three major classifications that parallel infant classifications: a secure category or one of two insecure categories ("dismissing" or "preoccupied"). There is also a fourth category related to traumas of loss and/or abuse.

Individuals classified as secure express a balanced view of attachment relationships, value those relationships, and view attachment-related experiences as influential in development. The narrative provides consistent, believable reports of parental behavior, such that general descriptions of parenting correspond well to specific memories of parental behavior. Because security is inferred from coherence, any kind of childhood experience may be associated with a secure classification.

The insecure classifications are associated with incoherent accounts, meaning that interviewees' overviews of experience with parents are not matched by descriptions of parental behavior. "Dismissing" adults deny the impact of attachment relationships on development, have difficulty recalling specific events, and idealize experiences; that is, there is evidence of rejection in the context of an overarching assessment of loving parents. "Preoccupied" adults display confusion or oscillation about past experiences, and descriptions of relationships with parents are marked by active anger and/or passivity. The classification is associated with ratings of involving/role-reversing parenting. Individuals may also be classified as "unresolved" in addition to one of the major classifications when they report attachment-related traumas of loss and/or abuse, and manifest confusion and disorganization when discussing the trauma.

The construct and discriminant validities of the AAI are clearly established (Crowell et al., 2016). There is high stability of attachment classifications (78–90% for three classifications up to 13 years) (Booth-LaForce & Roisman, 2014; Crowell & Hauser, 2008; Crowell et al., 2002). The secure classification is especially stable, suggesting that it is very difficult to negatively impact a solid knowledge base/script.

Analyses of large numbers of AAIs suggest that coherent discourse in the AAI is distributed along two independent dimensions (Crowell et al., 2016): (1) variation in the degree to which adults freely evaluate their childhood experiences or are dismissing of them and (2) variation in preoccupation (see Raby, Fraley, & Roisman, Chapter 9, this volume).

AAI security is consistently associated with ratings of social adjustment, stress, and depression (Crowell et al., 2016). Clinical populations have a higher proportion of insecure classifications than the general population, but there are no specific relations between classifications and psychopathology. The unresolved group, not surprisingly, is overrepresented in clinical samples.

There is high correspondence between parent and infant attachment status (Crowell et al., 2016; Posada, Waters, Crowell, & Lay, 1995).

Observational studies find that mothers classified as secure, compared to those classified as insecure, are more responsive, cooperative, and sensitive to their children from infancy to adolescence (Crowell et al., 2016).

Meta-analysis of AAI attachment classifications of couples showed modest concordance between partners' AAI classifications (Bakermans-Kranenburg & van IJzendoorn, 2009). AAI security and marital satisfaction are not highly correlated, but there are clear associations with secure base behaviors in couples' interactions and questionnaire reports of physical aggression. Analyses find that the correlation between coherence and behavioral interactions is largely due to secure base script knowledge (Waters et al., 2013). In other words, access to the secure base script both informs behavior and facilitates coherence of the narrative because the interview questions make sense to the individual, allowing for retrieval of relevant memories and providing structure for a full answer, a critical factor in scoring coherence.

There is compelling support that the AAI assesses a generalized representation rather than being specific to a particular attachment relationship (Crowell et al., 2016). In contrast, the CRI is a narrative measure that draws on AAI scoring but focuses on the relationship with the romantic partner (Treboux, Crowell, & Waters, 2004). It differs from the AAI in that it is a concurrent interview, not retrospective, so accounts of events may be quite recent and emotionally charged. Like the AAI, the coherence score is based on consistency between and believability of the general overview of the relationship and accounts of specific experiences. Scoring specifically addresses the secure base concept, drawing on descriptions of the self and the partner's behavior. Security is defined by the concept that the partnership functions to support both the development of the individuals and the well-being of the relationship.

Coherence scores of the AAI and CRI are significantly correlated but not redundant, $r = .47$ ($p \leq .01$). Interactions among AAI and CRI security, and stressful life events were predictive of individuals' feelings and behavior in marriage, including divorce within the first 6 years (Treboux et al., 2004): 34% of individuals classified as secure AAI/insecure CRI divorced, with the next highest risk group for divorce being insecure AAI/insecure CRI individuals at 23%.

Self-Report Questionnaires

Hazan and Shaver (1987) noted that many emotional and behavioral dynamics of infant–mother attachment relationships characterize adult romantic relationships. Specifically, they argued that the infant patterns of attachment are similar to romantic attachment patterns observed among adults. To assess this hypothesis, they developed brief multisentence descriptions of three attachment types. Participants were asked to think about their history of romantic relationships and indicate which description best captured the way they generally experienced and acted in those relationships. These self-reported attachment styles related to a number of theoretically relevant variables, including beliefs about love and recollections of experiences with parents (Mikulincer & Shaver, 2016).

There were clear limitations of a categorical system, such as that test–retest stability was not robust (Crowell et al., 2016). Thus, a number of multi-item inventories were created to produce continuous attachment scores, and researchers quickly became overwhelmed by their sheer numbers. To address this problem, the distinct items of all known self-report measures were administered to over 1,000 undergraduates (Brennan et al., 1998). Analyses revealed two major factors of attachment: *anxiety* and *avoidance*.

These data were used to produce a new questionnaire, the Experiences in Close Relationships (ECR), using items that best captured the anxiety and avoidance dimensions. Each of the subscales predicted relevant outcomes, including emotions in an intimate context. The ECR and its variations are currently the most commonly used and recommended self-report measures of adult attachment.

With regard to normative continuity and change, a large-scale study indicated that attachment-related anxiety is highest among younger adults and lowest among middle-aged and older adults (Chopik, Edelstein, & Fraley, 2013). Avoidance shows less dramatic age differences, but is lowest in younger adults and highest among middle-aged adults. People in relationships report lower anxiety and avoidance compared to single individuals. Stability of self-reports of romantic relationships were weaker ($r \cong .65$) than those regarding parents ($r \cong .80$) (Fraley, Vicary, Brumbaugh, & Roisman, 2011). Thus, attachment styles may vary at different points in life and in different relationships, which matters in the interpretation of findings with the measure.

Individuals endorsing a secure style tend to have high self-esteem and are considered well adjusted, nurturing, and warm (Crowell et al., 2016). Adults with secure and dismissing styles report high levels of self-esteem, but "secure" adults derive self-esteem from internalized positive regard from others, whereas "dismissing" adults are more likely to derive self-esteem from abilities (Brennan & Morris, 1997). Adults with clinical disorders are more likely to report themselves as insecure (Mikulincer & Shaver, 2016).

Discussion

Measurement of adult attachment continues to present intriguing challenges. The AAI and the ECR methods have only a very weak association, $r = .09$, $n = 900$ (Crowell et al., 2016). Although both measures predict important aspects of close-relationship functioning in adulthood, they do not predict the same outcomes in the same ways.

AAI security appears to function as a general personal asset, that is, an outlook that values close relationships and a knowledge base/script for how to effectively use a secure base, that is, the degree to which an individual "knows" the benefits and has the capacity to use attachment relationships both in times of distress and under ordinary circumstances. It is a rich and well-validated autobiographical measure that provides considerable information about perceived childhood experiences. Nevertheless, the AAI is expensive, challenging to learn, and difficult to score.

The ECR and its modifications assume that people can accurately describe their feelings and behaviors in close relationships. They are used effectively in conjunction with psychophysiological, behavioral, and cognitive techniques to explore intrapsychic processes and behavior in close relationships.

What is clear is that *the AAI and ECR are not substitutes for each other.* Researchers should consider (1) the assumptions underlying each type of measure and the conceptual connection between measure and theory and (2) the relationship domain to be investigated (e.g., parents, partners). We can consider that AAI security reflects a knowledge base and the internal structure of the attachment system as it has developed since infancy in response to attachment experiences. This contrasts with the self-report of "what am I doing/feeling" with respect to relationships, which may be influenced concurrently by the nature of those relationships (present/ absent; parent/partner; happy/distressed) and the developmental stage of the individual. Both knowledge of and feelings about attachment clearly influence attachment behavior, but as is often the case, knowledge and feelings may lead to quite distinct outcomes. In light of the substantial differences among these measures, caution must be taken in how research findings are presented and the conclusions that are drawn.

REFERENCES

Bakersman-Kranenburg, M., & van IJzendoorn, M. (2009). The first 10,000 Adult Attachment Interviews: Distributions of adult attachment representations in clinical and non-clinical groups. *Attachment and Human Development, 11*(3), 223–263.

Booth-LaForce, C., & Roisman, G. I. (Eds.). (2014). The Adult Attachment Interview: Psychometrics, stability and change from infancy, and developmental origins. *Monographs of the Society for Research in Child Development, 79,* 1–316.

Bowlby, J. (1988). *A secure base: Parent–child attachment and healthy human development.* New York: Basic Books.

Brennan, K., Clark, C., & Shaver, P. (1998). Self-report measurement of adult attachment: An integrative overview. In J. A. Simpson & W. S. Rholes (Eds.), Attachment theory and close relationships (pp. 46–76). New York: Guilford Press.

Brennan, K. A., & Morris, K. A. (1997). Attachment styles, self-esteem, and patterns of seeking feedback from romantic partners. *Personality and Social Psychology Bulletin, 23*(1), 23–31.

Bretherton, I. (1985). Attachment theory: Retrospect and prospect. In I. Bretherton & E. Waters (Eds.), Growing points of attachment theory and research. *Monographs of the Society for Research in Child Development, 50*, 3–35.

Chopik, W., Edelstein, R., & Fraley, R. (2013). From the cradle to the grave: Age differences in attachment from early adulthood to old age. *Journal of Personality, 81*(2), 171–183.

Crowell, J., Fraley, R., & Roisman, G. (2016). Measurement of individual differences in adolescent and adult attachment. In J. Cassidy & P. R. Shaver (Eds.), *Handbook of attachment: Theory, research and clinical applications* (pp. 598–635). New York: Guilford Press.

Crowell, J., & Hauser, S. (2008). Attachment in adult relationships: Secure base behavior with a partner in community and high risk adults. In H. Steele & M. Steele (Eds.), *Clinical applications of the Adult Attachment Interview* (pp. 223–244). New York: Guilford Press.

Crowell, J., Treboux, D., & Waters, E. (2002). Stability of attachment representations: The transition to marriage. *Developmental Psychology, 38*, 467–479.

Fraley, R., Vicary, A., Brumbaugh, C., & Roisman, G. (2011). Patterns of stability in adult attachment: An empirical test of two models of continuity and change. *Journal of Personality and Social Psychology, 101*, 974–992.

Hazan, C., & Shaver, P. (1987). Romantic love conceptualized as an attachment process. *Journal of Personality and Social Psychology, 52*, 511–524.

Main, M., Goldwyn, R., & Hesse, E. (2003). *Adult attachment scoring and classification system*. Unpublished manual, University of California at Berkeley.

Main, M., Kaplan, N., & Cassidy, J. (1985). Security of infancy, childhood, and adulthood: A move to the level of representation. In I. Bretherton & E. Waters (Eds.), Growing points of attachment theory and research. *Monographs of the Society for Research in Child Development, 50*(1–2, Serial No. 209), 66–104.

Mikulincer, M., & Shaver, P. R. (2016). *Attachment in adulthood: Structure, dynamics, and change* (2 ed.). New York: Guilford Press.

Posada, G., Waters, E., Crowell, J., & Lay, K. (1995). Is it easier to use a secure mother as a secure base?: Attachment Q-sort correlates of the Adult Attachment Interview. In E. Waters, B. Vaughn, G. Posada, & K. Kondo-Ikemura (Eds.), Caregiving, cultural, and cognitive perspectives on secure-base behavior and working models: New growing points of attachment theory and research. *Monographs of the Society for Research in Child Development, 60*, 133–145.

Treboux, D., Crowell, J., & Waters, E. (2004). When "new" meets "old": Configurations of adult attachment representations and their implications for marital functioning. *Developmental Psychology, 40*, 295–314.

Waters, T., Brockmeyer, S., & Crowell, J. (2013). AAI coherence predicts caregiving and care seeking behavior: Secure base script knowledge helps explain why. *Attachment and Human Development, 15*, 316–331.

CHAPTER 12

The Dual-Function Model of Attachment Security Priming

Omri Gillath
Ting Ai

Priming is a well-validated social-cognitive research technique that allows researchers to study causality and directionality. In the attachment domain, researchers often use priming to activate the sense of attachment security or insecurity and examine the outcomes of such activation and its interactions with people's attachment style (i.e., trait-like levels of attachment anxiety and avoidance). In the current chapter, we provide a brief review of the attachment priming literature. We start by defining key concepts and follow with a concise review of attachment-related priming findings and a new model that explains these findings. We conclude with a discussion of the main contributions and limitations of this literature.

Priming

Priming is the activation of a particular mental representation or association in one's memory. Psychologists studying priming are often interested in the effects of these activated representations on a specific subsequent action or task (e.g., Tulving & Schacter, 1990), or on the activation of stored knowledge (Higgins & Eitam, 2014). For example, in a lexical decision task where participants are asked to decide whether letter strings are proper English words or not, exposure to the word *chair* (the prime) makes the identification of the letter string *table* (the target) easier and faster to process as compared with exposure to the word *phone*. Priming can occur following a conscious or an unconscious exposure to a cue (supraliminal vs. subliminal priming), with the person being either aware or unaware of the prime and the priming procedure. Priming can also operate at a presemantic level (i.e., before a meaning is inferred; Tulving & Schacter, 1990).

The proposed mechanisms underlying priming effects have two components: (1) the "excitation" of representations in memory by a process of spreading activation through a semantic network of associations and (2) the use of these excited (more accessible) representations to facilitate encoding information in a subsequent task (Molden, 2014). Human memory is often depicted as a semantic network of constructs associated to each other (Meyer & Schvaneveldt, 1971). When people are exposed to one construct (prime), other constructs (targets) that are associated with it become more accessible or salient in one's stream of thoughts. This cognitive accessibility increases the chances that the related constructs (or schemas) will be used in succeeding tasks (Higgins & Eitam, 2014).

Priming in Attachment

Interactions with primary caregivers or, as Bowlby (1982) called them, *attachment figures* are consolidated over time into internal working models (IWMs; Gillath, Karantzas, & Fraley, 2016). After they were internalized, these IWMs (or mental representations) can be activated in the laboratory using priming methods. Once activated, researchers can examine the outcomes of activation and the interaction of activation with people's chronic attachment style.

Priming methods have become increasingly common in the study of attachment (e.g., Baldwin, Keelan, Fehr, Enns, & Koh-Rengarajoo, 1996). They allow researchers not only to study issues related to directionality and causality of attachment processes in relatively controlled settings but also to overcome some of the limitations of other research methods (e.g., observational assessments, self-reports, and interviews), such as social desirability biases, positive self-presentations biases, and the inability to access people's unconscious processes or shed light on their mentalization abilities (i.e., the ability to understand the mental state of oneself or others).

Attachment-Related Schemas

IWMs, representing the self (as worthy of being loved or not) and others (as likely to provide help in times of need or not), can be positive or negative and are incorporated within long-term memory along with particular emotions, motives, goals, and behaviors that, collectively, underlie a person's attachment style (e.g., Gillath et al., 2016). Repeated encounters with sensitive and responsive attachment figures are likely to result in the formation of a secure attachment style, whereas interactions with inconsistent, insensitive, intrusive, or unresponsive attachment figures are likely to result in the development of an insecure attachment style. According to Baldwin and his colleagues (1996), most people experience a variety of relational interactions, situations, and relationship histories throughout their lives, which can make them feel secure, anxious, or avoidant at different points in time. Hence, everyone should have mental representations of secure and insecure experiences available in their long-term memory—memories that can be activated in the laboratory. Researchers can take advantage of these preexisting IWMs to prime a sense of attachment security, anxiety, or avoidance in study participants. For example, Baldwin and colleagues primed participants with different types of attachment experiences (security, anxiety, or avoidance) and found it influenced participants' attraction to dating partners who displayed a particular attachment style. Likewise, Birnbaum, Simpson, Weisberg, Barnea, and Assulin-Simhon (2012) primed attachment insecurity and showed it affected the reported content of participants' sexual fantasies.

The Methods of Priming

Different methods have been used to prime attachment security. These methods include (but are not limited to): (1) exposing people (subliminally or supraliminally) to security-related words (e.g., love, hug, affection, support) or the names of security-providing attachment figures via different tasks (e.g., a crossword puzzle); (2) exposing people to pictures representing attachment security (such as a mother hugging a child); (3) visualization by asking people to recall memories of being loved and supported by attachment figures; or (4) guided imagery by asking people to imagine such scenarios or relationships.

Priming Effects

According to attachment theory (Bowlby, 1982), among adults, the attachment behavioral system serves three main functions: (1) provision of *safe haven* (providing support, comfort, reassurance, and relief), (2) provision of *secure base* (facilitating exploration and supporting autonomy), and (3) proximity seeking/maintenance[1] (maintaining the individual's safety

---

[1] In adulthood, the fulfillment of proximity seeking/maintenance does not necessarily entail physical proximity because adults do not need to maintain physical proximity for safety. Instead, priming attachment security can lead to felt security, which simulates the effects of proximity to an attachment figure.

and security through contact with an attachment figure, which is more direct and common between infants and caregivers). An attachment figure is someone who fulfills these functions (Gillath et al., 2016), serving as either a safe haven, a secure base, or both. Given that priming should activate felt security in a similar way to that experienced in the actual presence of a security-providing attachment figure, one would expect that priming attachment security would activate both safe haven and secure base.[2]

For safe haven, security priming should result in an increase in positive emotions such as relaxation and a reduction in feelings of distress and anxiety. Indeed, security priming has been shown in multiple studies to increase positive emotions and to decrease negative emotions such as depression, hostility, prejudice toward outgroup members, and death anxiety. With regard to secure base, security priming should lead to more exploration, openness, and autonomy. Indeed, studies show that security priming leads to more creative problem solving, creativity, exploration, and openness (see Gillath et al., 2016, for a review).

Attachment security also facilitates the smooth operation of other behavioral systems, such as caregiving. When the sense of security is restored, people can perceive others not only as sources of security and support but also as human beings who need and deserve comfort and support themselves (Bowlby, 1982). Therefore, security priming can shift people's focus of attention from self to others. Indeed, studies show that following security priming people exhibit more compassion and altruism, and greater willingness to help others even while potentially risking themselves (see Gillath et al., 2016, for a review).

Although many studies show the effects of security priming to occur regardless of one's dispositional attachment style (e.g., Gillath & Shaver, 2007), some do reveal an interaction between security priming and attachment style. Gillath and Karantzas (2019) conducted a systematic review of recent studies related to security priming and its effects. They found that supraliminal priming has beneficial effects specifically for people high on attachment anxiety. Thus, supraliminal security priming may be especially effective in down-regulating the hyperactivating strategies of anxiously attached individuals. The same priming was not as effective among people high on attachment avoidance, perhaps due to their use of defense mechanisms. It may be that individuals high on attachment avoidance are more resistant to the beneficial effects of security priming, or that only subliminal priming may be able to bypass the cognitive-affective defenses of these individuals. The fact that in some studies security

---

[2]While both could be activated, we argue in our model presented later in the chapter that often one or the other will be activated, or the two functions are not activated to the same extent.

priming interacts with chronic attachment style and in others it does not, highlights the need to further explore factors that could moderate the effects of security priming (see Gillath et al., 2016, for a review).

Clinical Interventions

Due to the fact that security priming is relatively easy to administer, quick, and cheap, some researchers applied security priming or security-priming-based techniques to clinical intervention. For example, McGuire, Gillath, Jackson, and Ingram (2018) demonstrated that priming techniques could effectively reduce depressive symptoms among adolescents and emerging adults.

The Dual-Function Model: Stress Relief versus Mobilization

Based on the review of outcomes above, two distinct lines of outcomes associated with attachment security priming stand out: One relates to safe haven and the other to secure base. Accordingly, we propose the *Dual Function of Security Priming* (DFSP) model. On the one hand, when people encounter threat or stress and they need help, priming security activates the if–then scripts (Mikulincer, Shaver, Sapir-Lavid, & Avihou-Kanza, 2009; see also Waters, Waters, & Waters, Chapter 14, this volume). For example, *if* I encounter an obstacle or a threat, *then* I'll seek protection from my attachment figure, and he or she will be responsive and support-ive. If indeed support is provided, stress should abate and security should be regained. This script is a good depiction of the safe haven aspect of security, and the stress relief component of our model.

On the other hand, in a neutral context with no immediate threat (e.g., the stress level is low or there is no obvious threat), security prim-ing is likely to activate the sense of secure base, and contribute to what Mikulincer and Shaver (2004) refer to as the *broadening and building cycle* of attachment security. They suggest that security increases a person's resilience and expands his or her perspectives, and coping flexibility and capabilities. Priming security under these circumstances activates a dif-ferent script than the if–then script, a script according to which the world is safe, attachment figures will be there when called upon, and one can devote attention and effort to personal growth, self-development, or the needs of others. This represents the secure base aspect of our model.

The secure base function of security priming mobilizes people into action. The mobilization may psychologically signal individuals to actively engage with the environment. It may also physiologically activate meta-bolic processes to prepare the body for action and provide the energy to do so (Mendoza, 2017). Indeed, studies have shown that security-related primes result in feeling greater energy (Luke, Sedikides, & Carnelley, 2012) as well as higher blood glucose levels and greater heart-rate variability (Stanton, Campbell, & Loving, 2014).

Our dual-function model is in line with Feeney's (2004) Circle of Security model, according to which when a support-receiver experiences and perceives life stressors, a support-provider can fulfill the safe haven function by providing help and support that reduce the receiver's stress. Conversely, when a receiver encounters an exploration opportunity, the provider can engage in secure base behaviors to help the receiver's exploration. The Circle of Security model highlights the partner's support in romantic relationships. The dual-function model builds on Feeney's model by suggesting that security priming is similar to a partner providing either stress relief or mobilization, depending on the circumstances.

Both the dual-function model we propose and Feeney's (2004) Circle of Security model suggest that the functions of attachment security (or attachment figures) change in line with the context, specifically the level of stress imposed by the environment (e.g., social context). This is consistent with Tomaka, Blascovich, Kelsey, and Leitten (1993), who suggested that people may appraise context as either a threat or a challenge. When environmental demands are perceived as exceeding one's resources or ability to cope, people feel threatened and respond with high negative affect and inadequate or disorganized mobilization of resources. Conversely, when environmental demands are appraised as being within one's resources or ability to cope, people feel challenged and respond with positive affect and efficient, organized mobilization of resources. When people feel threatened, the main function that security priming serves is to relieve negative affect and restore physiological and psychological functioning (safe haven). In contrast, lower levels of demands/stress are likely to be associated with people feeling a challenge, so the main function of security priming is to facilitate the mobilization of resources and engagement with the challenge (secure base).

The literature on security priming is characterized by an interesting duality. Some studies show security priming leads people to relax and calm down; other studies show that security priming leads people to feel energized and ready for action. The DFSP model helps to explain this duality.

Concluding Remarks

Security priming increases people's sense of attachment security and, at least temporarily, makes them feel, think, and behave like securely attached individuals. The findings reviewed above further suggest that security priming procedures do not simply create a semantic connection between a positive stimulus and resulting positive affect, but result in a multitude of outcomes (affective, cognitive, and behavioral) that resemble the correlates of attachment security (e.g., stress relief, exploration, and prosocial behaviors). Our new DFSP model, according to which security priming can simulate safe haven or secure base functions, depending on the circumstances, helps explain the duality in the reviewed findings. With further empirical support the model could provide a framework for improving the understanding of the diverse effects of security priming and guide future studies. Finally, our model could increase the confidence in the priming literature more generally by illuminating the importance of potential interactions between priming and context.

REFERENCES

Baldwin, M. W., Keelan, J. P. R., Fehr, B., Enns, V., & Koh-Rangarajoo, E. (1996). Social-cognitive conceptualization of attachment working models: Availability and accessibility effects. *Journal of Personality and Social Psychology, 71,* 94–109.

Birnbaum, G. E., Simpson, J. A., Weisberg, Y. J., Barnea, E., & Assulin-Simhon, Z. (2012). Is it my overactive imagination?: The effects of contextually activated attachment insecurity on sexual fantasies. *Journal of Social and Personal Relationships, 29,* 1131–1152.

Bowlby, J. (1982). Attachment and loss: Retrospect and prospect. *American Journal of Orthopsychiatry, 52,* 664–678.

Feeney, B. C. (2004). A secure base: Responsive support of goal strivings and exploration in adult intimate relationships. *Journal of Personality and Social Psychology, 87,* 631–648.

Gillath, O., & Karantzas, G. (2019). Attachment security priming: A systematic review. *Current Opinion in Psychology, 25,* 86–95.

Gillath, O., Karantzas, G. C., & Fraley, R. C. (2016). *Adult attachment: A concise introduction to theory and research.* London: Academic Press.

Gillath, O., & Shaver, P. R. (2007). Effects of attachment style and relationship context on selection among relational strategies. *Journal of Research in Personality, 41,* 968–976.

Higgins, E. T., & Eitam, B. (2014). Priming . . . shmiming: It's about knowing when and why stimulated memory representations become active. *Social Cognition, 32,* 225–242.

Luke, M. A., Sedikides, C., & Carnelley, K. (2012). Your love lifts me higher!: The energizing quality of secure relationships. *Personality and Social Psychology Bulletin, 38,* 721–733.

McGuire, A., Gillath, O., Jackson, Y., & Ingram, R. (2018). Attachment security priming as a potential intervention for depressive symptoms. *Journal of Social and Clinical Psychology, 37,* 44–68.

Mendoza, S. P. (2017). Social stress: Concepts, assumptions, and animal models.

In D. W. Pfaff & M. Joels (Eds.), *Hormones, brain, and behavior* (pp. 261–284). Oxford, UK: Academic Press.

Meyer, D. E., & Schvaneveldt, R. W. (1971). Facilitation in recognizing pairs of words: Evidence of a dependence between retrieval operations. *Journal of Experimental Psychology, 90,* 227–234.

Mikulincer, M., & Shaver, P. R. (2004). Security-based self- representations in adulthood: Contents and processes. In W. S. Rholes & J. A. Simpson (Eds), *Adult attachment: Theory, research, and clinical implications* (pp. 159–195). New York: Guilford Press.

Mikulincer, M., Shaver, P. R., Sapir-Lavid, Y., & Avihou-Kanza, N. (2009). What's inside the minds of securely and insecurely attached people?: The secure-base script and its associations with attachment-style dimensions. *Journal of Personality and Social Psychology, 97,* 615–633.

Molden, D. C. (2014). Understanding priming effects in social psychology: What is "social priming" and how does it occur? *Social Cognition, 32,* 1–11.

Stanton, S. C., Campbell, L., & Loving, T. J. (2014). Energized by love: Thinking about romantic relationships increases positive affect and blood glucose levels. *Psychophysiology, 51,* 990–995.

Tomaka, J., Blascovich, J., Kelsey, R. M., & Leitten, C. L. (1993). Subjective, physiological, and behavioral effects of threat and challenge appraisal. *Journal of Personality and Social Psychology, 65,* 248–260.

Tulving, E., & Schacter, D. L. (1990). Priming and human memory systems. *Science, 247,* 301–306.

THE NATURE AND FUNCTION OF INTERNAL WORKING MODELS

- What are internal working models?

- How do they operate?

CHAPTER 13

In the Service of Protection from Threat
Attachment and Internal Working Models

Jude Cassidy

Protection from threat is a foundational necessity of all organisms. When faced with threat, rabbits freeze, foxes run to their dens, turtles withdraw into their shells, cobras spread their impressive hoods. Each organism must solve the same quandary: how to best enhance reproductive fitness *given the threats (and resources) existing in the environmental context in which it finds itself.*

In some species, the attachment behavioral system evolved as a central means of protection from threat. Attachment, in fact, can be viewed as a primate infant's central "threat protection device." Certainly this is how Bowlby (1969/1982), basing his revolutionary approach on evolutionary theory, originally viewed attachment—as the best solution to the most basic need of the human infant. Bowlby talked of the principal biological function of attachment as protection from threat.

Humans, like other animals, draw on all possible means to protect themselves. The evolution of the cognitive capacities that allow for the development of what Bowlby termed *internal working models* (IWMs) can be viewed as an adaptation providing increased protection from threat. Because of the significance of attachment to evolved threat protection, it is consideration of IWMs *within the context of threat* that is the focus of this chapter.

Following a brief description of the definition and properties of IWMs, I consider two key questions: (1) How do IWMs develop within the context of threat? and (2) How do IWMs influence later functioning within the context of threat? I move beyond Bowlby's initial consideration of protection from predators and consider protection from threats to reproductive fitness more broadly—a conceptualization that continues to include protection from predators (both nonhuman and human) and includes threats to social connections, resource and goal attainment, and self-regulation (see Simpson & Belsky, 2016, for discussion of modern evolutionary approaches to attachment). As such, I view the context of threat and that of distress as closely intertwined, occurring in a wide variety of contexts at multiple levels of intensity (e.g., physical abuse; a large, looming carnivore; misplacement of a valued teddy bear; playground bullying). These examples share a subjective experience of threat and distress.

Definition and Characteristics of IWMs

Bowlby (1973, 1980) believed that individuals create mental representations (IWMs) that provide them models of the workings, characteristics, and behavior of what he called *attachment figures* (typically parents in the case of children), and of the self, others, and relationships. These models, containing both cognitive and affective components, are similar to cognitive maps that permit successful navigation of an organism's environment, yet are active constructions rather than static representations. Bowlby proposed that IWMs, which often exist outside of consciousness, are quite stable and become increasingly resistant to change (see also Main, Kaplan, & Cassidy, 1985).

Bowlby framed the core content of IWMs within the secure base construct: Confidence in the responsiveness of the attachment figure in times of threat (the parent as a safe haven) supports the child's exploration of the environment (the parent as a secure base from which to explore). The intertwined secure base/safe haven functions enhance the child's reproductive fitness by allowing the child to maximize safety while learning about the environment. Children who are securely attached have an IWM reflecting confidence in the attachment figure as providing a secure base in the absence of threat and a safe haven in times of threat.

IWMs enhance protection from threat because the ability to anticipate the attachment figure's likely behavior across contexts allows the child to plan how to obtain needed protection while simultaneously conserving energy for other activities that enhance reproductive fitness.

How Do IWMs Develop within the Context of Threat?

Perhaps the most central conceptualization related to IWMs is that they develop, starting in the first year of life, in response to attachment-related experiences with individual attachment figures (see Thompson, Chapter

16, this volume, for the importance of considering developmental processes in IWM formation). Through repeated daily experiences, infants begin to acquire event-based knowledge of their attachment figures' tendencies to be available, responsive, and sensitive to their needs (Ainsworth, Bell, & Stayton, 1971; Bowlby, 1973). Bowlby theorized that this knowledge likely emerged through the formation of mental structures representing the realistic reproduction, or "mental simulation," of previous interactions with attachment figures.

These interactions, according to Bretherton (1985, 1990), create cognitive structures called scripts, which Waters and Waters (2006) labeled secure base scripts. These scripts are considered to provide infants with if–then contingencies of the ways in which attachment-related events typically unfold (e.g., "If I am hurt, then I go to my mother and she comforts me"). Bretherton (1990) described secure base scripts as the "building blocks" from which more complex IWMs develop. According to Main and colleagues (1985), "infants whose attempts to gain proximity to the caregiver are consistently accepted will develop different internal working models of relationships than do infants whose attempts to gain proximity are consistently blocked or are accepted only unpredictably" (p. 77). Children develop IWMs not only of caregivers' likely responses to their needs but also of themselves. Bowlby (1973, pp. 204–205) noted that although it is "logically indefensible," the child's model of the self is closely intertwined with IWMs of attachment figures.

The contexts of threat and safety are central to IWM development. Because the child's safety depends on access to the attachment figure when threatened, it is essential that the child have an accurate working model of this person's likely behavior *particularly in such times.* As such, the experiences from which IWMs of attachment develop are not random, nor do all experiences contribute equally. It is contexts that provide the infant with information about the parent's likely behavior when threatened (i.e., in response to activation of the infant's attachment system following threat), rather than all contexts, that are central. Bowlby (1969/1982) described the relevant contexts as "fall[ing] into two classes: those that indicate the presence of potential danger or stress (internal or external) and those concerning the whereabouts and accessibility of the attachment figure" (p. 373). Especially during the early years of life, both of these circumstances are likely to be associated with infant distress. Converging indications that maternal response to infant distress is more predictive of secure IWMs than maternal response to nondistress has emerged from several studies of infant attachment (e.g., Leerkes, Weaver, & O'Brien, 2012; see Thompson, 1997).

Although it is readily understandable that a child's representations about parental response to threat and distress come largely from parental behavior during such moments, it would be most efficient if such information could come from certain times of relative calm as well. In other words, it is possible that in times free of immediate threat, the child none-theless gathers information about the parent's response to the child when threatened. Surely humans of all ages sometimes approach an attachment figure for connection and physical contact in the absence of threat—just for a cuddle—an initiation that may reflect attachment system activation in the absence of another initiating factor (e.g., bids for play or food). If children are indeed biologically predisposed to make such initiations in the absence of threat—why do they do so? What are children learning that contributes to the development of their IWMs about likely response to distress? It may be that the child learns about the ready availability of the attachment figure—the extent to which he or she is sufficiently attentive so that if threat arose, he or she could be helpful. Other salient experiences may be those that involve shared attention to the importance of the relationship, including times of mutual delight in the relationship (e.g., as opposed to engagement with toys or teaching), particularly those initiated by the child (Woodhouse, Scott, Hepworth, & Cassidy, 2020).

How Do IWMs Influence Later Functioning within the Context of Threat?

Just as the level and nature of contextual threat is such a central *precursor* to IWM development, it is reasonable to assume that the *influence of IWMs on subsequent functioning* will also vary as a function of contextual threat. As noted above, the attachment behavioral system is the best solution to the most immediate need of protection for primate infants, and certainly the evolutionary processes that allowed for the development of experience-based IWMs in humans are helpful for creating strategies to maximize protection. The cascade of processes through which child IWMs influence later functioning is presented in Figure 13.1 and is discussed here within the context of threat.

   The concept of conditional behavioral strategies is central to under-standing how IWMs influence later functioning because the concept spec-ifies the biological basis for the range of ways infants obtain protection when the attachment system is activated in the face of threat. According to Main (1990), just as other organisms are genetically endowed to be flexibly responsive to the range of physical environments in which they may find themselves, so too does the infant possess the biologically based flexibility to adapt to a range of caregiving environments through strate-gic tailoring of the attachment behavior system in the service of protec-tion. These strategies are thought to be automatically employed and need not be conscious.

   Main (1990) proposed that experience-based IWMs of the self and others serve as the foundations from which strategies are constructed

(Figure 13.1, paths a and b). Main argued that the number of potential strategies for achieving protection when threatened is not infinite, but instead is comprised of only three options for responding to threat-related activation of the attachment system. For children who have sufficient confidence in the parent's availability when distressed, the child's strategy is simple: Explore when safe and seek care from the responsive caregiver when needed (considered a secure strategy). In contrast, when the caregiving context precludes an IWM of caregiver responsiveness, alternative child strategies (considered insecure) instead emerge to either minimize or maximize attachment behavior as a "response to a caregiver stressing either exaggerated offspring independence or dependence" (p. 52). As noted in Figure 13.1, strategies in turn provide the mechanism through which IWMs influence children's cognitions and emotions (i.e., children's information processing and emotion regulation; path c), which in turn influence more distal psychosocial functioning (path d). Protection from threat is central because these strategic calibrations of attachment behavior help to ensure protection given the nature of the parent's likely behavior in response to environmental events (see also Slade, 2014).[1]

I now describe the pathways that involve the two insecure strategies of minimizing and maximizing. For a child whose (threat-related) distress has led to repeated experiences of rejection, IWMs emerge of the

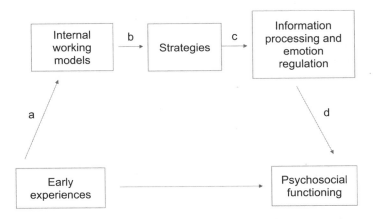

FIGURE 13.1. The role of IWMs in the link between early experiences and later psychosocial functioning.

---

[1] For children whose IWMs reflect the attachment figure as the source of threat, there is no effective strategy (Hesse & Main, 2006), and the IWMs of these children contribute to their psychosocial functioning, yet without involving an organized strategy. Neither these children, labeled insecure/disorganized, nor secure children are considered further in this brief report.

attachment figure as rejecting of distress and of the self as unable to elicit desired care. For these children, expressions of attachment behavior may have dangerous consequences. If the child overtly expresses the anger associated with rejected attachment behaviors (Bowlby, 1973), he or she might risk alienating the attachment figure. If the child makes further demands, he or she might risk being rebuffed altogether. Thus, working models that motivate expressing distress and seeking care are unlikely to succeed and the increased danger that results could reasonably lead the child to a strategy to cut off, repress, or falsify the expression of distress, thereby reducing arousal and preventing the direct expression of negative affect to the attachment figure. Moreover, as Main (1990) noted, by not alienating the attachment figure, the child who uses this strategy can maintain sufficient proximity to the attachment figure to be protected in times of severe threat.

The next step for individuals using a minimizing strategy involves regulation across multiple systems by reducing the likelihood that attachment behaviors will be activated (e.g., turning attention away from stimuli that might activate attachment; see Cassidy, 1994; Dykas & Cassidy, 2011). When IWMs contribute to a minimizing strategy in relation to a specific attachment figure, the short-term positive benefits bring a negative outcome of limiting access to help from others. When these patterns of restricting expression of distress and limiting bids for care become entrenched and carried into new relationships, they can have negative outcomes (e.g., Gross, 2015, provides extensive data on correlates of emotion suppression).

A different cascade emerges in response to a parent who is inconsistently responsive to bids for care in the face of threat. A child in this situation is likely to develop IWMs of the parent and self that lead to an understandable strategy of increasing bids for attention by exhibiting extreme dependence on the attachment figure. Main and Solomon (1986) noted that "in its heightened display of emotionality and dependence upon the attachment figure, this infant successfully draws the attention of the parent" (p. 112). This strategy is an adaptive response to the caregiving environment because, given an inconsistently responsive attachment figure who cannot be relied on for protection, maintaining proximity in the absence of threat increases the likelihood of protection during actual threat. An adaptive strategy of maximizing attachment behavior entails enlisting attention, memory, and interpretation in the search for and early detection of threat. Emotion experience and expression are also heightened because they alert others of the need for care (see Cassidy & Berlin, 1994). When IWMs contribute to strategies of maximizing activation of the attachment system, the short-term benefit of increasing the likelihood of protection also brings with it a negative outcome of preventing the child from attending to other developmentally appropriate tasks.

The child's subjective experience is also undermined (e.g., fearfulness may result from limited familiarity and success with the environment). Moreover, the child who must resort to extremes of affective signaling with unpredictable success is poorly equipped to understand and organize affective experiences. All of these sequelae of long-term maximizing contribute to the poor emotion-regulation skills and biased information-processing patterns that underlie many forms of psychopathology.

Summary

IWMs are central to understanding the ways that humans protect themselves. With increases in cognitive capacities afforded through evolution, humans gained an additional mechanism through which we are protected from threat. A focus on IWMs as mechanisms to enhance protection is a reminder of Bowlby's foundation in evolutionary theory.

REFERENCES

Ainsworth, M. D. S., Bell, S., & Stayton, D. (1971). Individual differences in Strange-Situation behaviour of one-year-olds. In H. R. Schaffer (Ed.), *The origins of human social relations* (pp. 17–58). Oxford, UK: Academic Press.

Bowlby, J. (1973). *Attachment and loss: Vol. 2. Separation.* New York: Basic Books.

Bowlby, J. (1980). *Attachment and loss: Vol. 3. Loss, sadness and depression.* New York: Basic Books.

Bowlby, J. (1982). *Attachment and loss: Vol. 1. Attachment* (2nd ed.). New York: Basic Books. (Original work published 1969)

Bretherton, I. (1985). Attachment theory: Retrospect and prospect. In I. Bretherton & E. Waters (Eds.), Growing points of attachment theory and research. *Monographs of the Society for Research in Child Development, 50*(1–2, Serial No. 209), 3–38.

Bretherton, I. (1990). Open communication and internal working models: Their role in the development of attachment relationships. In R. A. Thompson (Ed.), *Nebraska Symposium on Motivation: Vol. 36. Socioemotional development* (pp. 59–113). Lincoln: University of Nebraska Press.

Cassidy, J. (1994). Emotion regulation: Influences of attachment relationships. In N. Fox (Ed.), The development of emotion regulation. *Monographs of the Society for Research in Child Development, 59*(2–3, Serial No. 240), 228–249.

Cassidy, J., & Berlin, L. J. (1994). The insecure/ambivalent pattern of attachment: Theory and research. *Child Development, 65,* 971–991.

Dykas, M. J., & Cassidy, J. (2011). Attachment and the processing of social information across the lifespan: Theory and evidence. *Psychological Bulletin, 137,* 19–46.

Gross, J. J. (Ed.). (2015). *Handbook of emotion regulation* (2nd ed.). New York: Guilford Press.

Hesse, E., & Main, M. (2006). Frightened, threatening, and dissociative parental behavior in low-risk samples: Description, discussion, and interpretations. *Development and Psychopathology, 18,* 309–343.

Leerkes, E. M., Weaver, J. M., & O'Brien, M. (2012). Differentiating maternal sensitivity to infant distress and non-distress. *Parenting: Science and Practice, 12,* 175–184.

Main, M. (1990). Cross-cultural studies of attachment organization: Recent studies, changing methodologies, and the concept of conditional strategies. *Human Development, 33,* 48–61.

Main, M., Kaplan, N., & Cassidy, J. (1985). Security in infancy, childhood, and adulthood: A move to the level of representation. In I. Bretherton & E. Waters (Eds.), Growing points in attachment theory and research. *Monographs of the Society for Research in Child Development, 50*(1–2, Serial No. 209), 66–104.

Main, M., & Solomon, J. (1986). Discovery of an insecure-disorganized/disoriented attachment pattern. In T. B. Brazelton & M. W. Yogman (Eds.), *Affective development in infancy* (pp. 95–124). Westport, CT: Ablex.

Simpson, J., & Belsky, J. (2016). Attachment theory within a modern evolutionary framework. In J. Cassidy & P. R. Shaver (Eds.), *Handbook of attachment: Theory, research, and clinical applications* (3rd ed., pp. 93–116). New York: Guilford Press.

Slade, A. (2014). Imagining fear: Attachment, threat, and psychic experience. *Psychoanalytic Dialogues, 24,* 253–266.

Thompson, R. A. (1997). Sensitivity and security: New questions to ponder. *Child Development, 68,* 595–597.

Waters, H. S., & Waters, E. (2006). The attachment working models concept: Among other things, we build script-like representations of secure base experiences. *Attachment and Human Development, 8,* 185–197.

Woodhouse, S. S., Scott, J. R., Hepworth, A. D., & Cassidy, J. (2020). Secure base provision: A new approach to links between maternal caregiving and attachment. *Child Development, 91,* 249–265.

CHAPTER 14

From Internal Working Models to Script-like Attachment Representations

Harriet S. Waters
Theodore E. A. Waters
Everett Waters

The idea that we know something best when we know it from its beginning has a long history in philosophy and the natural sciences. For Aristotle, to know something is to have its *archae* (ἀρχή), its origin, its foundations, ever in mind. In psychology, this entails describing the course of development in detail and also identifying plausible mechanisms of action and developmental change. This chapter focuses on the roles of script-like representations of secure base experience in attachment behavior and development. Scripts are not the only mode of mental representation in play during attachment interactions and development, but they illustrate the descriptive and explanatory roles ordinary (as opposed to attachment-specific) cognitive processes can play in attachment theory and research.

Freud's emphasis on the enduring influence of early experience was one of the distinctive features of his theory. John Bowlby considered this an important insight with great significance for both prevention and adult psychotherapy. In his view, the origins of attachment lie in countless experiences of using the primary caregiver as a secure base from which to explore and as a haven of safety. These experiences lead to expectations about caregiver availability and responsiveness and eventually to internal working models (IWMs), which, in turn, help guide behavior and emotion, and help simulate possible courses of action in close relationships.

While acknowledging the heuristic value of the IWM concept, Hinde (1989) felt compelled to note that "in the very power of such a model lies a trap: It can easily explain everything" (p. 378). That is, an attachment theory built upon an overly broad IWM concept lacks definition and risks becoming the theory that "all good things go together." Attachment theorists' sensitivity to this problem is evident in recent reviews (e.g., Bretherton & Munholland, 2008). However, the problem is more than a matter of clear definition. For example, it is not obvious that all the functions attributed to IWMs require anything as complex as a mental model. Moreover, humans are not particularly good at manipulating any but the simplest mental models in real time (Epstein, 2014). Thus, on almost any formulation, IWMs would likely require too much information and effort (not to mention being too slow) to play the roles Bowlby had in mind in ongoing attachment interactions. Here, we propose exploring additional modes of mental representation that might be relevant to attachment interactions and relationships—returning to IWMs once we know better what can be explained without them.

Using Basic Cognitive Processes to Explicate Attachment Representation

Cognitive psychologists have investigated a wide range of representational processes that bear on encoding, retrieving, and responding to real-world experiences. These include verbal associations, concepts, narrative structures such as scenes and episodes, schemas, plans, prototypes, expectations, and even sensory and visual imagery. Each of these can play a role in how we represent, retrieve, and revise attachment-related experiences and how they bear on current and future affect, cognition, and behavior in relationships.

In cognition, as in other domains, parsimony suggests looking to ordinary, well-studied mechanisms before proposing new, domain-specific ones. Approaching the "attachment representation" or IWM concept in terms of specific modes of mental representation gives students of attachment access to the rich toolkit and library of empirical results cognitive psychologists have assembled. Working with concepts and results from cognitive psychology can help us to make specific predictions about how attachment-related experiences, representations, behaviors, memories, and emotions arise and interact. We expect that many of the functions currently covered by a very broadly drawn IWM concept can be explained in terms of specific modes of representation and processing that are already well known in cognitive psychology (e.g., Markman, 2013; Nelson & Fivush, 2004). To paraphrase Richard Dawkins (1998), this kind of rigor may seem like taking the beauty out of the rainbow. However, it is a valuable step toward ensuring the long-term good health of attachment study.

Defining and Measuring Script-like Representations of Attachment-Related Experience

Scripts are schematic representations of the temporal-causal structure and commonalities in recurring events. For example, Schank and Abelson (1977), suggested that repeated visits to a variety of dining establishments results in a restaurant script (look at menu, order food, eat, pay, leave). Scripts generate expectations and help prepare and organize ongoing behavior. They also have motivational significance, not because they have the power to impel behavior but because activating mental representations of goals lowers the threshold to enact behavior. Scripts also play an important role in reconstruction and retrieval processes when we recall past experiences (Abelson, 1981).

Bretherton (1991) pointed out the relevance of scripts as representations of attachment-related experiences. This raises the question, what kind of attachment-related experiences are likely to lead to significant script-like representations? Should we follow the lead of psychoanalysts who emphasized the importance of emergency responses, trauma, and the ensuing emotional distress? Or, following upon Bowlby's insights about the significance of ordinary (i.e., nontraumatic) experiences, focus on salient facets of everyday parent–child or adult–adult interactions?

Working from Ainsworth's ethological descriptions in Uganda and Baltimore, her (and our own) extensive experience with the Strange Situation Procedure (SSP), and our own home observations with the Attachment Q-set, we decided to focus specifically on the secure base concept. That is, on the key recurring elements in secure base excursions and returns to define a "secure base script" (Table 14.1).

With this in mind, Waters and Waters (2006) designed the Attachment Script Assessment (ASA) to determine whether an individual has summarized early attachment experiences in terms of a secure base script.

TABLE 14.1. Elements and Structure of the Secure Base Script

1. A child (or infant) and mother (or two adult attachment partners) are constructively occupied.
2. They are interrupted by an event or another actor. The infant (or one adult) is distressed.
3. There is a bid for help.
4. The bid for help is detected and help is offered.
5. The offer of help is accepted.
6. The help is effective in overcoming the difficulty.
7. The help includes effective comforting and affect regulation.
8. The pair return to (or initiate new) constructive interaction.

The ASA consists of several sets of 12–14 prompt words, each loosely suggesting the outline of a mother–child or adult–adult interaction. While supporting a wide range of possible stories, each prompt-word set implicitly suggests a secure base story line. If secure base organization was characteristic of an individual's attachment experiences, the prompt words will (implicitly) activate an underlying secure base script. This, in turn, establishes an interpretive set that shapes story production. Although first used with adult participants, the ASA has been adapted for use in adolescence and middle childhood, and across cultures.

Individuals are asked to review a prompt-word set and formulate a brief (typically 75–300 words) narrative passage, which is then recorded and transcribed. Passages are scored on a 7-point scale of secure base script organization. Scores from multiple prompt-word sets can be averaged to increase reliability. Unlike Adult Attachment Interview (AAI) scoring, which requires detailed attention to narrative structure and language use, ASA passages are simply scored in terms of the extent to which a passage is organized around the secure base script. Table 14.2 illustrates

TABLE 14.2. The Prompt-Word Outline Method

Doctor's Office prompt-word outline

Tommy	*hurry*	*mother*
bike	*doctor*	*toy*
hurt	*cry*	*stop*
mother	*shot*	*hold*

Example narrative with clear secure base script structure

Tommy was out riding, tumbles off his bike, and gets hurt. So he calls out for his mother and she says, "Let's hurry to the doctor to make sure that everything is OK." Meanwhile, Tommy is afraid of getting a shot and starts to cry. So mom calms him down and says, "Don't worry about getting a shot, the booboo will go away and you'll feel better." The mother holds Tommy while the doctor bandages his cut and gives him a shot. Afterward the mother says, "Let's get you a toy for being so brave." Tommy picks out a favorite action figure and they go home. Mom sits down with Tommy and tells him he'll be good as new.

Example narrative lacking secure base script structure

Tommy asks his mother if he could go outside to ride his bike. The mother said yes, and after a little time, she heard Tommy crying. She ran outside and saw that Tommy had gotten hurt. He was bleeding quite a bit, and she hurried to call the doctor. At the very least, he was going to need a tetanus shot. When they arrived at the doctor's office, the waiting room is full of children. Some were crying. Others were playing with toys. The doctor quickly stopped Tommy from bleeding with a bandage. He even let Tommy hold his stethoscope while he got his tetanus shot. This was a lot of excitement for one day, and Tommy and his mother were glad to get home.

(1) a narrative with extensive secure base organization and (2) an equally well-formed narrative that reflects little or no secure base structure—both produced from the same prompt-word set.

Validation Studies

Correlations reflecting convergent validity among and across mother–child and adult–adult prompt-word sets ranged from $r = .50$ to $r = .90$ (Waters & Waters, 2006). Confirmatory factor analysis in an independent sample confirmed that mother–child and adult–adult prompt-word sets assess a single, generalized secure base script (Waters et al., 2015).

ASA script knowledge scores have been linked to offspring's SSP classifications and secure base behavior at home (Tini, Corcoran, Rodrigues-Doolabh, & Waters, 2003; Vaughn et al., 2007). In addition, recent studies have shown that AAI coherence, ASA script knowledge, and early caregiving experiences are significantly correlated in a variety of samples (Schoenmaker et al., 2015; Steele et al., 2014). Finally, ASA scores based on culturally adapted prompt-word sets yield quite similar means and correlates in samples from the United States, Switzerland, Romania, Colombia, Zimbabwe, and Turkey, among others (see Waters & Roisman, 2019, and Waters & Waters, in press, for reviews of additional validation studies).

Looking Forward

The secure base script concept is a valuable tool for highlighting, clarifying, and helping resolve issues surrounding attachment representations and the IWM concept. Consider several questions that would be hard to formulate or have proven intractable as questions about IWMs.

Is the Secure Base Concept Replaced by Narrative Coherence in Adulthood?

Current attachment theory is beset by something of a paradox (critics might call it a deep incoherence). Simply put, while infant attachment theory is explicitly built on the secure base concept, much of adult attachment theory and research in developmental psychology focuses on AAI "coherence." This raises two questions. First, where did the secure base concept go in adult attachment theory? Second, how can we justify instead focusing adult attachment theory and research on the coherence of AAI narratives.

Thinking that there must be at least some secure base content in adult attachment narratives, Waters and Facompré (in press) searched a set of AAI transcripts and found them replete with examples of secure base vignettes and secure-base-related expectations. Evidently, the salience and significance of the secure base concept *is not* diminished in adulthood. This should not be surprising in light of the demonstrated relevance of secure base use and support behaviors in adult marital interactions (Crowell et al., 2002). Moreover, the secure base script concept casts light on the mechanisms underlying AAI coherence, its link to Grice's (1975) maxims (quantity, quality, relation, manner), and its many correlates. From a cognitive perspective, script-like representation of secure base experience facilitates conformity with Grice's maxims—guiding content retrieval, orderly unfolding of the narrative, identifying key events to relate, and a sense for how much material is required for a complete explanation. Although narrative coherence remains a valuable lens through which to view AAI transcripts, it is useful to have in mind that it arises from and reflects, rather than replaces, representations of secure base experience. The secure base concept remains attachment theory's key descriptive insight and core organizing construct throughout development. This resolves what appeared to be a difficult paradox. It is also a promising step toward realizing Bowlby's (e.g., 1980, p. 37) goal of eventually replacing many abstract trait and psychodynamic concepts with more rigorous and empirically accessible explanations from the emerging field of cognitive psychology.

Should We Expect to Find Avoidant and Resistant Scripts?

Probably not. At least, Waters and Facompré (in press) found no evidence of avoidant or resistant scripts in their review of AAI transcripts for secure base script content and additional attachment scripts/schemas. In the infant SSP, avoidance and resistance are brief responses to particular moments in reunion episodes. In both groups, they point to diffusely unskilled secure base use and elevated patterns of fussing and negative affect. In brief, avoidance or resistance in SSP reunions does not point to trait-like "avoidant" or "resistant" behavior styles in the laboratory or at home. How then would they abstract avoidant or resistant scripts? Moreover, it is not clear that the kinds of avoidant or resistant behavior observed in the SSP have the kind of recurring elements and temporal-causal structure necessary to abstract script-like representations.

Can the Secure Base Script Formulation Clarify the Multiple Working Models Concept?

Beginning with Bowlby (1980), attachment theorists have pointed out that individuals often construct multiple, potentially inconsistent, working models of their primary attachment figures. Main (1991) and others have suggested that conflict among inconsistent (or incoherent) working models can help explain a wide range of anxiety and dissociative phenomena.

Scripts can cue both generalized and context-specific expectations. On occasion, this can result in incompatible expectations or behavioral options being activated concurrently. The same situation can arise when a given script generates different expectations in different contexts (e.g., caregiver will provide competent support during problem solving; caregiver often loses composure during emergencies). Although incompatible script-based expectations may shed some light on the multiple models concept, it is not clear that it can account for the wide range of relationship problems and anxiety attributed to conflict among multiple working models.

Does a Cognitive Approach Ignore Emotion?

On the contrary, a cognitive perspective can help formulate issues about attachment and emotion in a manner that is both clearer and more testable than current attachment/IWM formulations. Emotion theorists have long recognized that confirmations and violations of expectations are among the most frequent occasions for emotional experience and expression (e.g., Epstein, 2014). The ability of script-like representations to instantly and effortlessly generate/cue expectations about the self, others, and the environment makes them powerful prompts to emotion, action, and adaptation in everyday life.

Does the Secure Base Script Concept Have Implications for Clinical Applications?

By definition, evidence-based therapies offer well-established methods for effecting therapeutic change. However, their underlying theories do not always provide a strong rationale for what to target in therapy. In contrast, attachment theory provides a rich list of targets for intervention. These range from specific aspects of parenting and marital behavior to secure base and exploratory behavior across ages and contexts. The secure base script also suggests an interesting perspective on trust between patient and therapist and in patients' other relationships. Combining evidence-based intervention methods with work on the secure base script (and related ideas about attachment representations) suggests a promising direction for research and a valuable organizational/developmental framework within which to formulate assessment and intervention (e.g., Bosmans, 2016; Young, Klosko, & Weishaar, 2003).

Conclusion

John Bowlby's theoretical insights and Mary Ainsworth's ethological observations provide some of the most evocative images in developmental psychology. They are the *archae,* the foundations, for understanding attachment across age and cultures. Here we have suggested that contemporary cognitive psychology can advance the clarity and testability of attachment theory and research questions. Our work on the secure base script is but one inviting example. The prospects ahead seem brighter than ever.

REFERENCES

Abelson, R. P. (1981). Psychological status of the script concept. *American Psychologist, 36,* 715–729.

Bosmans, G. (2016). Cognitive behavior therapy for children and adolescents: Can attachment theory contribute to its efficacy? *Clinical Child and Family Psychology Review, 19,* 310–328.

Bowlby, J. (1980). *Attachment and loss: Vol. 3. Loss, sadness and depression.* New York: Basic Books.

Bretherton, I. (1991). New wine in old bottles. In M. Gunnar & L. A. Sroufe (Eds.), *Concepts of self: Minnesota symposia on child psychology* (Vol. 23, pp. 1–34). Hillsdale, NJ: Erlbaum.

Bretherton, I., & Munholland, K. A. (2008). Internal working models in attachment relationships: Elaborating a central construct in attachment theory. In J. Cassidy & P. R. Shaver (Eds.), *Handbook of attachment: Theory, research and clinical application* (2nd ed., pp. 102–127). New York: Guilford Press.

Crowell, J. A., Treboux, D., Gao, Y., Fyffe, C., Pan, H., & Waters, E. (2002). Assessing secure base behavior in adulthood: Development of a measure, links to adult attachment representations, and relations to couples' communication and reports of relationships. *Developmental Psychology, 38*(5), 679–693.

Dawkins, R. (1998). *Unweaving the rainbow: Science, delusion, and the appetite for wonder.* New York: Houghton Mifflin Harcourt.

Epstein, S. (2014). *Cognitive-experiential theory: An integrative theory of personality.* New York: Oxford University Press.

Grice, P. (1975). Logic and conversation. In P. Cole & J. Morgan (Eds.), *Syntax and semantics: 3. Speech acts* (pp. 41–58). New York: Academic Press.

Hinde, R. (1989). Continuities and discontinuities: Conceptual issues and methodological considerations. In. M. Rutter (Ed.), *Studies of psychosocial risk: The power of longitudinal data* (pp. 367–384). Cambridge, UK: Cambridge University Press.

Main, M. (1991). Metacognitive knowledge, metacognitive monitoring, and singular (coherent) vs. multiple (incoherent) models of attachment: Some findings and some directions for future research. In P. Marris, J. Stevenson-Hinde, & C. Parkes (Eds.), *Attachment across the life cycle* (pp. 127–159). New York: Routledge.

Markman, A. B. (2013). *Knowledge representation.* New York: Psychology Press.

Nelson, K., & Fivush, R. (2004). The emergence of autobiographical memory: A social cultural developmental theory. *Psychological Review, 111*(2), 486–511.

Schank, R., & Abelson, R. (1977). *Scripts, plans, goals, and understanding.* New York: Wiley.

Schoenmaker, C., Juffer, F., van IJzendoorn, M., Linting, M., van der Voort, A., & Bakermans-Kranenburg, M. (2015). From maternal sensitivity in infancy to adult attachment representations: A longitudinal adoption study with secure base script. *Attachment and Human Development, 17*(3), 241–256.

Steele, R. D., Waters, T. E. A., Bost, K. K., Vaughn, B. E., Truitt, W., Waters, H. S., Roisman G. I. (2014). Caregiving antecedents of secure base script knowledge: A comparative analysis of young adult attachment representations. *Developmental Psychology, 50,* 2526–2538.

Tini, M., Corcoran, D., Rodrigues-Doolabh, L., & Waters, E. (2003). *Maternal attachment scripts and infant secure base behavior.* Presentation from poster symposium "Script-Like Representations of Secure Base Experience: Evidence of Cross-Age, Cross-Cultural and Behavioral Links" at the biennial meeting of the Society for Research in Child Development. Tampa, FL.

Vaughn, B. E., Copolla, G., Verissimo, M., Monteiro, L., Santos, A. J., Posada, G., . . . Korth, B. (2007). Coordination between organization of mothers' secure base knowledge and children's secure base behavior at home in three social-cultural groups. *International Journal of Behavioral Development, 31,* 65–76.

Waters, H. S., & Waters, E. (2006). The attachment working models concept: Among other things, we build script-like representations of secure base experiences. *Attachment and Human Development, 8,* 185–197.

Waters, H. S., & Waters, T. E. A. (in press). Measuring attachment representations as secure base script knowledge: The prompt-word outline method in adulthood, adolescence, and middle childhood. In E. Waters, B. E. Vaughn, & H. S. Waters (Eds.), *Measuring attachment: Developmental assessment across the lifespan.* New York: Guilford Press

Waters, T. E. A., & Facompré, C. R. (in press). Measuring secure base script knowledge in the Adult Attachment Interview. In E. Waters, B. E. Vaughn, & H. S. Waters (Eds.), *Measuring attachment: Developmental assessment across the lifespan.* New York: Guilford Press.

Waters, T. E. A., Fraley, R. C., Groh, A. M., Steele, R. D., Vaughn, B. E., Bost, K. K., . . . Roisman, G. I. (2015). The latent structure of secure base script knowledge. *Developmental Psychology, 51*(6), 823–830.

Waters, T. E. A., & Roisman, G. I. (2019). The secure base script concept: An overview. *Current Opinion in Psychology, 25,* 162–166.

Young, J. E., Klosko, J. S., & Weishaar, M. E. (2003). *Schema therapy: A practitioner's guide.* New York: Guilford Press.

CHAPTER 15

Parental Insightfulness and Parent–Child Emotion Dialogues
Shaping Children's Internal Working Models

David Oppenheim
Nina Koren-Karie

The concept of internal working models (IWMs) is of particular significance in attachment theory because it reflects the importance Bowlby accorded both to the inner world of the child and to the child's actual experiences (Bowlby, 1988). By emphasizing such experiences, Bowlby wanted to correct what he saw as the overemphasis of the psychoanalysts of his day on the role of children's drives and emotions as shaping their internal world. However, he never ceased to see the importance of the child's representational world, and for this purpose he included IWMs as an integral part of attachment theory.

For Bowlby, IWMs were dynamic representational structures based on the child's actual experiences with the social world that, once consolidated, serve to guide their thoughts, feelings, and behavior and are relatively resistant to change. Bowlby also stressed that while in early infancy IWMs are based primarily on the direct experience of children with their social world, parent–child patterns of verbal communication assume increased importance with age in shaping children's IWMs (Bowlby, 1988). This dual focus—on the grounding of IWMs in children's caregiving experiences and on parent–child emotional communication—guided our work. Specifically, we focused on parental insightfulness, that is, the capacity of the parent to think about the inner world of the child and the thoughts, motives, and emotions underlying the child's behavior (Oppenheim & Koren-Karie, 2013), and on how parents guide emotion dialogues with their children (Oppenheim & Koren-Karie, 2009), as important influences on the development of the child's IWMs.

Our work was also inspired by the "move to the level of representation" introduced by Main and her colleagues (Main, Kaplan, & Cassidy, 1985). Main's work highlighted that working models are not only aggregate "maps" drawn from the child's experience but are also rules that govern attention and the processing of information related to attachment. In fact, in her work using the Adult Attachment Interview, Main discovered that these rules are more important than the events discussed. For example, a mother's capacity to speak openly, coherently, and objectively about her attachment history is more important for assessing her security than whether she recollects positive or negative memories from her childhood (Hesse, 2016). This constructivist viewpoint, with its emphasis on coherent emotional meaning-making (Oppenheim, 2006), inspired our approach for assessing both parental insightfulness and parent–child emotion dialogues.

Parental Insightfulness

Insightfulness involves the parent's capacity to think about the motives that underlie the child's behavior in an open, accepting, and complex way while linking these thoughts to the child's behavior (Koren-Karie & Oppenheim, 2018). It is based on Ainsworth's description of the sensitive mother as "seeing things from the child's point of view" (Ainsworth, 1969) and is assessed using a video-replay method in which parents are interviewed about "what went on in their child's head" after watching several video clips of the child. Parents are required to engage in a "dialogue" between what they know about their child based on their shared history, and the specific behaviors of the child as captured on video. Influenced by the idea that the rules governing the processing of information are of crucial importance, the Insightfulness Assessment (IA) focuses on *how* parents talk about the videos they observe and not on the behaviors they describe. For example, whether the video shows cooperative and compliant child behavior or disruptive and noncompliant behavior, the insightfulness of the parent is reflected in the parent's thinking about and accepting the possible motives that may drive the child's behavior.

An insightful orientation by the parent is thought to underlie sensitive parenting behavior (Oppenheim & Koren-Karie, 2013). Importantly, insightful parents are also open to considering indications that they misread the child and to change their understanding accordingly. Most significant is the flexibility of the parent, openness to feedback from the child, acceptance of challenging or disappointing child behavior, and differentiating the inner world of the child from the wishes and fears of the parent. Based on this parental orientation, children of insightful parents are thought to develop a secure attachment to the parent, knowing that their emotional signals and needs are read correctly, and if they are not, parents are likely to repair the rupture and recalibrate their understanding of the child according to the child's feedback.

Parental insightfulness is important because it is expressed in parenting behavior and presumed to shape children's IWMs, that is, their expectations regarding the availability of the attachment figure and the degree to which they feel that their thoughts, wishes, and feelings are understood and accepted. Children's IWMs also include conclusions they draw about themselves: whether they feel they are worthy of attention, care, and protection. Empirical support for these hypotheses comes from studies showing that insightful parents are more sensitive than noninsightful parents and their children are more likely to develop secure attachments (Koren-Karie, Oppenheim, Dolev, Sher, & Etzion-Carasso, 2002). This has been found both with regard to typically developing infants and with regard to young children with autism spectrum disorder (ASD; Oppenheim, Koren-Karie, Dolev, & Yirmiya, 2009) and intellectual disability (Feniger-Schaal, Oppenheim, & Koren-Karie, 2019). These findings are particularly significant because children with special needs can be more challenging than typically developing children and their signals are often more difficult to read. Nonetheless, insightfulness with respect to their experience is possible and is associated with the same outcomes (e.g., maternal sensitivity, secure attachment) as in typically developing children. Importantly, the insightfulness of mothers of children with ASD was unrelated, in our study, to children's level of functioning or the severity of their diagnosis, indicating that insightfulness is more an indicator of parental meaning-making processes with regard to the child than a simple reflection of the severity of the child's diagnosis or the child's cognitive level.

Additional important findings involve the long-term consequences of early maternal insightfulness. One study showed that early maternal insightfulness was associated with children's insightfulness toward their best friend 15 years later (Shahar-Maharik, Oppenheim, & Koren-Karie, 2018), whereas another study, this time with children with ASD, showed that early insightfulness increased the likelihood of more inclusive educational placements (Dolev, Oppenheim, Koren-Karie, & Yirmiya, 2014). Although understanding the mechanisms for these longitudinal associations requires more research, the findings are consistent with the idea that children who were recipients of insightful parenting develop secure IWMs, which in turn promote their socioemotional adjustment.

Researchers are also interested in parental insightfulness as a buffer that protects children against the effects of stressful events. An insightful parent takes into consideration the child's exposure to stress and is more likely to respond to the child's resulting distress (or the disruptive behavior it may engender) with empathy and appropriate limits and to support the child's coping. In one study, children of noninsightful mothers exposed to community violence showed relatively high levels of behavior problems, whereas those of insightful mothers who were similarly exposed showed relatively low levels of behavior problems not different from those of unexposed children (Gray, Forbes, Briggs-Gowan, & Carter, 2015). In another study, insightfulness similarly moderated the effects of stress, such that mothers who experienced stressful life events but who were insightful showed positive parenting behaviors with their infants, whereas those who similarly experienced stressful life events but were noninsightful showed lower levels of positive parenting behavior (Martinez-Torteya et al., 2018). These studies suggest that an insightful stance can help mothers read their children's signals correctly and respond to their need for comfort and protection, even under stressful circumstances experienced by themselves and/or their children.

Parent–Child Emotion Dialogues

If the assessment of insightfulness is based on how parents talk *about* their children, the assessment of emotion dialogues is based on how parents talk *with* their children. Such dialogues provide an opportunity to observe how parents and children co-construct narratives about children's emotional experience, including which emotions are accepted, which emotions should be emphasized and even overemphasized, and which should not be discussed. Following Bowlby (1988) we see such dialogues as reflecting a psychological secure base that promotes children's exploration of their internal world, knowing that the caregiver is available for support and is a source of comfort and confidence when recalling negative events (Oppenheim & Koren-Karie, 2009). Such conversations are thought to contribute to children's emotion understanding and communication skills and, importantly, to the development of coherent IWMs of themselves, others, and their emotional experiences.

In our research parent–child emotion dialogues are elicited by asking parents to help their children recall, sequentially, events involving one of four emotions (one positive and three negative) and talk about each of the events. As in the IA, the emphasis is not on the events discussed by the children but rather on the discussion process. In conversations that foster open and well-regulated exploration of the child's emotional experiences, parents sensitively guide the dialogues with their children. They accept the examples the child chooses, maintain the focus on the child's experience, are involved while structuring the conversation as needed, and help the child think of positive coping solutions when appropriate. As expected, associations have been found between security in infancy and more "secure" emotion dialogues in the preschool and early school years (Hsiao, Koren-Karie, Moran, & Baily, 2015; Oppenheim, Koren-Karie, & Sagi-Schwartz, 2007).

A focus of one group of studies was on the effects of maternal sensitive guidance on children's IWMs, their processing of emotional information, and their capacity to integrate and regulate emotional experiences. Maternal sensitive guidance was associated with the specificity of children's autobiographical memory (Valentino et al., 2014), their emotion regulation and inhibitory control (Speidel, Valentino, McDonnell, Cummings, & Fondren, 2019), and fewer behavior problems (Sher-Censor, Koren-Karie, Getzov, & Rotman, 2017). In a longitudinal study, maternal sensitive guidance during the preschool years predicted in early adolescence the coherence of children's narratives about their friends and family and their secure representations of the mother (Tamari, Aviezer, & Oppenheim, 2019). Supporting the emphasis on the *quality* of maternal input as opposed to the *quantity* of mothers' interventions, one study showed that sensitive guidance was more important in predicting children's autobiographical memory than the quantity of elaborative statements made by mothers (Valentino et al., 2014). Finally, and perhaps most important in highlighting the role of mothers in shaping mother–child dialogues, a randomized controlled trial of a reminiscing and emotion training intervention with mothers of maltreated children showed that the intervention enhanced mothers' sensitive guidance, levels of children's memories, and their emotional knowledge (Valentino et al., 2019). Taken together, these studies show that mothers' sensitive guidance promotes a range of positive child outcomes that are theoretically related to children's IWMs.

Several correlates of mothers' sensitive guidance have also been examined as possible contributors to this important capacity. Mothers who experienced childhood sexual abuse (Koren-Karie et al., 2004), interpersonal traumas (Overbeek et al., 2019), had children identified as maltreated (Speidel et al., 2019), or experienced psychopathology (Cimino et al., 2020) showed lower sensitive guidance than controls. More pertinent to the discussion of IWMs, one study showed that mothers designated secure on the Adult Attachment Interview displayed a higher level of sensitive guidance compared to insecure mothers (Hsiao et al., 2015). Taken together, studies on mother–child emotion dialogues show that they promote a range of child memory and socioemotional outcomes and that they are related to pertinent maternal factors.

Conclusion

While there may not be a consensus among attachment researchers about operational definitions of IWMs or about the psychological structures and processes they include, IWMs have proven to be highly important for attachment theory for at least two reasons. First, they have been of great heuristic value, spurring a wide range of assessments and methods that have yielded an enormous amount of research. This research has built upon the foundations of Ainsworth's observational infancy studies but broadened the theory and the research to include ever widening ages, populations, and research questions. The studies of parental insightfulness and parent–child dialogues described in this chapter are one example of this. Our research has primarily focused on childhood, although one study (Shahar-Maharik et al., 2018) demonstrated more far-reaching benefits of early insightfulness during adolescence and outside of the mother–child relationship. Future studies can explore our hypothesis that experiencing parental insightfulness and emotionally open and well-regulated communication provides children with a solid representational foundation. This may serve them in subsequent developmental stages and challenges and in close relationships both in and outside their family of origin.

Second, the concept of IWMs has helped bridge the gap between attachment research and clinical applications. Clinicians from a wide range of schools of thought accord a central place to the way past relationship experiences are stored, the way they shape how we perceive ourselves and others and how we react to them, and how these prisms promote or hinder development and emotional functioning. It is therefore not a surprise that as the number of studies of IWMs grew so did the interest of clinicians in attachment research. This, in turn, stimulated researchers to increase attention to clinical questions regarding the origins and developmental course of psychopathology as well as the effectiveness of attachment-based interventions.

Bowlby's creative and integrative mind sought to base clinical work on sound scientific knowledge. When we look back at close to 50 years of attachment research, there is no question that his concept of IWMs has made a particularly important contribution for this cause.

REFERENCES

Ainsworth, M. D. S. (1969). Maternal Sensitivity Scales. Retrieved from *www.psy.sunysb.edu/ewaters/senscoop.htm.*

Bowlby, J. (1988). *A secure base: Parent–child attachment and healthy human development.* New York: Basic Books.

Cimino, S., Cerniglia, L., Tambelli, R., Ballarotto, G., Erriu, M., Paciello, M., . . . Koren-Karie, N. (2020). Dialogues about emotional events between mothers with anxiety, depression, anorexia, nervosa, and no diagnosis and their children. *Parenting: Science and Practice, 20,* 69–82.

Dolev, S., Oppenheim, D., Koren-Karie, N., & Yirmiya, N. (2014). Early attachment and maternal insightfulness predict educational placement of children with autism. *Research in Autism Spectrum Disorders, 8,* 958–967.

Feniger-Schaal, R., Oppenheim, D., & Koren-Karie, N. (2019). Parenting children with intellectual disability: Linking maternal insightfulness to sensitivity. *Journal of Intellectual Disability Research, 10,* 1285–1289.

Gray, S. A. O., Forbes, D., Briggs-Gowan, M. J., & Carter, A. S. (2015). Caregiver insightfulness and young children's violence exposure: Testing a relational model of risk and resilience. *Attachment and Human Development, 17,* 615–634.

Hesse, E. (2016). The Adult Attachment Interview: Protocol, method of analysis, and selected empirical studies: 1985–2015. In J. Cassidy & P. R. Shaver (Eds.), *Handbook of attachment: Theory, research, and clinical applications* (3rd ed., pp. 553–597). New York: Guilford Press.

Hsiao, C., Koren-Karie, N., Moran, G., & Baily, H. (2015). It takes two to talk: Longitudinal associations among infant–mother attachment, maternal attachment representations, and mother–child emotion dialogues. *Attachment and Human Development, 17,* 43–64.

Koren-Karie, N., & Oppenheim, D. (2018). Parental insightfulness: Retrospect and prospect. *Attachment and Human Development, 20,* 223–236.

Koren-Karie, N., Oppenheim, D., Dolev S., Sher, E., & Etzion-Carasso, A. (2002). Mothers' insightfulness regarding their infants' internal experience: Relations with maternal sensitivity and infant attachment. *Developmental Psychology, 38,* 534–542.

Main, M., Kaplan, N., & Cassidy, J. (1985). Security in infancy, childhood, and adulthood: A move to the level of representation. In I. Bretherton & E. Waters (Eds.), Growing points of attachment theory and research. *Monographs of the Society for Research in Child Development, 50*(1–2, Serial No. 209), 66–104.

Martinez-Torteya, C., Rosenblum, K. L., Beeghly, M., Oppenheim, D., Koren-Karie, N., Muzik, M. (2018). Maternal insightfulness protects against the detrimental effects of postpartum stress on positive parenting among at-risk mother–infant dyads. *Attachment and Human Development, 20,* 272–286.

Oppenheim, D. (2006). Child, parent, and parent–child emotion narratives: Implications for developmental psychopathology. *Development and Psychopathology, 18,* 771–790.

Oppenheim, D., & Koren-Karie, N. (2009). Mother–child emotion dialogues: A window into the psychological secure base. In J. Quas & R. Fivush (Eds.), *Emotion and memory in development: Biological, cognitive, and social considerations* (pp. 142–165). New York: Oxford University Press.

Oppenheim, D., & Koren-Karie, N. (2013). The insightfulness assessment: Measuring the internal processes underlying maternal sensitivity. *Attachment and Human Development, 15,* 545–561.

Oppenheim, D., Koren-Karie, N., Dolev, S., & Yirmiya, N. (2009). Maternal insightfulness and resolution of the diagnosis are related to secure attachment in preschoolers with autism spectrum disorder. *Child Development, 80,* 519–527.

Oppenheim, D., Koren-Karie, N., & Sagi-Schwartz, A. (2007). Emotion dialogues between mothers and children at 4.5 and 7.5 years: Relations with children's attachment at 1 year. *Child Development, 78,* 38–52.

Overbeek, M. M., Koren-Karie, N., Ben-Haim, A. E., de Schipper, J. C., Dreier Gligoor, P. D., & Schuengel, C. (2019). Trauma exposure in relation to the content of mother–child emotional conversations and quality of interaction. *International Journal of Environmental Research and Public Health, 16*(5), 1–15.

Shahar-Maharik, T., Oppenheim, D., & Koren-Karie N. (2018). Adolescent insightfulness toward a close friend: Its roots in maternal insightfulness and child attachment in infancy. *Attachment and Human Development, 20,* 237–254.

Sher-Cenzor, E., & Koren-Karie, N., Getzov, S., & Rotman, P. (2017). Maternal sensitive guidance of emotional dialogues and adolescents' behavior problems: The mediating role of adolescents' representations of their mothers. *Journal of Research on Adolescence, 5,* 1–18.

Speidel, R., Valentino, K., McDonnell, C. G., Cummings, E. M., & Fondren, K. (2019). Maternal sensitive guidance during reminiscing in the context of child maltreatment: Implications for child self-regulatory processes. *Developmental Psychology, 55*(1), 110–122.

Tamari, R., Aviezer, O., & Oppenheim D. (2019, March). *Predicting adolescents' attachment representations from early and current mother-child emotional communication.* Paper presented at the biennial meeting of the Society for Research in Child Development, Baltimore, MD.

Valentino, K., Cummings, E. M., Borkowski, J., Hibel, L. C., Lefever, J., & Lawson, M. (2019). Efficacy of a reminiscing and emotion training intervention on maltreating families with preschool-aged children. *Developmental Psychology, 55*(11), 2365–2378.

Valentino, K., Nuttall, A. K., Comas, M., McDonnell, C. G., Piper, B., Thomas, T. E., & Fanuele, S. (2014). Mother–child reminiscing and autobiographical memory specificity among preschool-age children. *Developmental Psychology, 50*(4), 1197–1207.

CHAPTER 16

Internal Working Models as Developing Representations

Ross A. Thompson

The concept of mental working models that are relationally based, affectively colored, dynamic, and integrative is one of the most generative concepts of attachment theory. It is also one of its most difficult. The generativity of this concept is reflected in how important it is to theoretical explanations for the association between the security of attachment and its correlates, the stability of security over time, and intergenerational consistency in attachment. Attachment researchers frequently use internal working models (IWMs) as their explanation for research findings. In light of these applications, it seems surprising that Bowlby did not devote greater attention to elucidating the concept of IWMs in his writings, perhaps leaving this to his followers. And therein lies the difficulty. Without a well-developed theoretical account of the nature and development of IWMs to guide their inquiry, attachment researchers have created a variety of conceptualizations to fit different theoretical and empirical needs. More than 30 years ago, Hinde (1988) stated the problem succinctly: "In the very power of such a model lies a trap: it can too easily explain anything" (p. 378), and since then IWMs have been enlisted to "explain" the association of attachment with political ideology, math achievement, and many other phenomena (see Thompson, 2016). Attachment theory has not been well served by a core theoretical concept that is so vaguely defined and flexibly applied.

In writing about IWMs, Bowlby wove together theoretical strands from diverse fields that had not been previously integrated. From his psychoanalytic background he reworked concepts from object relations theory and a rich legacy of thinking about psychological defenses. From developmental psychology he enlisted Piagetian concepts to explain changes in IWMs with increasing age. He also used concepts from cognitive psychology to describe mental representation and its functioning. Fifty years later, attachment researchers inhabit a much richer theoretical climate within which to clarify the meaning and applications of IWMs. But the task is not easy: The theoretical currents Bowlby integrated are not wholly consistent with each other, and attachment theory presents other vexing problems, such as understanding how IWMs combine influences from multiple attachment relationships (see Girme & Overall, Chapter 17, this volume). But currently there are promising efforts to clarify the concept of IWMs in light of contemporary psychological science, such as script theory (see Waters, Waters, & Waters, Chapter 14, this volume), and more should follow. In the end, attachment theory will have difficulty proceeding coherently without a clear concept of IWMs with well-defined boundaries to guide future research. As a contribution to this effort, this chapter discusses IWMs as developing representations and how this occurs in relation to other aspects of psychological growth.

Toward a Developmental Approach

In Bowlby's outline, IWMs have predictive, interpretive, and self-regulatory functions owing, in part, to their influences on attention and memory. Early in infancy, they are primarily concerned with expectations regarding the behavior of attachment figures, especially how these people serve protective safe haven and secure base functions. But IWMs also concern the self, particularly representations of one's characteristics and capabilities and one's acceptability in the eyes of attachment figures (Bowlby, 1973, p. 203). IWMs also provide guidance for how to relate to others, such that people choose new partners and interact with them in ways that are based on, and thus help to perpetuate, the models developed from earlier attachment relationships (e.g., Sroufe & Fleeson, 1986). These mental representations, which have unconscious elements but are also consciously accessible (Bowlby, 1969, p. 83), help children and adults navigate their environment of relationships and develop a sense of self, and they contribute in other ways to social and personality development.

These mental representations are developing representations. They are shaped by allied cognitive, social, and emotional capabilities and thus evolve with broadened experience and with the unfolding of other aspects of psychological development. Whereas Bowlby made reference to the decline of egocentrism in his developmental theory of IWMs, contemporary attachment theorists have a much wider range of concepts and can draw on a broader research literature to elaborate his developmental view (see Thompson & Winer, 2014, for a fuller survey). Here are some examples:

• Expectations for the behavior of attachment figures are central to IWMs, and there is growing evidence that generalized expectations for the behavior of adults toward infants (e.g., that adults will comfort rather than ignore a crying baby) emerge early in the first year, with some suggestion that 1-year-olds varying in attachment security also vary in this expectation (Jin, Houston, Baillargeon, Groh, & Roisman, 2018). Statistical learning may provide an explanation for these rapidly developing and evolving relational expectations (see Xu & Kushnir, 2013).

• Research on early memory shows that toddlers begin constructing generalized event representations, or scripts, which provide a scaffold for their memories of specific experiences. Bretherton and Munholland (2016) argued that similar processes also may contribute to the development of generalized relational representations that are central to IWMs. These relational scripts may help to scaffold representations of specific attachment-related experiences in memory.

• Studies of autobiographical memory and other emergent self-system processes (such as self-esteem) portray early childhood as the period when an enduring and valenced self-understanding begins to emerge. In particular, and in a manner reminiscent of Mead's "looking-glass self," this work shows that how young children appraise themselves derives from how they are appraised by people who matter to them, particularly attachment figures. Emergent autobiographical memory after age 3 may be especially important, furthermore, to constructing a continuing narrative of the self in relation to attachment figures, and of the behavior of the people to whom the child is attached (Nelson & Fivush, 2004).

• Developing understanding of "how to relate to others" derives from multiple lines of social-cognitive growth in early childhood, including developing emotion understanding, conflict resolution skills, psychological trait concepts, social domain understanding, social problem-solving capacities, conscience development, and many other aspects of social cognition that are relevant to developing working models of relationships. Because of their IWMs, securely attached children should differ on many of these social-cognitive skills compared to insecurely attached children and, as discussed below, research shows that they do. These social-cognitive skills also contribute to the development of the "goal-corrected partnership" that Bowlby viewed as an important development in attachment and IWMs.

Beyond these developmentally emergent components of IWMs in early childhood, Bowlby's theory also draws on many other concepts that have also been the focus of considerable research, such as work on constructive memory processes, prototypical knowledge systems, expectancy bias and confirmation bias, self-schemas, causal attribution biases, "hot" versus "cold" cognitive processes, and many others (see, e.g., Murray, Holmes, & Collins, 2006). It is reasonable to expect that IWMs incorporate many of these cognitive processes and are influenced by others, even though Bowlby's concept certainly also extends beyond these consciously accessible cognitive and social-cognitive capacities to include unconscious (e.g., defensive) processes.

What are the theoretical benefits of expanding Bowlby's developmental model of IWMs by connecting it to allied developments in thinking and emotion? One benefit is that it helps to define the characteristics we would expect to see in IWMs in children of different ages and in adults. We would not ordinarily expect, for example, that young children would represent their attachment figures in their IWMs as emotionally ambivalent until a concept of mixed and conflicting simultaneous emotions has begun to emerge in emotion understanding. If young children appear to represent their attachment figures in this manner, it might inspire research into what this means. More broadly, attachment security may be developmentally most influential in certain domains when working models have matured sufficiently to be associated with domain-relevant features of psychological growth that are emerging at the same time. Attachment security in infancy is associated with many features of parent–child interaction; security in early childhood may be more strongly associated with developing peer group functioning than in infancy, but would not be expected to be a significant predictor of identity in adolescence. Considerable research is consistent with this view (Thompson, 2016).

Second, expanding Bowlby's developmental model in this way inspires testable hypotheses concerning how securely and insecurely attached children differ because of these developing features of their IWMs. There is already considerable evidence, for example, that children with secure and insecure attachments differ significantly in their representations of and expectations for their attachment figures, in self-concept, self-esteem, and other self-system beliefs, and in multiple aspects of "how to relate to others," including peer competence, emotion understanding and empathy, emotion regulation, social problem solving, conflict resolution skills, and conscience development (Thompson, 2016). These and other aspects of social-emotional development may be viewed as reflecting components of their developing IWMs rather than merely as correlates. Third, expanding Bowlby's developmental model to incorporate insights from contemporary developmental science makes the IWM

concept more comprehensible and potentially more useful to developmental researchers outside attachment theory as well as within it. This
has the potential of broadening the range of contributions to attachment
theory from other fields of study. Fourth, connecting developing IWMs
to allied developmental achievements highlights methodological avenues
to the age-appropriate assessment of IWMs. Research on IWMs is limited
until researchers achieve consensus on how these mental models can be
adequately measured at different ages.

Finally, and importantly, expanding Bowlby's developmental model
in this way potentially enlarges understanding of the processes by which
IWMs develop.

How Do IWMs Develop?

Bowlby was committed to characterizing IWMs as derivative of the child's
direct experience with attachment figures. Beyond primary representations of experience, however, Bowlby (1969, p. 354) also respected "the
powerful and extraordinary gift of language" that extends and changes
the preverbal working models of infancy. Subsequent researchers from
within and outside attachment theory have offered hypotheses for how
this occurs (e.g., Astington & Baird, 2005). They note that language lexi-
calizes elements of internal experience, providing terms and concepts for
mental states, including motivations, emotions, and other psychological
realities of attachment experience. Language builds on the young child's
preverbal knowledge systems and transforms them by incorporating them
into structures of semantic representation that are relative to language
and culture. In this way, the emergence of language begins the reconstruction of an infant's implicit understanding of attachment-related
experiences into enculturated explicit knowledge that can be the focus of
reflection and sharing. Language also contributes in this manner to the
child's appropriation of values, beliefs, and a sense of personhood that is
incorporated into the content of what is heard from others.

Language is particularly important, of course, as a medium for sharing experience and comparing perspectives on shared experience. In this
manner, language provides secondary representations that can influence, in complex ways, the primary representations that children derive
from direct experience. Developmental researchers have documented the
influence of concurrent and retrospective parental discourse on young
children's representations of experience, showing how the content and
richness of parental discourse influences young children's event representation and episodic memory, the quality and depth of autobiographical memory, and even children's anticipatory event representation (see,

e.g., Fivush, 2007; Reese, 2002). Even more germane to developing working models are studies documenting the influence of parental discourse on emotion understanding and empathy, emotion regulation, theory of mind, and conscience development (see review by Thompson & Winer, 2014). These studies suggest that the secondary representations afforded by parent–child discourse can constructively supplement and expand young children's direct representations of people, experiences, and even the self. But they can alternatively contribute to distortions and defensive exclusion of the kind that Bowlby (1980, 1988) frequently discussed as "knowing what you are not supposed to know and feeling what you are not supposed to feel." It would be reasonable to see these influences of parent–child discourse as formative of developing IWMs.

If this conclusion is true, we would expect to find that the adults to whom children are securely attached engage conversationally with them in distinctive ways, especially compared with those in insecure relationships. And indeed we do. Many studies (including my own) document the narratively richer, more elaborative manner that mothers in secure relationships talk about experiences in the recent past with their children, providing greater information, making more frequent emotion references, and providing supportive acceptance and validation of the child's perspectives (Thompson, 2016; Thompson, Laible, & Ontai, 2003; Thompson & Winer, 2014). Other studies document the sensitive insightfulness of parents in secure attachments engaged in emotion dialogues with their children as they create a "psychological secure base" in which they offer support for the child exploring potentially disturbing thoughts and feelings (see Oppenheim & Koren-Karie, Chapter 15, this volume). These findings are consistent with Bowlby's (1988, p. 130) portrayal of the more open, "free-flowing conversation laced with expressions of feeling" characteristic of secure parent–child partners that are part of the relational co-construction of these working models. These findings also contribute perspective to the intergenerational transmission of attachment security as an outgrowth both of the child's early relational experience and the relational representations shared by parent and child through the quality and content of conversational discourse. These findings also provide a developmental context to the communication patterns characteristic of secure, dismissing, and preoccupied patients in attachment-informed psychotherapy (see Talia & Holmes, Chapter 40, this volume).

This literature is consistent with expanding inquiry into the origins of differences in attachment security, in which researchers are including measures of parental insightfulness, mind-mindedness, and discourse-based assessments of elaborative and validational conversational quality along with maternal sensitivity in understanding why children become and remain relationally secure or insecure (Fearon & Belsky, 2016). In so doing, they recognize that relational responsiveness is not only a behavioral quality but also a conversational process, and that together they shape the development and updating of IWMs.

Concluding Comments

An updated concept of IWMs that is informed by advances in psychological science has the potential of invigorating inquiry into attachment as well as contributing attachment perspectives to other research domains. It will require, however, the concerted theoretical and empirical work of clearly defining the nature and functioning of these working models in developmentally graded ways that reflect the significant psychological advances of the years when attachment takes shape.

REFERENCES

Astington, J. W., & Baird, J. A. (Eds.). (2005). *Why language matters for theory of mind.* New York: Oxford University Press.

Bowlby, J. (1969). *Attachment and loss: Vol. 1. Attachment.* New York: Basic Books.

Bowlby, J. (1973). *Attachment and loss: Vol. 2. Separation.* New York: Basic Books.

Bowlby, J. (1980). *Attachment and loss: Vol. 3. Loss, sadness and depression.* New York: Basic Books.

Bowlby, J. (1988). *A secure base.* New York: Basic Books.

Bretherton, I., & Munholland, K. A. (2016). The internal working model construct in light of contemporary neuroimaging research. In J. Cassidy & P. R. Shaver (Eds.), *Handbook of attachment* (3rd ed., pp. 63–88). New York: Guilford Press.

Fearon, R. M., & Belsky, J. (2016). Precursors of attachment security. In J. Cassidy & P. R. Shaver (Eds.), *Handbook of attachment* (3rd ed., pp. 291–313). New York: Guilford Press.

Fivush, R. (2007). Maternal reminiscing style and children's developing understanding of self and emotion. *Clinical Social Work, 35,* 37–46.

Hinde, R. (1988). Continuities and discontinuities: Conceptual issues and methodological considerations. In M. Rutter (Ed.), *Studies of psychosocial risk* (pp. 367–383). New York: Cambridge University Press.

Jin, K., Houston, J. L., Baillargeon, R., Groh, A. M., & Roisman, G. I. (2018). Young infants expect an unfamiliar adult to comfort a crying baby: Evidence from a standard violation-of-expectation task and a novel infant-triggered-video task. *Cognitive Psychology, 102,* 1–20.

Murray, S. L., Holmes, J. G., & Collins, N. L. (2006). Optimizing assurance: The risk regulation system in relationships. *Psychological Bulletin, 132,* 641–666.

Nelson, K., & Fivush, R. (2004). The emergence of autobiographical memory: A social cultural developmental theory. *Psychological Bulletin, 111,* 486–511.

Reese, E. (2002). Social factors in the development of autobiographical memory: The state of the art. *Social Development, 11,* 124–142.

Sroufe, L. A., & Fleeson, J. (1986). Attachment and the construction of relationships. In W. W. Hartup & Z. Rubin (Eds.), *Relationships and development* (pp. 51–71). Hillsdale, NJ: Erlbaum.

Thompson, R. A. (2016). Early attachment and later development: Reframing the questions. In J. Cassidy & P. R. Shaver (Eds.), *Handbook of attachment* (3rd ed., pp. 330–348). New York: Guilford Press.

Thompson, R. A., Laible, D. J., & Ontai, L. L. (2003). Early understanding of emotion, morality, and the self: Developing a working model. In R. V. Kail (Ed.), *Advances in child development and behavior* (Vol. 31, pp.137–171). New York: Academic Press.

Thompson, R. A., & Winer, A. (2014). Moral development, conversation, and the development of internal working models. In C. Wainryb & H. Recchia (Eds.), *Talking about right and wrong: Parent–child conversations as contexts for moral development* (pp. 299–333). New York: Cambridge University Press.

Xu, F., & Kushnir, T. (2013). Infants are rational constructivist learners. *Current Directions in Psychological Science, 22,* 28–32.

A Functional Account of Multiple Internal Working Models
Flexibility in Ranking, Structure, and Content across Contents and Time

Yuthika U. Girme
Nickola C. Overall

Working models are mental representations about attachment figures that organize people's thoughts, feelings, goals, expectations, and behaviors within close relationships (Bowlby, 1973; Collins & Read, 1994). Working models guide the way people respond to attachment figures when they need a *safe haven* (a source of comfort during times of distress) and *secure base* (a source of support during exploration and growth; Bowlby, 1973). The existence and function of working models theoretically explain how the beliefs and expectations generated from attachment experiences can be carried "from the cradle to the grave" (Bowlby, 1969/1982, p. 208) by enlisting a cognitive map of the relational world that guides the way people navigate attachment relationships across the lifespan.

This central function of working models can generate a misconception that attachment experiences are only generalized into a global working model that summarizes people's beliefs and expectations across all attachment relationships. Yet, Bowlby (1980) theorized that working models are flexible and open to updating, which we (and others) believe involves an interconnected network of multiple working models. Indeed, attachment-related functions are served by a variety of attachment figures, including family members, friends, and romantic partners (e.g., Doherty & Feeney, 2004). These distinct relationship domains, and the specific relationships within each domain, also involve varying attachment needs, functions, and experiences (Collins & Read, 1994). Thus, to provide an accurate map of what to expect and how to get attachment needs met across an array of attachment contexts, people possess multiple working models that provide contextually relevant guidance in response to different attachment needs that arise across time (Overall, Fletcher, & Friesen, 2003).

This chapter presents a functional account of multiple working models that should help adaptively guide (1) who people draw upon during times of need or exploration (a hierarchical ranking of multiple attachment figures) and (2) the ways people manage attachment needs with various attachment figures that likely respond differently in important attachment contexts (a hierarchical network of multiple working models). Our account also highlights that, in order to provide the most accurate and useful information within central attachment-relevant situations, the (1) ranking of multiple attachment figures and (2) relative activation and use of multiple working models should vary as people's experiences, networks, and needs vary across contexts and time. Our final section builds on the importance of flexibility across multiple working models to consider how people's multiple working models will also vary in content (beliefs, expectations, goals) across time in order to guide behavior in the changing reality of people's relationship landscapes.

Multiple Attachment Figures: Hierarchical Ranking That Varies across Context and Time

The bond between infants and mothers has been a principal focus in understanding people's attachment security because mothers tend to be the primary source of comfort and security during infancy (Ainsworth, Blehar, Waters, & Wall, 1978). However, as people enter middle childhood, adolescence, and then adulthood, developmentally relevant relationships with familial and nonfamilial others, such as best friends and romantic partners, become increasingly important sources of support and care (Doherty & Feeney, 2004). By adulthood, people usually identify several important attachment figures that provide a secure base and safe haven in times of need, including mothers, fathers, siblings, romantic partners, and close friends (Doherty & Feeney, 2004).

People also hierarchically rank attachment figures according to who is the best source of security and safe haven (e.g., Doherty & Feeney, 2004), which should increase the likelihood that people reach out to those most likely to fulfill important attachment functions. Recent examinations of the functions of multiple attachment figures provide behavioral evidence that people actually turn to primary attachment figures during times of need above other nonattachment, but proximal, others (e.g., roommates, work colleagues). By tracking daily support seeking to attachment and nonattachment figures in response to stressful events, Kammrath and colleagues (2020) illustrated that the odds of seeking support from an attachment figure (partner, mother, friend, but *not* father) was about 12 times higher than the odds of seeking support from a nonattachment figure.

Of course, hierarchical rankings of attachment figures vary across time as people's attachment needs and networks change, which is exactly what should occur if working models guide people's most adaptive responses to attachment needs. Mothers tend to be the primary attachment figures throughout infancy (Ainsworth et al., 1978), but mothers rank as a close second to romantic partners after people have developed committed intimate relationships in adolescence and adulthood (Doherty & Feeney, 2004). These rankings also vary across developmental phases. Adolescents may use friends more often as a safe haven compared to mothers (Markiewicz, Lawford, Doyle, & Haggart, 2006), and feel greater need fulfilment with best friends compared to mothers, fathers, and romantic partners (La Guardia, Ryan, Couchman, & Deci, 2000).

The relative ranking of attachment figures within the same developmental phase also varies according to context. Despite romantic partners typically becoming people's primary attachment figures in adulthood, adults are still more likely to seek mothers' safe haven when experiencing very serious stressors (Kammrath et al., 2020) or when mothers provide unique attachment-relevant support, such as when people are raising children of their own and mothers provide child care guidance, cooking, and babysitting (Deave, Johnson, & Ingram, 2008). Attachment figures and functions can also reverse later in life when parents have to rely on their children for caregiving (Karantzas, Evans, & Foddy, 2010).

Multiple Working Models: Hierarchical Networks That Differentiate Distinct Relationships and Domains

To determine which attachment figure to draw upon across different situations, and to assess how attachment needs can be best met across diverse relationships, people also need to accurately represent relationship-specific information across their multiple attachment figures (La Guardia et al., 2000). Accordingly, people likely possess an interconnected network of working models that differentiate across different types of relationships that fulfill different needs and generate different attachment concerns and expectations (Collins & Read, 1994). Research specifically measuring the content of working models across different domains and relationships has found that people hold distinct relationship-specific models of each attachment figure (e.g., mother, best friend, romantic partner), which combine to create general representations specific to the needs and qualities of different attachment domains (familial, friendships, romantic relationships; see Overall et al., 2003). Overall and colleagues (2003) also found evidence that different relationship- and domain-specific representations may contribute to a global working model summarizing beliefs and expectations people have developed across relationships, but theorized that relationship- and domain-specific representations are likely to be more influential in guiding attachment behavior.

A hierarchical network of relationship- and domain-specific models should be adaptive because it provides more precise and accurate information about what to expect in specific attachment domains and relationships, and therefore how people can manage their attachment needs across contexts. If this functional account is correct, then domain-specific or relationship-specific working models should be most predictive of attachment behavior and outcomes in corresponding domains and relationships. Providing support for this idea, people's working models of the romantic relationship domain predict the quality of relationship interactions with romantic partners, but not with nonromantic others, such as family or friends (Sibley & Overall, 2008). Similarly, working models of specific romantic partners predict satisfaction and commitment within that specific relationship more strongly than do working models of other relationships, such as those concerning family or friends (Fraley, Heffernan, Vicary, & Brumbaugh, 2011).

Nonetheless, these working models are not wholly independent because it should be adaptive to encode and apply experiences that are shared across domains. These shared connections should allow people to draw upon expectations, goals, and behavioral strategies that effectively guide responses in different, but related, attachment relationships and contexts. For example, working models with early caregivers include contextually relevant information about how to navigate attachment relationships in adulthood, especially in regard to caregiving. Accordingly, people with more secure working models of parents are more easily calmed by their romantic partners and provide more responsive support to their partners during stressful situations (e.g., Simpson, Winterheld, Rholes, & Oriña, 2007).

Working models of new relationships will also generate from existing attachment representations that provide a foundation for understanding relationships in specific domains. For example, working models of parents provide foundational information about caregiving that should be used as a basis for attachment relationships with one's own children. Providing evidence for this, mothers' maternal sensitivity during their children's first three years of life predicts those children's own later supportive parenting behavior with their children (Raby et al., 2015). These shared components across multiple working models may be activated to guide parent–child dynamics differentially depending on the relevance to the current situation, even as working models with parents versus children become more differentiated across time.

In sum, research supports that relationship- and domain-specific models are most influential in guiding attachment behavior in specific contexts, but applications of working models across domains allows the use of experiential knowledge as people encounter new situations or relationships. Such across-domain applications could introduce inconsistencies if the attachment conditions across domains are incongruent, such as when insecure models of parents undermine caregiving within more secure romantic or parenting relationships. Yet, consistent with our functional account, continued experiences within secure relationships may reduce how much other insecure models intrude into those relationships, especially given that relationship-specific models should be relatively more influential.

Revisions to Multiple Working Models: Variation in Content across Time

Multiple working models that are flexibly activated and applied to provide the most accurate and useful guidance within attachment-relevant situations will be most functional if the shared and distinct information across working models reflects people's changing reality. Thus, working models should flexibly vary in content to capture changes in people's relational environments. Some of these revisions arise from dramatic violations of beliefs and expectations, such as when major stressors or life transitions contradict people's existing working models. For example, the likelihood of attachment insecurity increases when children experience major life stress, when romantic relationships dissolve, or when couples fail to support one another during the transition to parenthood (see Scharfe, 2003).

Working models should also change in more routine and modest ways in order to ensure representations precisely diagnose what to expect from attachment figures in the immediate context. Indeed, relationship-specific working models of partners, mothers, or fathers can fluctuate across the span of days, weeks, and months (Fraley, Vicary, Brumbaugh, & Roisman, 2011; Girme et al., 2018). These fluctuations in attachment security likely reflect normative adjustments as relationships, and the attachment challenges people are facing, change across time, such as when couples' sexual intimacy changes in response to chronic stress, illness, or parenting demands. Such fluctuations may stabilize once attachment difficulties or specific challenges are managed, and thus occur independently of stability in the general content of working models (Khan et al.,

2020). For example, when children experience greater parent–child stress than usual, they also report greater attachment anxiety and avoidance at that time point, but these fluctuations are independent of the development of children's anxiety and avoidance across time (Khan et al., 2020). Alternatively, fluctuations may culminate to produce larger revisions to relationship- and domain-specific working models if changes in attachment environments mean that expectations, beliefs, and behavioral strategies should be amended to more accurately reflect people's relationship reality. When parents' depression produces more constant parent–child stress, for example, then children are more likely to have higher anxiety and avoidance at later time points (Khan et al., 2020).

Revisions to working models should be adaptive but may pose difficulties for relationships. Greater within-person fluctuations in working models of romantic partners predict increases in relationship distress over time, but primarily for people whose working models lead them to expect relationships to be stable (Girme et al., 2018). Of course, such incongruence between working models and the reality of specific relationships should produce changes in relationship evaluations if working models are functioning to ensure that people are tracking their attachment safety and security. Such fluctuations in working models of romantic partners, however, should not affect the entire network of working models (e.g., models involving friends and family). Thus, multiple working models enable the flexibility required to represent changes in particular attachment contexts, without impeding the ability to obtain attachment goals across people's attachment networks.

Summary

People's attachment experiences, and resulting expectations, beliefs, goals, and behavioral strategies, are likely stored in a hierarchical network of multiple working models. Such a network should provide the most accurate and useful information needed for people to achieve their attachment goals across diverse and varying attachment contexts. Consistent with this functional account, people's representations of attachment figures include rankings of who can be relied on and when, and these rankings vary according to development phases and contextual needs. Multiple working models of multiple attachment figures involve both interconnections representing similar information across different domains along with distinct relationship-specific information to provide the precision needed to navigate the different needs, goals, and conditions of different relationships. Finally, this hierarchical network provides a way of flexibly revising specific working models in response to changes in attachment conditions, which should generalize as people's experiences are consolidated within and across relationships across time. This flexible network of multiple working models necessarily matches the flexibility needed to manage the attachment relationships we live in.

REFERENCES

Ainsworth, M. D. S., Blehar, M., Waters E., & Wall S. (1978). *Patterns of attachment: A psychological study of the Strange Situation.* Hillsdale, NJ: Erlbaum.

Bowlby, J. (1973). *Attachment and loss: Vol. 2. Separation.* New York: Basic Books.

Bowlby, J. (1980). *Attachment and loss: Vol. 3. Loss, sadness and depression.* New York: Basic Books.

Bowlby, J. (1982). *Attachment and loss: Vol. 1. Attachment* (2nd ed.). New York: Basic Books. (Original work published 1969)

Collins, N. L., & Read, S. J. (1994). Cognitive representations of attachment: The structure and function of working models. In K. Bartholomew & D. Perlman (Eds.), *Advances in personal relationships: Vol. 5. Attachment processes in adulthood* (pp. 53–90). London: Jessica Kingsley.

Deave, T., Johnson, D., & Ingram, J. (2008). Transition to parenthood: The needs of parents in pregnancy and early parenthood. *BMC Pregnancy and Childbirth, 8,* 30–41.

Doherty, N. A., & Feeney, J. A. (2004). The composition of attachment networks throughout the adult years. *Personal Relationships, 11,* 469–488.

Fraley, R. C., Heffernan, M. E., Vicary, A. M., & Brumbaugh, C. C. (2011). The experiences in close relationships—Relationship Structures Questionnaire: A method for assessing attachment orientations across relationships. *Psychological Assessment, 23,* 615–625.

Fraley, R. C., Vicary, A. M., Brumbaugh, C. C., & Roisman, G. I. (2011). Patterns of stability in adult attachment: An empirical test of two models of continuity and change. *Journal of Personality and Social Psychology, 101,* 974–992.

Girme, Y. U., Agnew, C. R., VanderDrift, L. E., Harvey, S. M., Rholes, W. S., & Simpson, J. A. (2018). The ebbs and flows of attachment: Within-person variation in attachment undermine secure individuals' relationship wellbeing across time. *Journal of Personality and Social Psychology, 114,* 397–421.

Kammrath, L. K., Armstrong, B. F., III, Lane, S. P., Francis, M. K., Clifton, M., McNab, K. M., & Baumgarten, O. M. (2020). What predicts who we approach for social support?: Tests of the attachment figure and strong ties hypotheses. *Journal of Personality and Social Psychology, 118*(3), 481–500.

Karantzas, G. C., Evans, L., & Foddy, M. (2010). The role of attachment in current and future parent caregiving. *Journals of Gerontology Series B: Psychological Sciences and Social Sciences, 65,* 573–580.

Khan, F., Chong, J. Y., Theisen, J. C., Fraley, R. C., Young, J. F., & Hankin, B. L. (2020). Development and change in attachment: A multiwave assessment of attachment and its correlates across childhood and adolescence. *Journal of Personality and Social Psychology, 118*(6), 1188–1206.

La Guardia, J. G., Ryan, R. M., Couchman, C. E., & Deci, E. L. (2000). Within-person variation in security of attachment: A self-determination theory perspective on attachment, need fulfillment, and well being. *Journal of Personality and Social Psychology, 79*, 367–384.

Markiewicz, D., Lawford, H., Doyle, A. B., & Haggart, N. (2006). Developmental differences in adolescents' and young adults' use of mothers, fathers, best friends, and romantic partners to fulfill attachment needs. *Journal of Youth and Adolescence, 35*, 121–134.

Overall, N. C., Fletcher, G. J., & Friesen, M. D. (2003). Mapping the intimate relationship mind: Comparisons between three models of attachment representations. *Personality and Social Psychology Bulletin, 29*(12), 1479–1493.

Raby, K. L., Lawler, J. M., Shlafer, R. J., Hesemeyer, P. S., Collins, W. A., & Sroufe, L. A. (2015). The interpersonal antecedents of supportive parenting: A prospective, longitudinal study from infancy to adulthood. *Developmental Psychology, 51*, 115–123.

Scharfe, E. (2003). Stability and change of attachment representations from cradle to grave. In S. M. Johnson & V. E. Whiffen (Eds.), *Attachment processes in couple and family therapy* (pp. 64–84). New York: Guilford Press.

Sibley, C. G., & Overall, N. C. (2008). The boundaries between attachment and personality: Localized versus generalized effects in daily social interaction. *Journal of Research in Personality, 42*, 1394–1407.

Simpson, J. A., Winterheld, H. A., Rholes, W. S., & Oriña, M. M. (2007). Working models of attachment and reactions to different forms of caregiving from romantic partners. *Journal of Personality and Social Psychology, 93*, 466–477.

TOPIC 4

STABILITY AND CHANGE IN THE SECURITY OF ATTACHMENT

- Should we expect attachment security to remain consistent over time?

- Is there evidence for stability in attachment security?

CHAPTER 18

The Consistency of Attachment Security across Time and Relationships

R. Chris Fraley
Keely A. Dugan

Should we expect attachment security to remain consistent across time, relationships, or developmental periods, and, if so, to what degree? This question is a central one in attachment theory and research. Answering it clearly, however, requires unpacking several hidden assumptions about what "attachment security" means and how it should be measured. In this chapter, we review these assumptions and explain their implications for understanding consistency in attachment across time and relationships. Along the way, we summarize research that is able to speak to these issues and outline some directions for future work. We note from the outset that our focus is largely on adolescent and adult attachment, but some of the points we make may also be relevant to the study of infant and child attachment.

What Is Attachment Security?

Attachment security has been conceptualized and assessed in various ways by attachment scholars. For example, developmental psychologists interested in assessing adult attachment tend to rely upon the Adult Attachment Interview (AAI), a semistructured interview in which people describe their early attachment experiences. One of the key constructs in this approach is "coherence of mind" or "coherence of discourse," which represents the extent to which a person is capable of describing his or her experiences in a way that conforms to Grice's (1975) maxims of discourse.

People who provide a coherent account of their experiences are often classified as secure or "autonomous" with respect to attachment.

When assessed using the AAI, security is typically conceptualized as a dispositional or global attribute, one that has implications for multiple domains (e.g., romantic relationships, mental health). For example, Main, Kaplan, and Cassidy (1985, p. 78) wrote that the AAI can be used "to assess the security of the adult's overall working model of attachment, that is, the security of the self in relation to attachment in its *generality* rather than in relation to any particular present or past relationship" (emphasis added). Despite this assumption, it is critical to note that the assessment of security is done in the context of adults' reflections on their relationships with their parents during childhood. People are *not* queried about their relationships with romantic partners, coworkers, siblings, or friends. Thus, we refer to the AAI as a measure of *parental attachment,* although we recognize that this framing is not compatible with the way the AAI is typically portrayed.

In social and personality psychology, attachment security is typically conceptualized as representing the extent to which people are comfortable depending on others and using them for attachment-related functions (e.g., proximity-maintenance, safe haven, and secure base functions). Although the specific details of how this is conceptualized has varied across the history of social-psychological research (see Crowell, Fraley, & Roisman, 2016), each of these approaches maintains that a prototypically secure person believes that others will not abandon him or her and is comfortable depending on others and using them as a safe haven during times of distress. Attachment security is typically assessed using self-report instruments designed to measure *attachment-related anxiety* (i.e., the extent to which people are worried about the availability and support of close others) and *avoidance* (i.e., the extent to which people are uncomfortable depending on others), under the assumption that individual differences in security will manifest themselves differently in the ways people think about and experience their relationships.

Although the AAI is typically understood to represent a "general" measure of attachment (see above), social and personality psychologists have focused both on general and relationship-specific ways of assessing attachment (e.g., Klohnen, Weller, Luo, & Choe, 2005). For example, the Experiences in Close Relationships scale (ECR) and its revised version (ECR-R) are typically used to assess attachment security in the context of "close relationships" broadly construed. Researchers have also used these and related instruments to assess security in the context of specific relationships (e.g., Doyle, Lawford, & Markiewicz, 2009). For example, the Relationship Structures questionnaire (ECR-RS) can be used to assess security in the context of adults' relationships with their mothers, fathers, romantic partners, and friends (Fraley, Heffernan, Vicary, & Brumbaugh, 2011).

Attachment across Relationships

These distinctions among different ways of conceptualizing and measuring attachment security might seem overly pedantic. Here is why they matter: When considering consistency in attachment across relationships, early research focused on examining the association between self-reported attachment and AAI classifications. Not surprisingly, associations between security as measured by the AAI and self-reports tend to be small, hovering around .09 (see Roisman et al., 2007). However, these associations do not simply reflect the consistency of attachment security across relationships; they also reflect differences in the constructs being measured (i.e., coherence of mind vs. anxiety/avoidance) and differences in the methods used to assess them (i.e., coded interviews vs. self-reports).

One way to address this problem is to equate measures and constructs when examining cross-relationship consistency. Some scholars have used interview-based methods that focus on coherence of mind to examine separately attachment in the parental (i.e., AAI) and romantic domains (Crowell & Owens, 1996). For example, Crowell and her colleagues developed the Current Relationship Interview (CRI; Crowell & Owens, 1996) as a way to assess the coherence of adults' narratives about their current romantic relationships. Crowell and her colleagues found that security scores, as assessed in the AAI and the CRI, correlated approximately 0.29 (Owens et al., 1995). Fraley, Heffernan, and colleagues (2011) have adopted a similar approach using self-report instruments designed to assess attachment-related avoidance and anxiety in distinct relationship domains. They found that attachment security in the context of parental relationships was correlated approximately 0.20 with security assessed in the context of romantic relationships.

Collectively, research that "holds the methods/constructs constant" suggests that there is some consistency in attachment patterns across relationships. This suggests that people who tend to be secure in one relationship domain also tend to be secure in other relationship domains, too. However, it is important to note that these associations do not approach unity. There are many people who exhibit different patterns of attachment across relationships. For example, some people are secure in their parental relationships but are less so in their romantic relationships.

One of the important directions for future attachment research is to understand the nature of these disparities. Given the strong socialization assumptions inherent in attachment theory, it seems likely that, even if people bring specific strengths and insecurities with them to new relationships, those new relationships will nonetheless be driven by the actual interactions that take place between those involved. Thus, if someone secure in their relationships with their parents enters a new romantic relationship, they may become insecure in that relationship if their partner is unresponsive, neglectful, or potentially abusive. To the best of our knowledge, researchers have yet to investigate the extent to which the security of parental attachments combines with actual interactions in newly developing relationships to predict the security of those new relationships.

Attachment across Time

How consistent is attachment security across time? Many writers tend to emphasize the consistency rather than the instability of attachment across time (e.g., Dinero, Conger, Shaver, Widaman, & Larsen-Rife, 2008; Zayas, Mischel, Shoda, & Aber, 2011). Attachment theory, however, describes mechanisms of both stability and change. For example, Bowlby called attention to the self-perpetuating nature of the assumptions that people hold about the world and close others. People view their social interactions through a self-confirming lens, leading them to understand the world in a way that is consistent with the beliefs they already hold. However, Bowlby also argued that people's working models are "tolerably accurate" reflections of the world. He argued that people develop working models on the basis of their actual experiences. This kind of socialization process suggests that people are open to change, especially early in their interpersonal histories when they do not have as much information available to ground their judgments.

Given these alternative mechanisms, we have argued previously that attachment theory does not make strong predictions about consistency across time (e.g., Fraley, 2019). Nonetheless, the question itself is an important one, and answering it well is crucial for refining the theory in critical ways. We now briefly address attachment stability within relationships, across relationships, and across developmental periods.

Within a relationship across time, attachment security appears to be relatively consistent. But different kinds of relationships reveal different degrees of consistency. For example, in our longitudinal research, we have found that the security of adults' relationships with their parents is highly stable when assessed using test–retest correlations. Over periods of time ranging from a few weeks to a year, we found that the test–retest stability of attachment avoidance with parents was approximately .80 or higher (Fraley, Vicary, Brumbaugh, & Roisman, 2011). This implies that the rank-order stability of parental attachment in the adult years is exceptionally high: People who are insecure with their parents today are highly likely to be insecure with their parents in the future.

Attachment in romantic relationships, however, is not as stable as attachment in parental relationships. We found that, although the rank-order stability of attachment avoidance in romantic relationships was high across short test–retest intervals (e.g., 0.70), it was lower (e.g., about 0.30) over periods of time ranging from 20 weeks to 54 weeks. This implies that adult romantic relationships are more fluid or dynamic than adults' relationships with their parents.

Why does the across-time consistency in parental and romantic relationships differ? There are at least two potential explanations. First, it is possible that the difference is due to the kind of relationship. There may be something inherently more dynamic about romantic relationships, for example. That is, new partners are in an active state of learning more about each other's needs, vulnerabilities, and strengths. This may require some calibration and adjustment and may lead people's preexisting assumptions about relationships to be challenged or refined. Second, these differences in consistency could be due to differences in the age or duration of these relationships. Adults in their 30s, for instance, have been interacting with their parents for decades and have likely settled into patterns of interaction that are relatively robust. The romantic relationships of those same adults, however, have not lasted as long and, for some people, may still be in the early phases.

The canalization principle in attachment theory and research (Bowlby, 1973) suggests that, early in the development of a relationship, socialization processes should dominate, making it easier for people to be shaped by their environments. Over time, however, selection processes begin to take over, leading to increased stability in relational patterns. Given that the relationships that adults have with their parents are well established, we should expect the test–retest stability of those attachment patterns to be higher than it is in romantic relationships, which have had a shorter lifespan.

Consistent with this principle, data indicate that the test–retest stability of attachment in parent–child relationships is less stable early in life than it is later on. In the study of child attachment, of course, different measures are used to assess attachment security at different ages, making it difficult to draw unambiguous conclusions about how stability varies with age. But, using common instruments (e.g., the ECR), it appears that the 5-year stability of attachment among adolescents is lower (approximately .35) than it is among their parents (approximately .70) over the same time frame (Jones et al., 2018).

How stable is attachment across developmental periods? This is difficult to address given that the way attachment is assessed across different periods tends to vary considerably. Recent meta-analytic work (Pinquart, Feußner, & Ahnert, 2013) has attempted to quantify the test–retest stability of measures of attachment in early childhood and later adolescence and adulthood (see also Groh et al., 2014). The findings of this work suggest that consistency across certain critical developmental periods (i.e., infancy and early childhood to early adulthood) is fairly low, even if stability within the adult years is high. The implication of such findings is that, if one is seeking to understand why some adults are more secure than others, the answer may not lie solely in the early years of life. Indeed, even if early life is emphasized in popular writing about attachment, attachment researchers have been careful to call attention to the accumulation of experiences, the updating of working models in light of ongoing experiences, and the plurality of factors that may shape attachment patterns (e.g., Simpson, Collins, & Salvatore, 2011).

Short Answers to the Core Questions

- Attachment security is highly stable within certain relationship domains (e.g., within parental relationships) in adulthood.

- Attachment security is more stable in some relationship contexts (e.g., adult parental relationships) than others (adult romantic relationships).

- Commonly used measures of adult attachment (e.g., the ECR and the AAI) emphasize different relational domains (e.g., peers vs. parents), using different methods (e.g., self-reports vs. interviews), and using different theoretical concepts. Thus, answering questions about consistency by comparing different measures is suboptimal.

- Attachment security appears to be less stable in childhood and adolescence than in adulthood, at least based on research that attempts to equate the assessment methods used.

- Consistency in attachment across relationship domains appears to be modest in adulthood. Adults who have insecure relationships with their parents are more likely to have insecure relationships with peers, but there are many exceptions to this pattern.

REFERENCES

Bowlby, J. (1973). *Attachment and loss: Vol. 2. Separation*. New York: Basic Books.
Crowell, J. A., Fraley, R. C., & Roisman, G. I. (2016). Measurement of individual differences in adult attachment. In J. Cassidy & P. R. Shaver (Eds.), *Handbook of attachment: Theory, research, and clinical applications* (3rd ed., pp. 598–635). New York: Guilford Press.
Crowell, J. A., & Owens, G. (1996). *Current Relationship Interview and scoring system* Unpublished manuscript, State University of New York at Stony Brook.
Dinero, R. E., Conger, R. D., Shaver, P. R., Widaman, K. F., & Larsen-Rife, D. (2008). Influence of family origin and adult romantic partners on romantic security. *Journal of Family Psychology, 22*(4), 622–632.
Doyle, A. B., Lawford, H., & Markiewicz, D. (2009). Attachment style with mother, father, best friend, and romantic partner during adolescence. *Journal of Research on Adolescence, 19*(4), 690–714.

Fraley, R. C. (2019). Attachment in adulthood: Recent developments, emerging debates, and future directions. *Annual Review of Psychology, 70*(1), 401–422.

Fraley, R. C., Heffernan, M. E., Vicary, A. M., & Brumbaugh, C. C. (2011). The Experiences in Close Relationships—Relationship Structures questionnaire: A method for assessing attachment orientations across relationships. *Psychological Assessment, 23*(3), 615–625.

Fraley, R. C., Vicary, A. M., Brumbaugh, C. C., & Roisman, G. I. (2011). Patterns of stability in adult attachment: An empirical test of two methods of continuity and change. *Journal of Personality and Social Psychology, 101*(5), 974–992.

Grice, H. P. (1975). Logic and conversation. In P. Cole & J. L. Morgan (Eds.), *Syntax and semantics: Vol. 3. Speech acts* (pp. 41–58). New York: Academic Press.

Groh, A. M., Roisman, G. I., Booth-LaForce, C., Fraley, R. C., Owen, M. T., Cox, M. J., & Burchinal, M. R. (2014). Stability of attachment security from infancy to late adolescence. In C. Booth-LaForce & G. I. Roisman (Eds.), The Adult Attachment Interview: Psychometrics, stability and change from infancy, and developmental origins. *Monographs of the Society for Research in Child Development, 79*(3), 51–66.

Jones, J. D., Fraley, R. C., Ehrlich, K. B., Stern, J. A., Lejuez, C. W., Shaver, P. R., & Cassidy, J. (2018). Stability of attachment style in adolescence: An empirical test of alternative developmental processes. *Child Development, 89*, 871–880.

Klohnen, E. C., Weller, J. A., Luo, S., & Choe, M. (2005). Organization and predictive power of general and specific attachment models: One for all, and all for one? *Personality and Social Psychology Bulletin, 31*(12), 1665–1682.

Main, M., Kaplan, N., & Cassidy, J. (1985). Security in infancy, childhood, and adulthood: A move to the level of representation. In I. Bretherton & E. Waters (Eds.), Growing points of attachment theory and research. *Monographs of the Society for Research in Childhood Development, 50*(1–2, Serial No. 209), 66–104.

Owens, G., Crowell, J. A., Pan, H., Treboux, D., O'Connor, E., & Waters, E. (1995). The prototype hypothesis and the origins of attachment working models: Adult relationships with parents and romantic partners. *Monographs of the Society for Research in Child Development, 60*(2–3), 216–233.

Pinquart, M., Feußner, C., & Ahnert, L. (2013). Meta-analytic evidence for stability in attachments from infancy to early adulthood. *Attachment and Human Development, 15*(2), 189–218.

Roisman, G. I., Holland, A., Fortuna, K., Fraley, R. C., Clausell, E., & Clarke, A. (2007). The Adult Attachment Interview and self-reports of attachment style: An empirical rapprochement. *Journal of Personality and Social Psychology, 92*(4), 678–697.

Simpson, J. A., Collins, W. A., & Salvatore, J. E. (2011). The impact of early personal experiences on adult romantic relationship functioning: Recent findings from the Minnesota Longitudinal Study of Risk and Adaptation. *Current Directions in Psychological Science, 20*(6), 355–359.

Zayas, V., Mischel, W., Shoda, Y., & Aber, J. L. (2011). Roots of adult attachment: Maternal caregiving at 18 months predicts adult attachment to peers and partners. *Social Psychological and Personality Science, 2*(3), 289–297.

CHAPTER 19

Stability and Change in Attachment Security

Cathryn Booth–LaForce
Glenn I. Roisman

Attachment theory (Bowlby, 1969/1982) has inspired decades of empirical work, modification, and synthesis. In so doing, it has become one of the most well-validated theories in developmental science. Bowlby focused on the biological, evolutionary, and psychological bases of the child's tie to the mother, but also addressed individual differences in the quality of attachment. Specifically, a central tenet of attachment theory is that the quality of early experiences with the primary caregiver (i.e., caregiver's sensitivity and availability) form the basis for the child to develop a relatively secure or insecure specific attachment to that caregiver, which then generalizes to an internal representation of attachment that guides future relationships and social-emotional development. Ainsworth and her colleagues (Ainsworth, Blehar, Waters, & Wall, 1978) advanced this work on individual differences in attachment quality, and inspired decades of subsequent research on the sources of these individual differences and their developmental consequences.

Because of Bowlby's background and focus on the earliest manifestations of attachment as reflecting both biological and psychological processes, and because Ainsworth's validated assessment of attachment security (the Strange Situation) was designed for the infancy period, most of the early empirical work in this area addressed attachment security in infancy and its sequelae in early childhood. That said, a lifespan perspective was a fundamental aspect of Bowlby's and Ainsworth's work. In the past few decades, a growing number of researchers have focused on attachment in middle childhood, adolescence, and adulthood, made possible by the development of assessments and procedures pertaining to these older age periods.

These assessments have made it feasible to evaluate the extent to which attachment security remains consistent across time, relationships, and developmental periods, and to test a central premise of attachment theory. In fact, it was not until the beginning of the 21st century that long-term longitudinal data became available to address questions about whether, or to what extent, early attachment security remains stable across time into late adolescence and early adulthood. However, before addressing these empirical results, it is worth stating why we expect attachment security to remain consistent across time, relationships, or developmental periods.

Bowlby's Theory

As noted, according to attachment theory, children's early experiences with primary caregivers form the basis for the development of a generalized internal working model of attachment, which is an outgrowth of the security of the infant's specific attachment to the primary caregiver. This model is reinforced under conditions of relative stability in parent–child relationship quality over time. With developmental change, the model is hypothesized to be updated but is still theorized to be relatively stable due to the increasing automatization of caregiver–child interaction patterns and the child's positive or negative perceptual biases arising from these habitual patterns (Bowlby, 1969/1982). In other words, security of attachment in infancy is purported to be relatively stable across time due to primary caregivers' stable quality of care and due to the child's developing sense of self in relation to others as well as expectations about what should be anticipated and sought from close relationships and the social world.

Of particular note in this regard is that Bowlby was influenced by (and in turn, influenced) the emerging field of ethology. In particular, he was strongly attracted to the idea of imprinting in very young animals as the basis for affectional bonds with their mothers, and this idea influenced his concept of the development of attachment in humans as a phenomenon with lifelong consequences for the individual. Bowlby's investigations of mental health issues in homeless children and the early backgrounds of juvenile thieves supported his initial ideas (van der Horst, van der Veer, & van IJzendoorn, 2007).

Of course, children are neither inoculated in infancy with a large bolus of security that will last a lifetime, nor infected with an equally long-lasting dosage of insecurity. As Bowlby theorized, continuing security (or insecurity) is dependent on the relative stability in the caregiving environment; that is, the continuing availability and responsiveness (or lack thereof) of the primary caregiver, as well as the increasing automatization of caregiver–child interaction patterns and the child's positive or negative perceptual biases arising from these patterns. But to what extent would we expect such continuity and under what specific circumstances? We now turn to the evidence, accumulated over many studies and many decades.

The Evidence for Stability

Rank-order stability in attachment became possible to estimate once post-infancy assessments of attachment were developed and validated. But it was not until the turn of the 21st century that findings from a number of long-term longitudinal studies were published, with mixed results regarding the stability of attachment security from infancy through adulthood. Generally, these studies had relatively modest sample sizes (n = 30–125). As such, consequent variation in results was not surprising. However, a meta-analysis (Pinquart, Feußner, & Ahnert, 2013) evaluating both the short-term and long-term stability of attachment security in 127 studies did find evidence of moderate stability over time (r = .39), but it varied depending on a number of factors. Specifically, stability decreased as the intervals between assessments increased and stability was also lower if different types of attachment assessments were used (i.e., observational vs. representational measures). Likewise, stability was higher in middle-class (low-risk) normative samples than in at-risk samples. Moreover, in lower-risk samples, secure attachment was more stable than was insecure attachment, but in higher-risk samples, insecure attachment was more stable. These meta-analytic results support a central tenet of attachment theory, namely, that continuity in attachment security is dependent on stability in the caregiving environment—either supportive or unsupportive.

It is worth noting that attachment stability *from infancy to adulthood* in the Pinquart and colleagues (2013) meta-analysis of generally small samples was r = .14. Remarkably, in the largest longitudinal analysis of attachment security to date in a normative-risk sample (National Institute of Child Health and Human Development [NICHD] Study of Early Child Care and Youth Development [SECCYD], n = 857; see Booth-LaForce & Roisman, 2014), the stability from infancy to age 18 was quite similar—r = .12, a statistically significant yet relatively weak effect (Groh et al., 2014). Similar findings have also been found in the largest *high*-risk longitudinal study of attachment stability, the Minnesota Longitudinal Study of Risk of Adaptation (MLSRA; Raby, Cicchetti, Carlson, Egeland, & Collins, 2013).

To us, it is not surprising to find some evidence of attachment stability from infancy to adulthood, but it is also not surprising that it is relatively weak—due to the number of years between assessments, the differences in the types of assessments, and the likelihood of changing circumstances, environments, and relationships during the life of the developing child. Moreover, the reliance on just a few minutes of coded behavior from the Strange Situation may underestimate stability in attachment from infancy to adulthood. Indeed, in the SECCYD, we found that observed maternal and paternal sensitivity in early childhood, compared with Strange Situation classifications, were more strongly related to late-adolescent AAI states of mind (Haydon, Roisman, Owen, Booth-LaForce, & Cox, 2014).

The Evidence for Lawful Change

Of equal importance to the attachment stability discussion is the identification of circumstances under which attachment security would be expected to change over time. As noted, Bowlby maintained that attachment security or insecurity should be reinforced by both the likelihood of consistency in the caregiving environment and the child's consolidation of the internal working model of self in relation to others. But this also means that the quality of attachment security should not be immutable, especially if significant changes occur during the child's life. For example, caregiving sensitivity could decrease in the face of stressful life changes that could alter the child's expectation of the parent's availability as well as the parent's actual availability, thereby leading to a change from security to insecurity. As indicated in the Pinquart and colleagues (2013) meta-analysis, such change may be more likely when the child is already in an at-risk environment. Similarly, improvements in the primary caregiver's sensitivity and availability, perhaps as a result of a positive change in life circumstances, would be expected to potentiate a change from insecurity to security. Such a change would be more likely in a lower-risk environment, according to Pinquart and colleagues.

In long-term longitudinal studies with relatively small samples, a number of proximal and distal factors were identified as possible sources of change in attachment security from infancy to late adolescence/early adulthood (see Booth-LaForce et al., 2014). Among these were the high-risk or low-risk nature of the sample (Fraley, 2002; Pinquart et al., 2013), trauma directly experienced by the participant (e.g., death of a parent), changes in life experiences in the family environment, parental depression, presence or absence of the father in the home, and changes in the quality of caregiver–child interactions.

Although these studies yielded mixed results, they provided a road-map for further analyses of NICHD SECCYD data. As a follow-up study to the NICHD SECCYD (see NICHD Early Child Care Research Network,

2005), which spanned the period from birth through age 15 years, we assessed participants at age 18 years with the Adult Attachment Interview (AAI). Mother–child attachment had been assessed three times in the infancy/preschool period (Strange Situation procedure at age 15 months, Attachment Q-Sort at age 24 months, and modified Strange Situation procedure at age 36 months), from which we derived a measure of the number of times the child was secure during this period. The wealth of data from the SECCYD provided the opportunity for us to assess the role of a variety of factors in maintaining or altering security/insecurity from early childhood to late adolescence.

First, we affirmed that participants who remained insecure, compared with those who remained secure, had mothers who were less sensitive over time, who were less likely to have a father present in the home, and whose fathers had more depressive symptoms. Then, comparing participants who remained secure with those who changed from secure to insecure between early childhood and late adolescence, we found the following: As hypothesized, we observed that those who became insecure had experienced a larger increase in negative life events and a greater decline in observed maternal sensitivity, and they were less likely to be living with their fathers. We also compared those who remained insecure with those who changed from insecurity to security and found that those in the latter group had experienced a higher level of maternal sensitivity in the years between early childhood and late adolescence (Booth-LaForce et al., 2014).

These results support both principles of attachment theory and prior research on sources of continuity and discontinuity in attachment security over time in the largest sample to date in which attachment security was assessed during infancy and late adolescence. An additional source of evidence in this regard comes from the literature on attachment security in adoptive and foster families. For children with a history of maltreatment or institutional rearing, substantial improvement in attachment quality with adoptive caregivers has been found, presumably from positive changes in sensitive caregiving (see Raby & Dozier, 2019). Additionally, in the Bucharest Early Intervention Project, in which orphaned institutionalized children were randomly assigned to care as usual versus foster care, those placed in foster care before age 24 months improved markedly in their security of attachment compared with controls (Smyke, Zeanah, Fox, Nelson, & Guthrie, 2010).

Other Considerations

Of course, there is always room for additional research, and not all of the questions about the stability of attachment security have been answered.

For example, no studies have addressed how attachment stability may be related to consistency in internal working models over time, despite the centrality of this concept in attachment theory. Another issue is we do not know enough about the stability of *sub-categories* of insecurity or the extent to which individuals may change from one to another—or the factors driving such changes. Also, the majority of the extant research (but see Groh et al., 2014) has considered the stability of attachment categories (secure, insecure), rather than adopting a dimensional approach to the measurement of attachment security (see Fraley & Roisman, 2014). The latter approach is worth greater exploration.

Conclusions

We began this chapter by asking whether attachment security should be expected to remain consistent over time, and if so, why and to what degree? The answer to the first part of this question is yes—from both a theoretical perspective and from the empirical evidence to date. But this conclusion is tempered by the size of the effect. We know, from both a meta-analysis of 127 studies and from the largest study to date of attachment security from infancy onward, that the association between early and later attachment security is relatively small in magnitude and may depend on the time between assessments and the nature of the assessments themselves. Moreover, it is clear that consistency should only be expected under conditions of stability in caregiving quality and other aspects of the rearing environment, whereas change from security to insecurity (or the reverse) can be lawfully attributed, in part, to improvement or deterioration in these factors.

REFERENCES

Ainsworth, M. D. S., Blehar, M. C., Waters, E., & Wall, S. (1978). *Patterns of attachment: A psychological study of the Strange Situation*. New York: Erlbaum.

Booth-LaForce, C., Groh, A. M., Burchinal, M. R., Roisman, G. I., Owen, M. T., & Cox, M. J. (2014). V. Caregiving and contextual sources of continuity and change in attachment security from infancy to late adolescence. *Monographs of the Society for Research in Child Development, 79*, 67–84.

Booth-LaForce, C., & Roisman, G. I. (Eds.). (2014). The Adult Attachment Interview: Psychometrics, continuity and change from infancy, and developmental origins. *Monographs of the Society for Research in Child Development, 7*(3, Serial No. 314).

Bowlby, J. (1982). *Attachment and loss: Vol. 1. Attachment* (2nd ed.). New York: Basic Books. (Original work published 1969)

Fraley, R. C. (2002). Attachment stability from infancy to adulthood: Meta-analysis and dynamic modeling of developmental mechanisms. *Personality and Social Psychology, 6*, 123–125.

Fraley, R. C., & Roisman, G. I. (2014). III. Categories or dimensions?: A taxometric analysis of the Adult Attachment Interview. *Monographs of the Society for Research in Child Development, 79*, 36–50.

Groh, A. M., Roisman, G. I., Booth-LaForce, C., Fraley, R. C., Owen, M. T., Cox, M. J., & Burchinal, M. R. (2014). IV: Stability of attachment security from infancy to late adolescence. *Monographs of the Society for Research in Child Development, 79*, 51–66.

Haydon, K. C., Roisman, G. I., Owen, M. T., Booth-LaForce, C., & Cox, M. J. (2014). VII. Shared and distinctive antecedents of AAI state of mind and inferred experience dimensions. *Monographs of the Society for Research in Child Development, 79*, 108–125.

NICHD Early Child Care Research Network. (Eds.). (2005). *Child care and child development.* New York: Guilford Press.

Pinquart, M., Feußner, C., & Ahnert, L. (2013). Meta-analytic evidence for stability in attachments from infancy to early adulthood. *Attachment and Human Development, 15*, 189–218.

Raby, K. L., Cicchetti, D., Carlson, E. A., Egeland, B., & Collins, W. A. (2013). Genetic contributions to continuity and change in attachment security: A prospective, longitudinal investigation from infancy to young adulthood. *Journal of Child Psychiatry and Psychology, 54*, 1223–1230.

Raby, K. L., & Dozier, M. (2019). Attachment across the lifespan: Insights from adoptive families. *Current Opinion in Psychology, 25*, 81–85.

Smyke, A. T., Zeanah, C. H., Fox, N. A., Nelson, C. A., & Guthrie, D. (2010). Placement in foster care enhances quality of attachment among young institutionalized children. *Child Development, 81*, 212–223.

van der Horst, F. C. P., van der Veer, R., & van IJzendoorn, M. H. (2007). John Bowlby and ethology: An annotated interview with Robert Hinde. *Attachment and Human Development, 9*, 321–335.

CHAPTER 20

Beyond Stability
Toward Understanding the *Development* of Attachment Beyond Childhood

Joseph P. Allen

Our efforts to understand the development of attachment beyond childhood have led us to reconsider the value of the field's longstanding quest to assess stability in attachment over time (see, e.g., Benoit & Parker, 1994; Groh et al., 2014; Vaughn, Egeland, Sroufe, & Waters, 1979; Waters, Hamilton, & Weinfield, 2000). Much as adolescence transforms family interactions, exploring attachment in adolescence has upended our thinking about whether stability is even the right construct to be exploring beyond childhood. This rethinking has led to the following six principles, which we now see as central to building a truly developmental, lifespan theory of the workings of the attachment system and attachment relationships, illustrated in part by Figure 20.1.

Principle 1: The question "Is there *stability* in attachment security across time and contexts?" is often logically flawed. Early excitement at the strikingly robust long-term correlations between the infant Strange Situation and functioning later in childhood (e.g., to independent preschool teachers' ratings of competence; Sroufe, 1983) and strong relation between the Adult Attachment Interview (AAI) and offspring attachment (e.g., correlations as high as $r = .62$; Main, Kaplan, & Cassidy, 1985) gave rise to the idea that something remarkably powerful and stable was being assessed. No doubt, remarkable processes were indeed being assessed. Yet the construct of stability logically presumes that *the same thing* is being measured at different times. Moving from the relationship level (e.g., the Strange Situation) to the functional level or the intrapsychic level (e.g.,

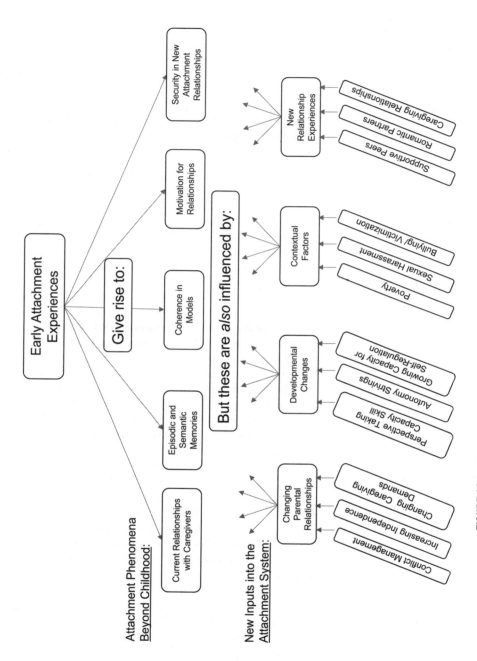

FIGURE 20.1. The development of the attachment system beyond childhood.

states of mind in the AAI), we may or may not reveal striking continuities, but *stability* is logically the wrong thing to be looking for.

Notably, even within infancy, neither Bowlby nor Ainsworth presumed that there would necessarily be consistency from one attachment relationship to another (i.e., infant–mother to infant–father). So, in most cases, stability will be the wrong target, but something equally interesting, yet more theoretically challenging—continuity—will be. This shift in perspective, however, quickly gives rise to an additional question: Continuity to *what*? As the individual moves from childhood through adolescence and numerous developmental transformations take place, a range of new facets of attachment relationships and attachment-related cognitions and emotions emerge. Thus, rather than a single "stability" question, we now have a multitude of distinct and important questions about continuity to consider, as Principle 2 outlines.

Principle 2: Beyond childhood, we can and should address the continuity question with regard to *many* distinct attachment-related phenomena. The relative simplicity of single attachment relationships in infancy gives way to a far more complex set of experiences (both relational and intrapsychic) as the individual develops. Thus, the roots of early attachment bonds with a primary caregiver give rise to *many* different branches in adolescence and beyond, as illustrated in the top half of Figure 20.1. These include:

1. The degree of security in *current* attachment relationships with caregivers
2. The *content* of an individual's episodic and semantic memories of past attachment experiences
3. Coherence in *processing* memory and affect related to attachment in a way that will lead to secure caregiving (i.e., the secure states of mind that the AAI assesses)
4. *Expectations* of one's own behavior and of others' behavior in new attachment relationships
5. *Motivation* to be in (or avoid) close relationships
6. The degree of security in the *peer* and *romantic* relationships that are rapidly coming to take on aspects of full-fledged attachment relationships

This partial list makes clear why strong continuities from one facet of attachment to another might be at times difficult to find—there are simply too many other moving pieces in play. This observation in turn gives rise to the third key principle.

Principle 3: The attachment system is open and dynamic and should be studied as such. Bowlby's (1980) recognition that qualities of working models of attachment often operate outside of conscious awareness and that individuals will tend to recreate past relationship patterns has often been misinterpreted to imply that attachment phenomena are unlikely to change. Given the importance of the attachment system and of supportive relationships to human survival across the lifespan (Holt-Lunstad, Smith, & Layton, 2010), the idea that the attachment system would be highly unresponsive to environmental inputs beyond infancy, though vaguely consistent with Freudian theory, would seem both implausible and quite dysfunctional. Rather than view what is captured by the Strange Situation as some sort of homunculus that resides intact within the individual to pop up in various forms throughout the lifespan, it is far more precise to view Strange Situation behavior as a reflection of a *single experience* of caregiving with one caregiver, an important input to be sure, but one of many as development progresses. In the past 15 years we've learned a great deal about the extent to which even implicit and unconscious associations can be altered by new relationship experiences and metacognitive monitoring (Dasgupta & Asgari, 2004; Monteith, Ashburn-Nardo, Voils, & Czopp, 2002), and as outlined below, both become central features of development as adolescence progresses.

So, even as we make an appropriate move from a focus on stability to a focus on continuities, what we need is not an intensive effort to identify simple continuities from infancy onward (or even continuities within adolescence or adulthood), but rather to develop a model that accounts for the *multiple* inputs to the operation of the attachment system, explaining both continuities and discontinuities, as individuals move through the lifespan. In short, we need to move from a fixed personality perspective (viewing security as an enduring intrapsychic trait) to a true social-developmental perspective. The final three principles presented below and illustrated in the bottom half of Figure 20.1 make clear why even simple continuities may be hard to find given how much changes during development. More importantly, however, these principles also provide an initial enumeration of some of the key inputs that we need to examine to fully understand the development of the attachment system beyond childhood.

Principle 4: The attachment system will be influenced by individual development and the broader social context. To the extent the attachment system evolved to both assure the infant's safety and to provide a sufficient sense of security as to allow exploration in the absence of significant threat, development is bound to bring major changes in the system's operation. For example, from infancy to adolescence, the individual develops dramatically enhanced capacities for self-regulation and self-soothing. In addition, normative autonomy drives push the adolescent to use these new capacities to seek emotional independence from attachment figures so as to prepare for successful functioning as an adult. These two phe-nomena combine to decrease the extent to which adolescents need (or want) to turn to their attachment figures when distressed. Inevitably, this alters the nature of the adolescent–parent attachment relationship.

Similarly, both the emergence of strong perspective-taking skills, as cognitive development progresses, and increasing autonomy vis-à-vis attachment figures provide a greater opportunity to revisit and alter exist-ing states of mind regarding attachment. These skills and this autonomy then influence the likelihood that, to use just one example, an individual with a history of insecure relationships might ultimately come to what Main, Goldwyn, and Hesse (2002) have termed an autonomous and valu-ing state of mind with respect to attachment.

Finally, larger social contextual factors take on a much more direct role with development. Adolescents are potentially exposed to threats such as sexual assault, aggression, and bullying to an extent not hereto-fore experienced. Poverty and racism are now likely to affect the adoles-cent in myriad new ways as they move more independently into the larger society. These factors, and no doubt many other similar social contextual factors, all have the potential to overwhelm the attachment system, pro-viding stressors that attachment figures cannot address and leading to a range of less adaptive responses in turn. Alternatively, they may in some instances be met by adolescents reaching still higher levels of adaptation and coping.

Principle 5: Attachment processes will be influenced by changing family relationships. Although many factors can affect the quality of attachment relationships in infancy, beginning in adolescence a major new source of change arrives as many of the *fundamental tasks* of parental caregiving change. Primary caregivers' principal/key task changes from 24/7 sensitive responsiveness and soothing of an infant to a much more intermittent, but equally important, focus on promotion of self-soothing and autonomy on the part of the adolescent. A frequent challenge for parents of adolescents is the experience that "My teen no longer seems to need or want my help." Neither is true, of course, but what *is* true is that the adolescent no longer needs the parent in the same way as they did in infancy or childhood. Hence, a key input to the adolescent's attachment system becomes the capacity of the parent to manage this relatively new task. If the infant's working model of self-in-relationship asks, "Can I get help from my caregiver when I'm threatened or distressed," the adoles-cent's model likely adds an element: "Can I get help when I need it *in a way that doesn't threaten my growing need for autonomy?*" This challenge also appears at earlier stages of development, of course, but the balance changes radically in adolescence in ways that can be either helpful or harmful. Parents who are comfortable with the intensity and intimacy involved in nurturing an infant may find the more distant, inconsistent needs of adolescents to be highly disconcerting. Conversely, parents who were overwhelmed by their infant's intense, omnipresent needs may find this relative distance to be a relief and may now easily handle the give and take involved.

Parents must also now manage adolescent attachment needs while also potentially handling significant *conflict* in their relationship with their teens. Although the "storm and stress" view of adolescence was always overstated, even routine conflicts take on a new level of intensity. Managing toddler anger is challenging, but for most parents it is not personally threatening; adolescents, in contrast, have the capacity to directly challenge parents in ways that are far more likely to leave parents off-balance. A secure attachment relationship certainly aids in handling these conflicts well, but how they are ultimately managed is influenced by multiple other drives and systems as well, including dominance drives, and cognitive and perceptual systems for detecting and responding to conflict, anger, and hostility. Even though the conflict system is distinct from the attachment system, failure to manage it well can make it difficult for the adolescent to approach the parent with attachment needs and/or for the parent to respond helpfully.

Principle 6: The attachment system will be influenced by new relationships. Although Bowlby (1980) notes that we tend to re-create relationships based on our existing models, we *also* fall into relationships in ways over which we have little control or are influenced by factors unrelated to attachment. Proximity, similarity of interests, sexual attraction, and compatibility, among other factors, all influence our choice of companions and will routinely leave us interacting with others who have far different attachment strategies than our own, adding new and powerful inputs to the development of attachment working models. Furthermore, adult attachment relationships can and do change radically over time, as evident in unfortunate marital relationships that devolve from deep and satisfying to alienated and bitter.

In addition, one of the largest developmental changes of adolescence is the emergence of peer and romantic relationships that gradually begin to take on the characteristics of full-fledged attachment relationships. Indeed, in their drive to attain emotional autonomy vis-à-vis parents, adolescents will often turn to peers and then to romantic partners for comfort in situations where these partners are likely to be highly variable in their capacity to provide it. Adolescence is also a period during which teens are uniquely primed to learn from and internalize peer experiences (Blakemore & Mills, 2014; Dahl & Hariri, 2005). Some teens may successfully turn to peers and romantic partners for support in coping with parental dysfunction; others may find that close, supportive peer relationships are a frustrating chimera in social Darwinian adolescent (and adult) peer worlds in which social success is viewed as a zero-sum contest and social survival as a group member is never fully secured. Ultimately, for some adolescents and most adults, new caregiving relationships introduced through becoming parents themselves or caring for siblings or elders will also powerfully stir up attachment-related memories and cognitions with great potential to alter the attachment system.

Toward a Developmental Contextual Model of the Attachment System Beyond Childhood

Even this very cursory overview of factors likely to influence attachment models, behaviors, and relationships beyond childhood should make clear that we can do much better than simply trying to identify levels of continuity (let alone stability) in attachment phenomena over time. The current examples are from adolescence, but further transformations occur as individuals move into adulthood. The problem is not that searching for continuity from a single relationship is likely to lead to limited success, it is that doing so distracts from the far more productive task of seeking to understand the many factors that go into influencing attachment cognitions, behavior, and relationships as these develop across the lifespan.

REFERENCES

Benoit, D., & Parker, K. C. H. (1994). Stability and transmission of attachment across three generations. *Child Development, 65,* 1444–1456.

Blakemore, S.-J., & Mills, K. L. (2014). Is adolescence a sensitive period for sociocultural processing? *Annual Review of Psychology, 65,* 187–207.

Bowlby, J. (1980). *Attachment and loss: Vol. 3. Loss, sadness and depression.* New York: Basic Books.

Dahl, R. E., & Hariri, A. R. (2005). Lessons from G. Stanley Hall: Connecting new research in biological sciences to the study of adolescent development. *Journal of Research on Adolescence, 15*(4), 367–382.

Dasgupta, N., & Asgari, S. (2004). Seeing is believing: Exposure to counterstereotypic women leaders and its effect on the malleability of automatic gender stereotyping. *Journal of Experimental Social Psychology, 40*(5), 642–658.

Groh, A. M., Roisman, G. I., Booth-LaForce, C., Fraley, R. C., Owen, M. T., Cox, M. J., & Burchinal, M. R. (2014). IV. Stability of attachment security from infancy to late adolescence. *Monographs of the Society for Research in Child Development, 79*(3), 51–66.

Holt-Lunstad, J., Smith, T. B., & Layton, J. B. (2010). Social relationships and mortality risk: A meta-analysis. *PLOS Medicine, 7*(7), 1–20.

Main, M., Goldwyn, R., & Hesse, E. (2002). *Adult Attachment Scoring and*

Classification Systems, Version 7.1. Unpublished manuscript, University of California at Berkeley.

Main, M., Kaplan, N., & Cassidy, J. (1985). Security in infancy, childhood, and adulthood: A move to the level of representation. In I. Bretherton & E. Waters (Eds.), Growing points in attachment theory and research. *Monographs of the Society for Research in Child Development, 50*(1–2, Serial No. 209), 66–104.

Monteith, M. J., Ashburn-Nardo, L., Voils, C. I., & Czopp, A. M. (2002). Putting the brakes on prejudice: On the development and operation of cues for control. *Journal of Personality and Social Psychology, 83*(5), 1029.

Sroufe, L. A. (1983). Infant–caregiver attachment and patterns of adaptation in preschool: The roots of maladaptation and competence. In M. Perlmutter (Ed.), *Minnesota Symposium on Child Psychology: Vol. 16. Development and policy concerning children with special needs* (pp. 41–83). Hillsdale, NJ: Erlbaum.

Vaughn, B. E., Egeland, B. R., Sroufe, L. A., & Waters, E. (1979). Individual differences in infant–mother attachment at twelve and eighteen months: Stability and change in families under stress. *Child Development, 50*(4), 971–975.

Waters, E., Hamilton, C. E., & Weinfield, N. S. (2000). The stability of attachment security from infancy to adolescence and early adulthood: General introduction. *Child Development, 71*(3), 678–683.

CHAPTER 21

Stability and Change in Adult Romantic Relationship Attachment Styles

Ramona L. Paetzold
W. Steven Rholes
Tiffany George

Adult attachment styles reflect Bowlby's notion of a lifespan approach to attachment theory (Bowlby, 1979). These attachment styles reflect internal working models (IWMs), which Bowlby (1979) observed as relatively stable, observing that

> whatever [IWMs] . . . an individual builds during his [*sic*] childhood and adolescence . . . tend to persist relatively unchanged into and throughout adult life. As a result he tends to assimilate any interactions with any new person with whom he may form a bond, such as spouse or child . . . to an existing model . . . and often continue to do so despite repeated evidence that the model is inappropriate. (p. 141)

At the same time, Bowlby (1980) saw IWMs as subject to change. He noted that

> there is certain information . . . that we find hard to process [such as] information that is incompatible with our existing [IWMs]. In general, when new information clashes with established models . . . an old model may be replaced by a new one. (pp. 230–231)

He noted that this change could be barely perceptible or appear as a major shift in IWM when major life events of attachment significance—for example, marriage, divorce, birth of a child—occur. Thus, Bowlby saw

IWMs as both resistant to change (assimilation view) but potentially subject to change under appropriate circumstances (accommodation view).

In this chapter, we review evidence of change and stability in adulthood, primarily concerning the transition to parenthood, an attachment-related time of significance in an individual's life. We also briefly raise new questions about stability and change that have not been addressed in this literature.

Major Life Events and Stability and Change in Romantic Adult Attachment Styles

First, relationship status is important in examining attachment security. Davila, Karney, and Bradbury (1999) examined Bowlby's accommodation notion, finding that marital satisfaction among newlyweds is associated with a change toward greater attachment security (using the Revised Adult Attachment Scale; Collins & Read, 1990). Scharfe and Cole (2006) observed that young adults graduating from college experienced greater stability in attachment if they stayed in the same romantic relationships (i.e., relationship status moderated attachment stability) (using the Relationship Scales Questionnaire; Bartholomew & Horowitz, 1991). On the other hand, Kirkpatrick and Hazan (1994) found that dissolution of a premarital romantic relationship could affect security (using Hazan & Shaver's [1987] three-category measure). In a 4-year study, they found that 90% of secure people who continued their relationships were secure 4 years later. Only 50% of initially secure people experiencing a relationship dissolution remained secure 4 years later.

Next, as expected, studies of the transition to parenthood, the period surrounding the birth of a couple's first child, illustrate that attachment style may change. Feeney, Alexander, Noller, and Holhaus (2003) used a matched-sample methodology to compare similar-age couples, allowing for comparisons between those couples going through the transition and those without children. Women undergoing the transition experienced less-stable attachment anxiety (as measured by the Attachment Style Questionnaire; Feeney, Noller, & Hanrahan, 1994) than other wives, as measured by comparing the second-trimester and 6-month-after-birth attachment styles (test–retest correlation = .54 vs. test–retest correlation = .72).

Simpson, Rholes, Campbell, and Wilson (2003) conducted a study that is one of the most direct tests of Bowlby's accommodation notion. The study hypothesized that information incongruent with an individual's avoidant and/or anxious attachment style (as measured by the Experiences in Close Relationships [ECR] scale; Brennan, Clark, & Shaver,

1998) would encourage change along a temporal continuum beginning at a prenatal testing session about 6 weeks before the birth of the couple's first child to 6 months after birth. It was first hypothesized that more anxious women who perceived higher levels of support and/or lower levels of anger from their husbands should become less anxious because the receipt of support and/or lower levels of anger would be inconsistent with wives' expectations based on their more anxious attachment style. The study also predicted that wives who sought support from their husbands would experience lower avoidance because of incongruence with their more avoidant IWMs. Finally, the authors hypothesized that giving support to a spouse would be incongruent with the avoidant IWM, thus leading husbands who provided more support to experience lower levels of avoidance. Evidence supported each of these hypotheses. Giving and seeking support led to declines in avoidance. Receiving support and encountering less anger from partners led to lower levels of anxiety.

More recently, Stern and colleagues (2018) investigated two kinds of attachment stability and change relevant to the transition to parenthood. They asked whether the average mother in their study became more or less secure during the transition (using the ECR to measure attachment style), finding no tendency of change in security levels on average. However, they found that some environmental variables were related to the amount and direction of change for some of the individuals across the transition. Depressive symptoms and levels of general psychological distress were moderating factors. Mothers exhibiting more depressive symptoms reported being more anxious and avoidant at Time 1 (with newborns) and became more anxious and avoidant over the 2-year course of the study. Mothers reporting more general psychological distress showed the same trend for anxiety, but not for avoidance. The authors also found tentative evidence that the level of social support provided to the mother by her own mother predicted decreases in levels of anxiety, but not depression. These findings are consistent with those of other studies that show that support and care by attachment figures can change attachment styles (Rholes, Eller, Simpson, & Arriaga, 2020; Simpson et al., 2003).

The most recent transition to parenthood work (Rholes et al., 2020) is a five-observation examination of change and stability in attachment IWMs. Married couples were observed five times, once about 6 weeks before the birth and then every 6 months until the infant was 24 months old. Three key variables were assessed for women and men: support seeking from their partner, receiving support from their partner, and giving support to their partner. Each of these behaviors was considered incongruent with the avoidant IWM. Attachment styles were measured using the ECR. Results showed that during any 6-month period in which husbands or wives reported receiving support from their partners, avoidance dropped at the next testing period. The same outcome was observed for support seeking and support giving. People who sought support from their partners or gave support to their partners also showed declines in avoidance over time. These latter two findings, particularly the one involving giving support to partners, demonstrate that individuals can be active agents in their movement from avoidance toward greater security.

Trait versus State Issues Addressed in the Literature

One question that remains for attachment researchers in social psychology is, given some evidence of change in attachment styles, how lasting is that change? Can an individual's IWM be permanently changed, or if not, how long can change last and under what conditions? Another way of framing the question would be to ask whether attachment style is a trait or a state.

The most influential work on the stability of self-reported romantic attachment styles has been conducted by Fraley and associates (Fraley, 2002; Fraley, Vicary, Brumbaugh, & Roisman, 2011). They examined test–retest correlations of within-individual attachment styles to determine whether a prototype or revisionist model provides a better representation of the stability versus change issue. The prototype model predicts that test–retest correlations should not approach zero over the long term (i.e., asymptotically). The revisionist model allows for the possibility of test–retest correlations approaching zero as the length of the test–retest interval increases. Empirical work suggests that the prototype model is a better representation of the data (Fraley et al., 2011). For example, people who are more avoidant, particularly with regard to their earlier attachment figures, tend to remain that way over time. Romantic partner attachment stability is lower than parental attachment, but still supports the prototype model. Overall, the prototype model suggests an underlying, stable factor for attachment style, even if it is relatively latent at some points in time (e.g., Roisman, Collins, Sroufe, & Egeland, 2005). In general, Fraley's trait versus state consideration is consistent with the idea that attachment style is both a trait and a state—for example, anxiety consists of a stable trait, an autoregressive trait that can slowly change over time, and a state reflecting change at each time of measurement (e.g., Fraley et al., 2011).

To date, stability and change have been examined on average (across study participants) and as test–retest correlations (within-participants in the study). As indicated by the studies, change is seen within participants, but not necessarily on average across participants (e.g., Simpson et al., 2003). This raises the question of whether there might be other ways of examining stability and change. For example, could probabilistic/stochastic modeling lend insights about stability and change?

New Considerations for Assessing Change and Stability

Stochastic processes could allow for within-person changes in attachment style to be examined at various points in time. To do this, the probabilistic notion of a "state" would be used to correspond to the attachment style notion of "relatively high" in avoidance or anxiety or "relatively low" in avoidance or anxiety. Stochastic modeling allows for consideration of questions that have not yet been addressed:

1. *Does an individual's current probabilistic "state" (i.e., existing attachment style) depend* only *on their preceding attachment style?* This is important, for example, because a person who has been relatively avoidant for a period of time, but then appears relatively secure, may have a different probability of shifting to a more anxious state than someone whose current more anxious state depends *only* on the fact that most recently, they appeared to be relatively secure. The existence of a "probabilistic memory" of shifts in attachment styles is important in answering this question.

2. *Is it possible for individuals to move with equal probability from one attachment state to another?* For example, are there circumstances in which a person who is relatively secure could just as easily become more avoidant as they could become more anxious? Alternatively, is that highly improbable, and under what circumstances?

3. *Is it likely that individuals cannot move from some attachment styles to others?* For example, can someone become highly avoidant if most recently they have been highly anxious? Or do they first need to become less avoidant (i.e., more secure) before high anxiety is a possibility?

4. *Once a probabilistic state is left, can it ever be entered again?* This consideration would be important, for example, when considering the efficacy of psychotherapy for attachment-related disorders or issues. The goal of psychotherapy would be to produce a lasting, more secure attachment style. Thus, a more avoidant or more anxious probabilistic state would, it would be hoped, not be entered again.

5. *Are some probabilistic states "absorbing" or "relatively absorbing"?* A probabilistic state is often referred to as absorbing if, once reached, it cannot ever be left. One application of this question would allow for consideration of those who have experienced major life events—such as a traumatic loss or a transition to parenthood—and have become more insecure as a result. Is it possible that, for at least some of those people, they will remain in their more insecure state forever? For example, will some parents never recover, in an attachment sense, from the death of a child?

Conclusion

In this chapter, we have presented both existing theory and evidence about stability and change of adult romantic attachment styles as well as consideration of questions that future research might try to address. We began with Bowlby's perspective, which made clear that attachment styles and their associated IWMs are resistant to change but, under some circumstances, should be capable of change. We next presented evidence of change, at least over relatively short periods of time (slightly over 2 years). The empirical evidence clearly demonstrated, particularly for the transition to parenthood, that individual attachment styles could become more secure, sometimes even through their own efforts. Then we briefly reviewed the existing literature indicating that a prototype model appears to underlie attachment style, which would suggest that although attachment style is likely a trait–state combination, a trait-like prototype makes attachment style resistant to change in the long run. Finally, we suggested an alternative way of looking at stability and change within individuals, using stochastic modeling. This approach would allow for consideration of questions that have not yet been answered in the attachment theory literature regarding stability and change, suggesting that it may have some advantages—or at least suggest alternatives—to the existing methodology for assessing stability and change.

REFERENCES

Bartholomew, K., & Horowitz, L. M. (1991). Attachment styles among young adults: A test of a four-category model. *Journal of Personality and Social Psychology, 61,* 226–244.

Bowlby, J. (1979). *The making and breaking of affectional bonds.* London: Routledge.

Bowlby, J. (1980). *Attachment and loss: Vol. 3. Loss, sadness and depression.* New York: Basic Books.

Brennan, K. A., Clark, C. L., & Shaver, P. R. (1998). Self-report measurement of adult romantic attachment: An integrative overview. In J. A. Simpson & W. S. Rholes (Eds.), *Attachment theory and close relationships* (pp. 44–76). New York: Guilford Press.

Collins, N. L., & Read, S. J. (1990). Adult attachment, working models, and relationship quality in dating couples. *Journal of Personality and Social Psychology, 58,* 644–663.

Davila, J., Karney, B. R., & Bradbury, T. N. (1999). Attachment change processes in the early years of marriage. *Journal of Personality and Social Psychology, 76,* 783–802.

Feeney, J., Alexander, R., Noller, P., & Holhaus, L. (2003). Attachment insecurity, depression, and the transition to parenthood. *Personal Relationships, 10,* 475–493.

Feeney, J. A., Noller, P., & Hanrahan, M. (1994). Assessing adult attachment. In M. B. Sperling & W. H. Berman (Eds.), *Attachment in adults: Clinical and developmental perspectives* (pp. 128–152). New York: Guilford Press.

Fraley, R. C. (2002). Attachment stability from infancy to adulthood: Meta-analysis and dynamic modeling of developmental mechanisms. *Personality and Social Psychology Review, 6,* 123–151.

Fraley, R. C., Vicary, A. M., Brumbaugh, C. C., & Roisman, G. I. (2011). Patterns of stability in adult attachment: An empirical test of two models of continuity and change. *Journal of Personality and Social Psychology, 101,* 974–992.

Hazan, C., & Shaver, P. R. (1987). Romantic love conceptualized as an attachment process. *Journal of Personality and Social Psychology, 52,* 511–524.

Kirkpatrick, L. A., & Hazan, C. (1994). Attachment styles and close relationships: A four-year prospective study. *Personal Relationships, 1,* 123–142.

Rholes, W. S., Eller, J., Simpson, J. A., & Arriaga, X. B. (2020). Support processes predict declines in attachment avoidance across the transition to parenthood. *Personality and Social Psychology Bulletin.* [Epub ahead of print]

Roisman, G. I., Collins, W. A., Sroufe, L. A., & Egeland, B. (2005). Predictors of young adults' representations of and behavior in their current romantic relationship: Prospective tests of the prototype hypothesis. *Attachment and Human Development, 7,* 105–121.

Scharfe, E., & Cole, V. (2006). Stability and change attachment representations during emerging adulthood: An examination of mediators and moderators of change. *Personal Relationships, 13,* 363–374.

Simpson, J. A., Rholes, W. S., Campbell, L., & Wilson, C. L. (2003). Changes in attachment orientations across the transition to parenthood. *Journal of Experimental Social Psychology, 39,* 317–331.

Stern, J. A., Fraley, R. C., Jones, J. D., Gross, J. T., Shaver, P. R., & Cassidy, J. (2018). Developmental processes across the first two years of parenthood: Stability and change in adult attachment style. *Developmental Psychology, 54,* 975–988.

CHAPTER 22

Change in Adult Attachment Insecurity from an Interdependence Theory Perspective

Ximena B. Arriaga
Madoka Kumashiro

Relationship partners who promote attachment security mutually influence each other (interdependence), generally maintain proximity, reciprocate caring and responsive behaviors, and thus rely on each other as a secure base from which to pursue goals and confront challenges (Feeney, 2004). Attachment patterns (in children) and orientations (in adults) develop as individuals encode key interactions into mental representations (internal working models). These mental models reflect self-worth (model of self) and beliefs about depending on others (models of others); they encapsulate expectations, salient memories, and easily accessed beliefs, and they guide automated emotional reactions and habitual behavioral responses (Collins & Feeney, 2004). Internal working models also provide the ingredients of attachment tendencies, including (1) comfort with closeness and resilience when confronting challenges (attachment security); (2) anxiety and concerns about being loved and valued, and uncertainty over one's ability to navigate challenges (attachment anxiety); and/or (3) avoidance of emotional intimacy that protects oneself from being hurt by others but also causes chronic, problematic self-reliance (attachment avoidance).

Adult attachment orientations change when new experiences challenge or revise existing working models, which may lead individuals to reassess their self-worth and reevaluate whether they can count on others. Interdependence theory, with its emphasis on the role of interactions in shaping relationship quality, personal motives, and personality traits (Kelley, 1983), offers insights into the interplay of partners during attachment-relevant experiences. The current chapter integrates interdependence and attachment perspectives to suggest interactions that may revise working models and change attachment orientations. We specifically focus on interdependent experiences that bring about greater security across time (see Mikulincer & Shaver, 2016, regarding the dynamics of insecurity).

Adult attachment orientations are not immutable; they change across time (Arriaga, Kumashiro, Finkel, VanderDrift, & Luchies, 2014) and vary across interaction partners (e.g., with romantic partners, relatives, friends; Fraley, Heffernan, Vicary, & Brumbaugh, 2011). Little is known if such natural changes occur intentionally or beyond awareness, but theory suggests that attachment tendencies, like other human tendencies, develop as "solutions" to a person's specific social circumstances (Kelley, 1983). Experiences with trusting a partner who is untrustworthy, depending on a friend who is unreliable, and seeking comfort from a neglectful family member, all suggest caution and self-protection (Murray & Holmes, 2009), either through increased vigilance of the person's dependability (anxiety) or by reducing dependence (avoidance). Thus, anxious and avoidant strategies reflect adaptations to repeated interactions with close others who have failed to foster a sense of security (Mikulincer & Shaver, 2016). Such adaptations can become self-fulfilling; even individuals who desire change may feel unable to break out of established patterns. It thus becomes important to understand the specific conditions and processes that bring about greater security.

How Do Adult Attachment Orientations Change?

What is the process through which individuals may feel, and eventually become, more secure? We briefly review research demonstrating change toward greater attachment security in romantic relationships,[1] and then present a theoretical model of enhancing security.

Can Romantic Partners Buffer Insecurity?

Romantic partners can function as allies in fostering a person's security. Partners mutually influence each other across time and interactions, and they provide a dynamic source of new beliefs and feelings that can be absorbed into working models.

A growing literature reveals that partners can mitigate the potentially damaging effects of attachment insecurity on relationships, and can

---

[1]Priming of attachment security induces short-term felt-security (e.g., Carnelley & Rowe, 2007), but it is unclear if this can be sustained over time.

avert interactions that reinforce insecurities (Simpson & Overall, 2014). Chronically attachment-anxious individuals exhibit less insecurity when their partner: provides affectionate touch during moments of jealousy (Jakubiak & Feeney, 2016); withholds criticism (Lemay & Dudley, 2011); or makes up for hurtful behavior by conveying guilt and strong commitment (Overall, Girme, Lemay & Hammond, 2014). Avoidant reactions to issues that trigger avoidance (e.g., being asked to change, feeling pressured to fulfill a request) are attenuated when partners acknowledge the magnitude of their requests and express confidence in the avoidant individual's ability to honor the request (Overall, Simpson, & Struthers, 2013).

Can Romantic Partners Enhance Security?

Individuals might encounter security-enhancing experiences on their own. However, these moments are more likely with an ally who warrants trust, and who is willing and able to provide novel ways of viewing oneself and others. Clinicians trained in emotion-focused therapy effectively address and revise deeply entrenched insecure patterns (Johnson, 2019). Not everyone, however, feels the need for psychotherapy or can afford it.

Change is challenging; internal working models can guide people into self-fulfilling relationships where they encounter situations that they have come to expect and that reinforce their insecurities (Fraley & Roisman, 2019). For example, an anxious person may be more likely than a relatively secure person to become suspicious and mistrustful when a partner arrives late from work; any accusations of infidelity will trigger conflict and distress in the partner and/or relationship.[2] Avoidant individuals who have a secure partner may avoid emotional intimacy; the partner is left yearning for more connection and becomes distressed. Even when a person has a security-enhancing partner and is motivated to change, adopting new responses takes time, patience, and a willingness to go outside of one's comfort zone.

The attachment security enhancement model (ASEM; Arriaga, Kumashiro, Simpson, & Overall, 2018) suggests specific pathways in nonclinical settings through which relationship partners can become security allies. According to the ASEM, greater security is likely to occur when partners utilize effective communication and interaction strategies that (1) mitigate immediate tension and destructive responses when attachment-related concerns arise; and (2) encourage long-term revisions to working models. The ASEM further suggests distinct partner responses and pathways to change chronic attachment anxiety versus avoidance.

---

[2]Anxiety would be a reasonable and adaptive response if the partner actually is unfaithful, as suggested above.

Changing Attachment Avoidance

For avoidant individuals who hold negative internal models of others (including romantic partners), the pathway to greater security is likely to involve new experiences with partners who instill trust (Arriaga et al., 2014). This can begin to occur when partners mitigate the negative impact of tense interactions by enacting "soft" strategies (e.g., acknowledging the desire for avoidance, but making requests with a reasonable tone of voice; see Arriaga et al., 2018; Overall et al., 2013). For example, in one study, avoidant individuals remained committed months later if their partner acknowledged and validated the avoidant individual's efforts to make a sacrifice (Farrell, Simpson, Overall, & Shallcross, 2016).

In addition to mitigating the negative effects of tense moments (e.g., efforts to resist partner influence), partners can pivot to situations that encourage positive beliefs, feelings, and expectations regarding the give-and-take of interdependent relationships. Simply engaging in fun and intimate activities (e.g., self-disclosure, touch) can cause declines in avoidance one month later (Stanton, Campbell, & Pink, 2017). However, more lasting change may require reducing dread and aversion regarding needing or providing support, and revising suppressed fear that harkens back to painful past experiences of depending on others (e.g., being neglected or shut out).

Relationships can also provide opportunities to revise beliefs about dependence. For example, in a sample of new parents, fathers who were attachment-avoidant, and probably wary of caregiving, exhibited greater security 1 year later if they found themselves in the role of providing effective support to their wives (Simpson, Rholes, Campbell, & Wilson, 2003). Avoidant reactions may soften when individuals form new positive mental associations with providing care; these new beliefs may chip away at the broader belief that dependence is aversive or painful. Figure 22.1 illustrates how this process might unfold, and the specific influence that partners can provide.

Changing Attachment Anxiety

Anxiously attached individuals tend to have a negative self-model that keeps them yearning for approval. Thus, the pathway for greater security is likely to involve new experiences that foster confidence and pride in one's personal qualities and abilities. Chronically anxious individuals tend to be preoccupied with their relationships. They may not attend to their own abilities and goals because they must first feel secure in their relationships. This can begin to occur when partners soothe an anxious person's worries and concerns by enacting "safe" strategies (e.g., providing

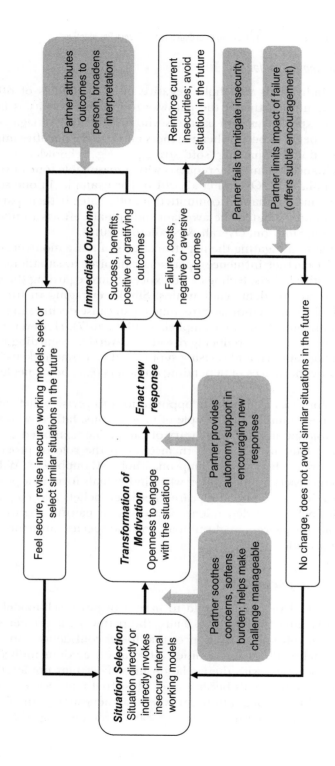

FIGURE 22.1. Partners as allies in interdependent interactions that enhance attachment security.

reassurance, conveying commitment, diffusing negative emotion through calming behavior; see Arriaga et al., 2018).

In addition to mitigating anxious thoughts and feelings, partners can encourage activities to bolster an anxious person's self-worth and self-efficacy. For example, in a sample of committed couples, anxiously attached individuals exhibited greater security one year later if they felt that their personal goals were supported and validated by their partner (Arriaga et al., 2014). Anxiously attached individuals also may feel more secure when they succeed in a personal task and their partners provide positive and honest feedback that amplifies the success; an immediate success can be interpreted in terms of its broader meaning about the anxiously-attached person's personal strengths and competence (cf. Marigold, Holmes, & Ross, 2007). Finally, if/when failure occurs, partners can provide a secure base by relying on safe strategies that limit reading too much into setbacks (see Figure 22.1).

Summary

The ASEM suggests different pathways to security. Attachment avoidance may be reduced when individuals' relationship contributions become worthy and valued by their partner, which fosters the belief that giving and receiving care in relationships need not be aversive. Attachment anxiety may be reduced as individuals encounter opportunities to gain self-confidence, which reduces the need to rely on or be preoccupied with one's relationship.[3]

Key Questions for Future Research

The dyadic journey to attachment security can be similar to a weekend-leisure drive: Some rides are smooth and others bumpy, and conditions may be optimal or treacherous; drivers may disclose the route and destination or make them a surprise; the destinations could be mundane, memorable, exhilarating, or disappointing; and looking back, some aspects of the ride, which at the time did not seem important, can become meaningful. Similarly, some security-fostering interactions are smooth, others stressful; the immediate (given) situation may be enjoyable or aversive; a partner may fully disclose ways they are trying to make the other more secure, while others may subtly encourage changes to resist

---

[3]This does not necessarily mean that a person becomes "as secure" as chronically secure individuals are, nor that one categorically changes one's essence to be "secure." The changes described above are *within individuals relative to their own selves,* rather than relative to others.

suspicion, skepticism, or resistance; a key interaction may immediately seem important or memorable, or it may become meaningful only upon further reflection and interpretation.

What factors contribute to a smoother and more rewarding security ride? Rather than prescribing specific behavior, the ASEM suggests processes that unfold in a variety of ways (e.g., there are multiple ways to improve confidence in one's personal or relational abilities and worth). Individuals may become more secure when ASEM (or other) processes emerge organically to meet the needs of each partner.

Although we know more now than 10 years ago about how attachment tendencies might change, there are many unanswered questions to be addressed in future research. For example, should efforts to help a person become more secure be within or beyond the person's awareness? Even among insecure individuals who are motivated to change, will they resist a partner's security-enhancing strategies? Should partners disclose that they are encouraging new responses, while also allowing interaction behavior to unfold naturally and organically? Can internal working models change following one interaction, or is it necessary to have repeated interactions that overwrite insecure tendencies? Even when an insecure person seems to have become more secure, do certain conditions (e.g., stressors) facilitate new security versus potentiate "regression" to more insecure working models? From a developmental perspective, can these relational processes be influential even among children, or do they require a more mature relational context? Finally, does there need to be a major experience that acts as a catalyst for change (e.g., a stressful experience, or "hitting rock bottom"), or can change occur gradually without any significant or turbulent events?

Conclusion

For deep-seated working models to change, individuals need to be confronted with experiences that foster a new appreciation of oneself, with respect to personal or relational abilities. If these experiences trigger insecurities, a trustworthy partner can be an ally to buffer insecurities and amplify positive outcomes. New experiences that contradict negative beliefs and assumptions, encourage new beliefs and assumptions, and lead to revisions of insecure working models, all may generate more lasting changes if they involve overcoming challenges. After all, some of the more memorable rides that have the potential to change a person are also those that seem precarious at the time; having a driving partner help navigate the "security ride" may be essential to arrive at a more secure destination.

ACKNOWLEDGMENTS

The writing of this chapter was supported by funding to both authors from the National Science Foundation (SBE/BCS No. 1531226) and the Economic and Social Research Council (No. ES/N013182/1).

REFERENCES

Arriaga, X. B. (2013). An interdependence theory analysis of close relationships. In J. A. Simpson & L. Campbell (Eds.), *The Oxford handbook of close relationships* (pp. 39–65). Oxford, UK: Oxford University Press.

Arriaga, X. B., Kumashiro, M., Finkel, E. J., VanderDrift, L. E., & Luchies, L. B. (2014). Filling the void: Bolstering attachment security in committed relationships. *Social Psychological and Personality Science, 5,* 398–405.

Arriaga, X. B., Kumashiro, M., Simpson, J. A., & Overall, N. C. (2018). Revising working models across time: Relationship situations that enhance attachment security. *Personality and Social Psychology Bulletin, 22,* 71–96.

Carnelley, K. B., & Rowe, A. C. (2007). Repeated priming of attachment security influences later views of self and relationships. *Personal Relationships, 14,* 307–320.

Collins, N. L., & Feeney, B. C. (2004). Working models of attachment shape perceptions of social support: Evidence from experimental and observational studies. *Journal of Personality and Social Psychology, 87*(3), 363–383.

Farrell, A. K., Simpson, J. A., Overall, N. C., & Shallcross, S. L. (2016). Buffering the responses of avoidantly attached romantic partners in strain test situations. *Journal of Family Psychology, 30,* 580–591.

Feeney, B. C. (2004). A secure base: Responsive support of goal strivings and exploration in adult intimate relationships. *Journal of Personality and Social Psychology, 87,* 631–648.

Fraley, R. C., Heffernan, M. E., Vicary, A. M., & Brumbaugh, C. C. (2011). The Experiences in Close Relationships-Relationship Structures questionnaire: A method for assessing attachment orientations across relationships. *Psychological Assessment, 23,* 615–625.

Fraley, R. C., & Roisman, G. I. (2019). The development of adult attachment styles: Four lessons. *Current Opinion in Psychology, 25,* 26–30.

Jakubiak, B. K., & Feeney, B. C. (2016). A sense of security: Touch promotes state attachment security. *Social Psychological and Personality Science, 7,* 745–753.

Johnson, S. (2019). Attachment in action—changing the face of 21st century couple therapy. *Current Opinion in Psychology, 25,* 101–104.

Kelley, H. H. (1983). The situational origins of human tendencies: A further reason for the formal analysis of structure. *Personality and Social Psychology Bulletin, 9,* 8–30.

Lemay, E. P., Jr., & Dudley, K. L. (2011). Caution: Fragile! Regulating the interpersonal security of chronically insecure partners. *Journal of Personality and Social Psychology, 100,* 681–702.

Marigold, D. C., Holmes, J. G., & Ross, M. (2007). More than words: Reframing compliments from romantic partners fosters security in low self-esteem individuals. *Journal of Personality and Social Psychology, 92,* 232–248.

Mikulincer, M., & Shaver, P. R. (2016). *Attachment in adulthood: Structure, dynamics, and change* (2nd ed.). New York: Guilford Press.

Murray, S. L., & Holmes, J. G. (2009). The architecture of interdependent minds: A motivation-management theory of mutual responsiveness. *Psychological Review, 116,* 908–928.

Overall, N. C., Girme, Y. U., Lemay, E. P., Jr., & Hammond, M. T. (2014). Attachment anxiety and reactions to relationship threat: The benefits and costs of inducing guilt in romantic partners. *Journal of Personality and Social Psychology, 106,* 235–256.

Overall, N. C., Simpson, J. A., & Struthers, H. (2013). Buffering attachment-related avoidance: Softening emotional and behavioral defenses during conflict discussions. *Journal of Personality and Social Psychology, 104,* 854–871.

Simpson, J. A., & Overall, N. C. (2014). Partner buffering of attachment insecurity. *Current Directions in Psychological Science, 23,* 54–59.

Simpson, J. A., Rholes, W. S., Campbell, L., & Wilson, C. L. (2003). Changes in attachment orientations across the transition to parenthood. *Journal of Experimental Social Psychology, 39,* 317–331.

Stanton, S. C., Campbell, L., & Pink, J. C. (2017). Benefits of positive relationship experiences for avoidantly attached individuals. *Journal of Personality and Social Psychology, 113,* 568.

THE CONTINUING INFLUENCE OF EARLY ATTACHMENT

- What domains of later behavior should early attachment relationships predict, and why?

- For what domains should we not expect an association with early security?

- What are, in other words, the boundary conditions for the influence of early attachment?

CHAPTER 23

The Legacy of Early Attachments
Past, Present, Future

Glenn I. Roisman
Ashley M. Groh

Research on the legacy of early attachments might profitably be construed in terms of three relatively distinct, even if partially overlapping, phases of scholarly inquiry. The first phase was initiated by two watershed moments in attachment research in the 1960s and 1970s: First and most crucially, Mary Ainsworth's development of the Strange Situation Procedure (SSP; Ainsworth, Blehar, Waters, & Wall, 1978); and second, the subsequent launching of a prospective, longitudinal investigation focused on the sequelae of early attachments built on that innovative methodological foundation, the Minnesota Longitudinal Study of Risk and Adaptation (MLSRA; Sroufe, Egeland, Carlson, & Collins, 2005).

A second phase, which has been ongoing for the last two decades, has been marked by both meta-analytic review of the now multitudinous smaller sample longitudinal studies focused on the consequences of early attachments (Groh, Fearon, Van IJzendoorn, Bakermans-Kranenburg, & Roisman, 2017) and the emergence of more adequately powered investigations of individual differences in early attachment, including the NICHD Study of Early Child Care and Youth Development (SECCYD; NICHD Early Child Care Research Network, 2005). In this second phase, scientific efforts to probe seminal insights about the consequences of early attachments were scaled up and, in some instances, early orthodoxies were challenged (Fraley & Spieker, 2003; Groh, Roisman, et al., 2014; Groh et al., 2017).

The third and most recent phase is one where we perceive that a tension has begun to mount. On the one hand, a major effort is clearly well under way to disseminate key insights from initial studies of the legacy of early attachments in a variety of clinical, legal, and other high-stakes settings. Such important efforts necessarily assume that the early empirical discoveries and key methodological innovations in this area are sturdy enough to support such translational efforts. On the other hand, some scholars, including ourselves, have encouraged a reevaluation of both key methods and conclusions from the initial wave of research in this area in light of the findings from larger sample investigations, along with meta-analytic reviews. We discuss these three phases of attachment research and their implications for the future of attachment scholarship and translation in greater depth below.

A Program of Research Is Launched

The introduction of Ainsworth's SSP was a seminal moment in the history of developmental science. By demonstrating how it might be possible to distill an infant's expectations about the availability and responsiveness of the primary caregiver into just a few minutes of expertly coded separation and reunion behaviors, Ainsworth's painstaking observational work represented a clarion call for research examining to what extent differences in infant attachment quality were reflected in aspects of (mal)adaptation over development.

At the forefront of those early efforts was the MLSRA, an ongoing, landmark investigation of 267 mothers and their firstborn children. Byron Egeland, along with Amos Deinard (a pediatrician), began this prospective, longitudinal study to interrogate the intergenerational transmission of maltreatment in a sample of children born into poverty. Alan Sroufe soon partnered with Egeland and, together with crucial early input from their students (notably Brian Vaughn and Everett Waters—one of Ainsworth's undergraduates), the MLSRA early on expanded its focus to include the study of infant attachment. In so doing, both the high-risk Minnesota cohort, along with a lower-risk sample studied by Sroufe and his students (e.g., Matas, Arend, & Sroufe, 1978), helped generate some of the first and ultimately most influential evidence regarding the role of early attachments in shaping adaptation to the salient developmental tasks of childhood, adolescence, and beyond.

A complete cataloguing of the findings of the MLSRA regarding the sequelae of early attachments is beyond the scope of a brief essay (Sroufe et al., 2005). Nonetheless, this work might be understood as having helped the field reach three broad, interim conclusions. First, the findings of the MLSRA suggested that early attachments—though not deterministic in their role in shaping development—nonetheless are meaningfully associated with variation in socially skilled behavior outside the home and serve an important role in the development of externalizing and internalizing psychopathology. Second, Sroufe, Egeland, and Kreutzer (1990) persuasively argued that the legacy of early attachments is likely to endure over the life course in part because representations of early attachment experiences cannot be fully erased by subsequent experiences. Third, Sroufe viewed the MLSRA as providing

> some evidence for the distinctive correlates of the avoidant and resistant groups [in that] those in the resistant group [are] disadvantaged in situations involving novelty, high physical stimulation, and social complexity [whereas] . . . those in the avoidant group are particularly disadvantaged with regard to social intimacy and trust. They are self-isolated and/or exhibit hostile aggression in preschool . . . and later show conduct problems. (2003, p. 214)

Meta-Analytic Synthesis

The groundbreaking findings from the MLSRA in turn launched a wave of research on the legacy of children's early attachments for socioemotional development. Although many of these efforts produced findings consistent with the Minnesota studies, narrative reviewers found it difficult to draw firm conclusions about the developmental significance of early attachment from subsequent studies given the sheer number of publications, range of correlates examined, and diversity of samples investigated. Together with our colleagues, we therefore leveraged meta-analysis as a structured tool for addressing key questions concerning the predictive significance of early attachments. Guided by central conclusions of the MLSRA along with claims that a third form of insecurity—disorganization—was broadly disruptive of children's psychological development, we sought to (1) more precisely quantify to what extent early attachment (in)security is associated with (mal)adaptation within the domains of children's social competence with peers, externalizing behavior problems, and internalizing symptomatology; (2) examine whether these associations were enduring in the sense that the magnitude of meta-analytic effects did not wane as the age at which outcomes were assessed increased; and (3) investigate whether specific patterns of attachment insecurity and disorganization serve as distinctive diatheses for maladjustment within each developmental domain (Groh et al., 2017).

Overall, findings from our meta-analyses—comprising the most comprehensive set of quantitative reviews of this literature conducted to date—indicated that early attachment security is associated with greater social competence with peers ($r = .19$; Groh, Fearon, et al., 2014), fewer behavior problems ($r = -.15$; Fearon, Bakermans-Kranenburg, van

IJzendoorn, Lapsley, & Roisman, 2010), and fewer internalizing symptoms ($r = -.07$; Groh et al., 2012). Importantly, however, a formal comparison of the magnitude of these associations revealed that early attachment security was more strongly correlated with children's social competence with peers and fewer aggressive behavioral problems than with lower levels of internalizing symptoms. Moreover, in light of Cohen's (1988) criteria, associations between early security and peer competence/externalizing behavior would be characterized as modest in magnitude in the absolute sense, whereas the association between early attachment and internalizing symptoms was quite small, falling below the threshold for defining a weak effect (i.e., $r = .10$).

Findings from the meta-analyses also provided no evidence that the age at which socioemotional outcomes were assessed across studies reliably moderated study effect sizes. Thus, consistent with a central claim supported by the early studies of infant attachment, including the Minnesota work, these findings suggested that (even if modest) the significance of early security for children's socioemotional adjustment does not wane from infancy to early adolescence.

Finally, our program of meta-analytic research examined the shared and distinctive significance of specific patterns of insecurity and disorganization. Providing evidence consistent with expectations that all patterns of insecurity undermine children's social competence, early avoidant, resistant, and disorganized attachments were comparably associated with (modestly) lower levels of peer competence (avoidant: $r = -.09$; resistant: $r = -.14$; disorganized: $r = -.12$; Groh, Fearon, et al., 2014). However, findings provided mixed support for the expected differential significance of specific patterns of attachment insecurity and disorganization for externalizing and internalizing symptomatology (Fearon et al., 2010; Groh, Roisman, van IJzendoorn, Bakermans-Kranenburg, & Fearon, 2012). Specifically, early avoidant attachment was significantly, albeit weakly, associated with externalizing ($r = .06$) *and* internalizing ($r = .09$) symptomatology, whereas early resistant attachment was not associated with children's adjustment within either outcome domain. Indeed, perhaps the most striking result from these meta-analyses was that the association between resistant attachment and internalizing symptomatology was essentially nil ($r = .02$). Findings were also mixed concerning the role of disorganization in childhood emotional and behavior problems. Specifically, early disorganization was found to place children at greatest risk for externalizing problems (relative to other insecure categories; $r = .17$) but was not significantly associated with internalizing distress ($r = .04$).

Limitations of our meta-analytic program of research include that it relied on the aggregation of mostly underpowered studies and was not informed by recent methodological advances (e.g., individual participant data synthesis) that allow more complex models to be considered. For example, (1) it is not known to what extent the modest associations we observed between infant attachment and subsequent aspects of developmental (mal)adaptation might be accounted for by demographic and other confounders and (2) the meta-analytic tests of whether associations were consistent with an Enduring Effects model (i.e., Fraley, Roisman, & Haltigan, 2013) were fairly low-resolution, between-study analyses that did not track the predictive significance of early attachments for each outcome domain within the same set of individuals over time.

As a separate matter, the absence of large sample studies in this area through the 1980s meant both that (1) basic psychometric work on the latent structure of individual differences as assessed by the SSP lagged for decades and (2) precise estimates of how strongly infant attachment as measured by the SSP is associated with different aspects of socioemotional development were unavailable. As discussed below, improvements on both fronts nonetheless followed.

The Modern Era: Generativity versus Stagnation

Beginning in the early 1990s, the emergence of a handful of larger sample studies of infant attachment, including the SECCYD, allowed attachment researchers to formally test basic assumptions about the measurement of early attachments using the SSP, including that (1) avoidant and resistant attachments are mutually exclusive attachment patterns, (2) disorganization and resistance represent distinct constructs, and (3) the individual differences studied by generations of researchers are, in fact, categorically distributed. Importantly, the handful of studies that now speak directly to these issues have thrown into doubt each of these claims. Indeed, such studies have shown that (1) avoidance and resistance tend to be weakly correlated (and thus not mutually exclusive), (2) indicators of disorganization and resistance load on a common latent factor, and (3) individual differences in infant attachment behaviors are more consistent with a continuous rather than categorical model (Fraley & Spieker 2003; Groh et al., 2019). It is too early to know whether the wider adoption of existing dimensional approaches would, on its own, serve to improve the predictive validity of the SSP (Raby, Fraley, & Roisman, Chapter 9, this volume). However, it is certainly possible that subtle misrepresentations of the latent structure of the SSP have made it more difficult to study the distinctive correlates of avoidance, resistance, and disorganization. For example, analyses of categorical infant attachment data rely on a measurement model that assumes that infants with avoidant relationships cannot also (simultaneously) share resistant relationships with their caregivers, thereby decreasing variation in resistance in particular, which is especially problematic given the low base rate of resistant attachments.

More importantly, larger sample studies like the SECCYD allowed a new generation of attachment scholars to estimate with far greater precision how strongly early attachments (as measured by the traditional coding system for the SSP) are associated with social and emotional development over time. These efforts have increasingly highlighted that the weak to modest associations between infant attachment and aspects of subsequent (mal)adaptation we reported meta-analytically are consistent with the returns from parallel analyses based on adequately powered studies (e.g., Haltigan & Roisman, 2015; McCartney, Owen, Booth, Clarke-Stewart, & Vandell, 2004). This consistency in results, combined with evidence that (1) the SSP has weak predictive significance for adult attachment states of mind ($r = .10–.15$; Groh, Roisman, et al., 2014), yet (2) these same assessments of adult attachment are notably more strongly associated with the observed quality of caregiving experienced in childhood ($r = ~.30$; Haydon, Roisman, Owen, Booth-LaForce, & Cox, 2014) should prompt attachment scholars to question whether innovations in the assessment of early attachments may now be necessary, particularly given that most attachment-based interventions and even some recent child custody recommendations rest on arguably outdated assumptions about the strengths and limitations of the SSP (Granqvist et al., 2017; Roisman & Cicchetti, 2017).

The question that now confronts the field is whether attachment researchers are, in fact, willing to revisit these fundamental methodological issues. On the one hand, it is possible that research on the legacy of early attachments has entered what van IJzendoorn and Tavecchio (1987) described decades ago (building on the concepts of the philosopher of science Imre Lakatos) as a period of *exhaustion,* in which theoretical and methodological rigidity are dominant features, and correspondingly as the field turns away from basic science toward translation—an obviously worthy goal. On the other hand, such a reappraisal might serve as a generative (and generational) reckoning regarding the degree to which acceptance of limited refinements in the measurement of early attachments over the past few decades along with a continued reliance on evidence drawn from underpowered studies (1) has slowed our basic scientific understanding of the legacy of early attachments and/or (2) might be hampering efforts to optimally translate what we know about the consequences of early attachments in support of children and families (Granqvist et al., 2017).

REFERENCES

Ainsworth, M. D. S., Blehar, M. C., Waters, E., & Wall, S. (1978). *Patterns of attachment: A psychological study of the Strange Situation.* Hillsdale, NJ: Erlbaum.

Cohen, J. (1988). *Statistical power analysis for the behavioral sciences* (2nd ed.). Hillsdale, NJ: Erlbaum.

Fearon, R. P., Bakermans-Kranenburg, M. J., van IJzendoorn, M. H., Lapsley, A., & Roisman, G. I. (2010). The significance of insecure attachment and disorganization in the development of children's externalizing behavior: A meta-analytic study. *Child Development, 81,* 435–456.

Fraley, R. C., Roisman, G. I., & Haltigan, J. D. (2013). The legacy of early experiences in development: Formalizing alternative models of how early experiences are carried forward over time. *Developmental Psychology, 49,* 109–126.

Fraley, R. C., & Spieker, S. J. (2003). Are infant attachment patterns continuously or categorically distributed?: A taxometric analysis of Strange Situation behavior. *Developmental Psychology, 39,* 387–404.

Granqvist, P., Sroufe, L. A., Dozier, M., Hesse, E., Steele, M., van IJzendoorn, M., . . . Duschinsky, R. (2017). Disorganized attachment in infancy: A review of the phenomenon and its implications for clinicians and policy-makers. *Attachment and Human Development, 19,* 534–558.

Groh, A. M., Fearon, R. P., Bakermans-Kranenburg, M. J., van IJzendoorn, M. H., Steele, R. D., & Roisman, G. I. (2014). The significance of attachment security for children's social competence with peers: A meta-analytic study. *Attachment and Human Development, 16,* 103–136.

Groh, A. M., Fearon, R. M. P., van IJzendoorn, M. H., Bakermans-Kranenburg, M. J., & Roisman, G. I. (2017). Attachment in the early life course: Meta-analytic evidence for its role in socio-emotional development. *Child Development Perspectives, 11,* 70–76.

Groh, A. M., Propper, C., Mills-Koonce, R., Moore, G., Calkins, S., & Cox, M. (2019). Mothers' physiological and affective responding to infant distress: Unique antecedents of avoidant and resistant attachments. *Child Development, 90,* 489–505.

Groh, A. M., Roisman, G. I., Booth-LaForce, C., Fraley, R. C., Owen, M. T., Cox, M. J., & Burchinal, M. R. (2014). Stability of attachment security from infancy to late adolescence. In C. Booth-LaForce & G. I. Roisman (Eds.), The Adult Attachment Interview: Psychometrics, stability and change from infancy, and developmental origins. *Monographs of the Society for Research in Child Development, 79*(3), 51–66.

Groh, A. M., Roisman, G. I., van IJzendoorn, M. H., Bakermans-Kranenburg, M. J., & Fearon, R. (2012). The significance of insecure and disorganized attachment for children's internalizing symptoms: A meta-analytic study. *Child Development, 83,* 591–610.

Haltigan, J. D., & Roisman, G. I. (2015). Infant attachment insecurity and dissociative symptomatology: Findings from the NICHD Study of Early Child Care and Youth Development. *Infant Mental Health Journal, 36,* 30–41.

Haydon, K. C., Roisman, G. I., Owen, M. T., Booth-LaForce, C., & Cox, M. J. (2014). Shared and distinctive antecedents of Adult Attachment Interview state-of-mind and inferred-experience dimensions. In C. Booth-LaForce & G. I. Roisman (Eds)., The Adult Attachment Interview: Psychometrics, stability and change from infancy, and developmental origins. *Monographs of the Society for Research in Child Development, 79*(3), 108–125.

Matas, L., Arend, R. A. & Sroufe, L. A. (1978). Continuity of adaptation in the second year: The relationship between quality of attachment and later competence. *Child Development, 49,* 547–556.

McCartney, K., Owen, M. T., Booth, C. L., Clarke-Stewart, A., & Vandell, D. L. (2004). Testing a maternal attachment model of behavior problems in childhood. *Journal of Child Psychology and Psychiatry, 45,* 765–778.

NICHD Early Child Care Research Network. (Eds.). (2005). *Child care and child development.* New York: Guilford Press.

Roisman, G. I., & Cicchetti, D. (2017). Editorial: Attachment in the context of atypical caregiving. *Development and Psychopathology, 29,* 331–335.

Sroufe, L. A. (2003). Attachment categories as reflections of multiple dimensions: Comment on Fraley and Spieker (2003). *Developmental Psychology, 39,* 413–416.

Sroufe, L. A., Egeland, B., Carlson, E. A., & Collins, W. A. (2005). *The development of the person: The Minnesota Study of Risk and Adaptation from Birth to Adulthood.* New York: Guilford Press.

Sroufe, L. A., Egeland, B., & Kreutzer, T. (1990). The fate of early experience following developmental change: Longitudinal approaches to individual adaptation in childhood. *Child Development, 61,* 1363–1373.

van IJzendoorn, M. H., & Tavecchio, L. W. C. (1987). The development of attachment theory as a Lakatosian research program: Philosophical and methodological aspects. In L. W. C. Tavecchio & M. H. van IJzendoorn (Eds.), *Attachment in social networks* (pp. 3–31). Amsterdam: Elsevier.

CHAPTER 24

Are Attachment Security and Disorganization Etched on the Brain?

Marinus H. van IJzendoorn
Anne Tharner
Marian J. Bakermans-Kranenburg

Are attachment security and disorganized attachment etched on the brain? If so, attachment differences would be prime predictors of later development across the lifespan in a broad range of domains (Groh, Fearon, van IJzendoorn, Bakermans-Kranenburg, & Roisman, 2017). One of the core assumptions of attachment theory is the inborn nature of attachment (Bowlby, 1969). Every newborn comes into the world with the innate bias to show proximity-seeking behavior such as vocalizing, crying, and laughter in order to trigger protective behavior in a parent or other caregiver. The babies' temperature modulation, their stress regulation, and their immune and metabolic systems are critically dependent on attachment figures (Gunnar, 2017). A few regular caregivers need to learn the crucial attachment signals and ways in which they can respond to those signals to provide a safe haven and at least a minimum of "good-enough" care (van IJzendoorn, & Bakermans-Kranenburg, in press). This contributes to survival of the infants and to their development to a relatively autonomous functioning and procreative age. Here we briefly discuss some studies on neural correlates of attachment security and disorganization to shed light on the question of whether and how individual differences in attachment get under the skin and become embodied in the brain, and what role genetics might play.

Adverse Childhood Experiences
Affect Structural Brain Development

A slow but persistent search for neural correlates of attachment security and disorganization is a necessary (but not sufficient) condition to understand how and why early childhood experiences may have long-term sequelae that cannot be explained by stability of the social environment. Impressive evidence for the enduring experiential effects on brain structure has been provided by the famous taxi drivers study (Maguire et al., 2000) showing that the posterior hippocampal volumes of experienced taxi drivers were significantly larger than those of their matched controls without this job that challenges spatial memory. Effects of adverse childhood experiences on brain morphology have also been observed. For example, cumulative maltreatment experiences have been linked to smaller hippocampal volume (Riem, Alink, Out, van IJzendoorn, & Bakermans-Kranenburg, 2015).

Structural neglect suffered by institutionalized children because of the 24/7 care regimen with frequent caregiver shifts and turnover has an equally large impact on brain growth (van IJzendoorn et al., 2020). Because newborns are hardwired to become attached, their physical and psychosocial development is jeopardized when they grow up in institutional care settings without stable attachment figures. Such an impersonal and neglectful regimen can have a grave impact on brain development, which in turn may have long-term detrimental consequences. For example, Bauer, Hanson, Pierson, Davidson, and Pollak (2009) found that 11-year-old children adopted to the United States from Russian and Romanian orphanages at 30 months after birth had a smaller cerebellum, which in turn predicted lower performance on memory and planning tasks compared to their peers without these adverse early years. In the randomized Bucharest Early Intervention Project, Sheridan, Fox, Zeanah, McLaughlin, and Nelson (2012) documented significant delays in grey matter development, indicating the number of cell bodies in the brain, about 7 years after the children were removed from institutional care and placed in foster care. In a meta-analysis of 20 studies on brain development in institutionalized children ($N = 2,042$ children) we found more than one standard deviation smaller head circumferences (assessed as a proxy for neural development) in institutionalized children but also an impressive recovery after transition into foster or adoptive families (van IJzendoorn et al., 2020). Whether similar effects on brain structures and basic (resting state) brain functions can be discovered in less extremely insensitive social environments and can be connected to attachment (in)security or disorganization is the next question to be addressed.

Is Structural Brain Development Affected by Typical Variation in Parental Sensitivity?

What influence does typical variation in parental sensitivity instead of structural neglect have on the development of brain structures? We examined this question in one of the largest longitudinal cohort studies in this area to date, the Generation R study. The Rotterdam cohort study of nearly 10,000 children has been investigated from fetal life to adolescence. In part of this sample, children's attachment and both parents' sensitivity were observed between 14 and 48 months. Brain imaging was carried out at 6 weeks using ultrasound assessments and between 6 and 10 years using magnetic resonance imaging (MRI).

In the first study on the relation between parental sensitivity and brain development, Kok and colleagues (2015) observed parental interactions with their toddlers at 1, 3, and 4 years of age ($N = 191$). At one year, mothers' sensitivity and cooperation were observed with their infants in a free-play session and during a psychophysiological assessment, each with a duration of about 5 minutes. At 3 and 4 years of age, supportive presence and intrusiveness were rated in two different interaction tasks of about 4 minutes, each designed to be slightly too difficult for the child to complete without parental support. Scores were aggregated across tasks and parents, as well as kept separate for mothers and fathers.

Controlling for 6-week head circumference, gender, age, and a series of other potential confounders, higher levels of combined but not individual parental sensitivity in early childhood predicted larger total brain volume and larger white matter volume assessed at 8 years of age, with effect sizes of around $r = .15$. In addition, both combined parental sensitivity and mothers' sensitivity predicted larger gray matter volume. Larger volumes at this age are considered markers of more optimal brain development. Associations were similar for earlier versus later sensitivity assessments, and they were not significantly different for maternal versus paternal sensitivity (Kok et al., 2015). Particularly strong effect sizes were found for the association between parental sensitivity and cortical thickness of the child's precentral frontal gyri, which show a high density of mirror neurons (neurons possibly implicated in the development of empathy). In contrast with a much smaller study ($N = 33$; Bernier et al., 2019), we did not find associations between parental sensitivity and specific subcortical volumes (right amygdala and bilateral hippocampus).

Next to associations with structural brain development, we also found that insensitive parenting might accelerate brain circuit development. Thijssen and colleagues (2017) used resting state MRI (rsMRI) in the absence of a specific task during scanning to assess amygdala–medial prefrontal cortex (mPFC) connectivity, that is, circuits or networks of coordinated neural activity of those two brain regions. The amygdala is suggested to be implicated in emotional states such as feeling threatened or anxious, whereas the mPFC is thought to play a role in cognitive modulation of such emotions. Using observational assessments of maternal and paternal sensitivity at 4 years of age (described above), lower combined parental sensitivity and especially lower maternal sensitivity predicted accelerated amygdala–mPFC connectivity in 8- to 10-year-old children (N = 124). This suggests that suboptimal parenting may prematurely activate the development of neural structures important for emotion regulation, enabling children in suboptimal caregiving circumstances to self-regulate and become independent of external regulation by parents at an earlier age. In a study of preschool children, Wang et al. (2019) found similar age-related shifts in associations between early parental sensitivity and an anterior hippocampal functional network. Both sets of findings are consistent with life-history theory, which predicts accelerated brain development in children from less privileged and more stressful family backgrounds because they have to be ready at an earlier stage to function without their protective caregivers (Hochberg & Belsky, 2013; see also Szepsenwol & Simpson, Chapter 27, this volume).

Structural Brain Development and Disorganized Attachment

Whereas differences in parental sensitivity may leave their trace in children's brains, it has also been argued that as a consequence, infant attachment would be hardwired into the brain. Here we focus on disorganized attachment as the presumably most atypical category of attachment. Disorganization of attachment is thought to indicate the infant's response to abusive, frightening, frightened, or dissociated parental behavior (Hesse & Main, 2006). Elevated percentages of disorganized attachment have also been associated with an accumulation of risk factors such as socioeconomic deprivation in the absence of major losses, family violence, or maltreatment (Cyr, Euser, Bakermans-Kranenburg, & van IJzendoorn, 2010). In the mildly stressful Strange Situation Procedure (SSP) disorganized attachment may be derived from sequential or simultaneous display of contradictory behaviors (e.g., distress and avoidance), stereotypical or anomalous movements, freezing or stilling, and expressions of fear, apprehension, or confusion regarding the parent (Main & Solomon, 1990). Disorganized infant attachment has been found to predict long-term elevated risks for symptoms of behavior problems, in particular externalizing issues, and psychopathological symptoms involving dissociative tendencies (Groh et al., 2017).

In the longitudinal Minnesota study, clear-cut evidence for neurobiological predictors of attachment quality seemed elusive, as maternal medical history, infant anomalies at birth, neonatal behavioral orientation response, or temperament were not implicated in attachment disorganization *in toto*. However, Padrón, Carlson, and Sroufe (2014) presented some tentative evidence that newborn emotion regulation might be a precursor of fearful or disoriented behaviors in the SSP. This finding converges with one of the earliest suggestions that an atypical behavioral orientation response in newborns, assessed with the Neonatal Behavioral Assessment Scale, may increase the risk of disorganized attachment (Spangler, Fremmer-Bombik, & Grossmann, 1996).

In the Generation R study, Tharner and colleagues (2011) used cranial ultrasound of 6-week-old infants to assess the diameter of their gangliothalamic ovoid, which comprises subcortical structures associated with goal-directed behavior such as the striatum. Infants with a larger gangliothalamic ovoid had a lower risk of attachment disorganization as assessed in the SSP at 14 months (N = 629; around 20% of the children were disorganized). Volume of the lateral ventricles (assessed as an index of general brain development) was not associated with attachment disorganization, so the prediction seems specific to the development of the limbic system, which is the "usual suspect" for neural studies on emotions.

Assuming brain structure and function to be potentially both cause and effect in bidirectional or transactional relations with the environment and with endophenotypic characteristics of the human organism, we also examined the predictive association between disorganized attachment at 14 months (N = 551) and brain morphology at age 10 years in Generation R data (Cortes Hidalgo et al., 2019). Children classified as disorganized in infancy had larger hippocampal volumes than those with (secure or insecure) organized attachment patterns, but, in contrast to the small study on adults of Lyons-Ruth, Pechtel, Yoon, Anderson, and Teicher (2016), disorganized attachment did not predict differences in the amygdala. Again, accelerated growth of brain regions related to memory and emotion might be evolutionary advantageous in adverse caregiving environments as suggested above (Szepsenwol & Simpson, Chapter 27, this volume; Thijssen et al., 2017). We did not find similar differences between the organized (avoidant, resistant, secure) attachment patterns, which might mean that even in large but nonclinical samples, atypical neural development can only be found in the most atypical attachment phenotype of disorganization.

Are Attachment Differences Rooted in Genes?

Long-term predictions from early parental sensitivity and children's attachment to later social-emotional and cognitive development might also be explained by a stable genetic foundation. This is a plausible complementary hypothesis to the idea that attachment becomes etched on the brain because brain structures have been shown to be partly heritable. In a twin sample (ages 7–9 years; $N = 512$), we found that surface area and cortical thickness of structures that are at the core of the so-called social brain are partly heritable (van der Meulen et al., 2020). We also found heritability of observed parental limit-setting in a child-based twin design study including 236 families with 4- to 5-year-old twins. However, effects of shared environmental factors on observed parental sensitivity and limit-setting were more substantial (Euser et al., 2020).

Twin studies of observed child attachment showed large environmental influences and no evidence for heritability (Bakermans-Kranenburg & van IJzendoorn, 2016). In adolescent twins however, Fearon, Shmueli-Goetz, Viding, Fonagy, and Plomin (2014) found substantial heritability in attachment assessed with the Child Attachment Interview, suggesting more genetic influence with growing age. In a combination of data from the Generation R study and the National Institute of Child Health and Human Development (NICHD) Study of Early Child Care and Youth Development (SECCYD), we explored the molecular genetics of infant attachment differences focusing on candidate genes, but we did not find convincing evidence. Next, a genomewide association study (GWAS) covering 2.5 million single-nucleotide polymorphisms (SNPs) was conducted in Generation R. Only a very small percentage of variance in attachment could be explained. Going beyond the hunt for attachment genes, it is fruitful to consider the role of genes in differential susceptibility to explain why some children are more influenced by parental (in)sensitivity, for better *and* for worse, whereas other children seem less impacted by parenting and stay secure or insecure whatever their circumstances. Children's genetic makeup is crucially important in gene-by-environment interaction, but it is difficult to see how genetics would explain attachment becoming embodied in the brain to determine long-term development (for a detailed discussion of the genetics of attachment, see Bakermans-Kranenburg & van IJzendoorn, 2016).

Conclusion

Looking for signs of attachment etched on the brain, we have only just scratched the rather impenetrable surface of this elusive association. There is no evidence for speculative "expansions" of attachment theory into a "regulation theory," with an unsubstantiated emphasis on the lateralized right brain, suggesting a hazardous etiological connection between attachment and autism (Schore, 2014). Using the Generation R study with one of the largest samples in this area, we could only arrive at some speculative predictive hypotheses. In this field of inquiry, we are just beginning

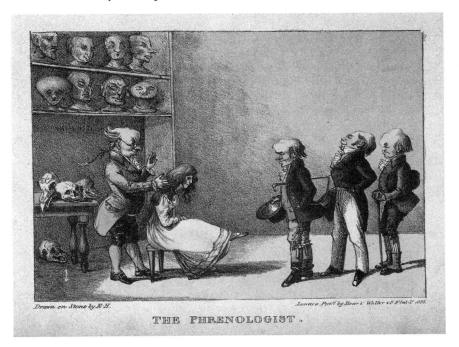

FIGURE 24.1. Franz Joseph Gall examining the head of a pretty young girl, while three gentlemen wait in line. Colored lithograph possibly by Edward Hull, 1825. Wellcome Collection Gallery.

to go beyond Gall's phrenology (see Figure 24.1) in creating robust and replicable findings to be used as a firm basis for theoretical speculation, and in the long run for clinical or policy applications (van IJzendoorn & Bakermans-Kranenburg, in press).

REFERENCES

Bakermans-Kranenburg, M. J., & van IJzendoorn, M. H. (2016). Attachment, parenting, and genetics. In J. Cassidy & P. R. Shaver (Eds.), *Handbook of attachment* (3rd ed., pp. 155–179). New York: Guilford Press.

Bauer, P. M., Hanson, J. L., Pierson, R. K., Davidson, R. J., & Pollak, S. D. (2009). Cerebellar volume and cognitive functioning in children who experienced early deprivation. *Biological Psychiatry, 66*(12), 1100–1106.

Bernier, A., Degeilh, F., Leblanc, E., Daneault, V., Bailey, H. N., & Beauchamp, M. H. (2019). Mother–infant interaction and child brain morphology: A multidimensional approach to maternal sensitivity. *Infancy, 24*(2), 120–138.

Bowlby, J. (1969). *Attachment and loss: Vol. 1. Attachment.* New York: Basic Books.

Cortes Hidalgo, A. P., Muetzel, R., Luijk, P. C. M., Bakermans-Kranenburg, M. J., El Marroun, H., Vernooij, M., . . . Tiemeier, H. (2019). Observed infant–parent attachment and brain morphology in middle childhood—a population-based study. *Developmental Cognitive Neuroscience, 40,* 100724.

Cyr, C., Euser, E. M., Bakermans-Kranenburg, M. J., & van IJzendoorn, M. H. (2010). Attachment security and disorganization in maltreating and high-risk families: A series of meta-analyses. *Development and Psychopathology, 22,* 87–108.

Euser, S., Bosdriesz, J. R., Vrijhof, C. I., van den Bulk, B. G., van Hees, D., De Vet, S. M., . . . Bakermans-Kranenburg, M. J. (2020). How heritable are parental sensitivity and limit-setting?: A longitudinal child-based twin study on observed parenting. *Child Development, 91,* 2255–2269.

Fearon P., Shmueli-Goetz, Y., Viding, E., Fonagy, P., & Plomin, R. (2014). Genetic and environmental influences on adolescent attachment. *Journal of Child Psychology and Psychiatry, 55,* 1033–1041.

Groh, A. M., Fearon, R. M. P., van IJzendoorn, M. H., Bakermans-Kranenburg, M. J., & Roisman, G. I. (2017). Attachment in the early life course: Meta-analytic evidence for its role in socioemotional development. *Child Development Perspectives, 11*(1), 70–76.

Gunnar, M. R. (2017). Social buffering of stress in development: A career perspective. *Perspectives on Psychological Science, 12,* 355–373.

Hesse, E., & Main, M. (2006). Frightened, threatening, and dissociative parental behavior in low-risk samples: Description, discussion, and interpretations. *Development and Psychopathology, 18*(2), 309–343.

Hochberg, Z. E., & Belsky, J. (2013). Evo-devo of human adolescence: Beyond disease models of early puberty. *BMC Medicine, 11*(1), 113.

Kok, R., Thijssen, S., Bakermans-Kranenburg, M. J., Jaddoe, V. W. V., Verhulst, F. C., White, T., . . . Tiemeier, H. (2015). Normal variation in early parental sensitivity predicts child structural brain development. *Journal of the American Academy of Child and Adolescent Psychiatry, 54,* 824–831.

Lyons-Ruth, K., Pechtel, P., Yoon, S. A., Anderson, C. M., & Teicher, M. H. (2016). Disorganized attachment in infancy predicts greater amygdala volume in adulthood. *Behavioural Brain Research, 308,* 83–93.

Maguire, E. A, Gadian, D. G., Johnsrude, I. S., Good, C., D., Ashburner, J., Frackowiak, R. S. J., & Frith, C. D. (2000). Navigation-related structural change in the hippocampi of taxi drivers. *Proceedings of the National Academy of Sciences of the USA, 97,* 4398–4403.

Main, M., & Solomon, J. (1990). Procedures for identifying infants as disorganized-disoriented during the Ainsworth Strange Situation. In D. C. M. T. Greenberg, D. Cicchetti, & E. M. Cummings (Eds.), *Attachment in the preschool years: Theory, research and intervention* (pp. 121–160). Chicago: University of Chicago Press.

Padrón, E., Carlson, E. A., & Sroufe, L. A. (2014). Frightened versus not frightened disorganized infant attachment. *American Journal of Orthopsychiatry, 84*(2), 201–208.

Riem, M. M. E., Alink, L. R. A., Out, D., van IJzendoorn, M. H., & Bakermans-Kranenburg, M. J. (2015). Beating the brain about abuse: Empirical and meta-analytic studies of the association between maltreatment and hippocampal volume across childhood and adolescence. *Development and Psychopathology, 27,* 507–520.

Schore, A. N. (2014). Early interpersonal neurobiological assessment of attachment and autistic spectrum disorders. *Frontiers in Psychology, 5,* 1049.

Sheridan, M. A., Fox, N. A., Zeanah, C. H., McLaughlin, K. A., & Nelson, C. A. (2012). Variation in neural development as a result of exposure to institutionalization early in childhood. *Proceedings of the National Academy of Sciences of the USA, 109*(32), 12927–12932.

Spangler, G., Fremmer-Bombik, E., & Grossmann, K. (1996). Social and individual determinants of infant attachment security and disorganization. *Infant Mental Health Journal, 17*(2), 127–138.

Tharner, A., Herba, C. M., Luijk, M. P. C. M., van IJzendoorn, M. H., Bakermans-Kranenburg, M. J., Govaert, P. P., . . . Tiemeier, H. (2011). Subcortical structures and the neurobiology of infant attachment disorganization: A longitudinal ultrasound imaging study. *Social Neuroscience, 6*(4), 336–347.

Thijssen, S., Muetzel, R. L., Bakermans-Kranenburg, M. J., Jaddoe, V. W. V., Tiemeier, H., Verhulst, F. C., . . . van IJzendoorn, M. H. (2017). Insensitive parenting may accelerate the development of the amygdala-medial prefrontal cortex circuit. *Development and Psychopathology, 29*(2), 505–518.

van der Meulen, M., Wierenga, L. M., Achterberg, M., Drenth, N., van IJzendoorn, M. H., & Crone, A. E. (2020). Genetic and environmental influences on structure of the social brain in childhood. *Developmental Cognitive Neuroscience, 44,* 100782.

Van IJzendoorn, M. H., & Bakermans-Kranenburg, M. J. (in press). Replication crisis lost in translation?: On translational caution and premature applications of attachment theory. *Attachment and Human Development.*

van IJzendoorn, M. H., Bakermans-Kranenburg, M. J., Duschinsky, R., Goldman, P. S., Fox, N. A., Gunnar, M. R., . . . Sonuga-Barke, E. J. S. (2020). Institutionalisation and deinstitutionalisation of children: 1. A systematic and integrative review of evidence regarding effects on development. *Lancet Psychiatry, 7*(8), 703–720.

Wang, Q., Zhang, H., Wee, C.-Y., Lee, A., Poh, J. S., Chong, Y.-S., . . . Qiu, A. (2019). Maternal sensitivity predicts anterior hippocampal functional networks in early childhood. *Brain Structure and Function, 224,* 1885–1895.

CHAPTER 25

Early Attachment and Later Physical Health

Katherine B. Ehrlich
Jude Cassidy

What is the lasting legacy of early attachment relationships? Researchers have been asking this question for decades, and the result of such curiosity has led to a rich accumulation of evidence that, collectively, suggests that the "long arm" of early attachment persists across the lifespan. Investigations of the lasting influence of infant–parent attachments have found that these early experiences are reliably associated with the quality of future close relationships, mental health, social cognition, and personality (see Thompson, 2016). Other studies have even identified links to more distal outcomes, including academic performance and IQ, that can be explained by individual differences in the extent to which children are able to recruit assistance from parents and support from others, and develop self-regulatory capacities that facilitate learning in the classroom (e.g., West, Mathews, & Kerns, 2013). After over 40 years of research on the consequences of early attachment experiences, it is clear that attachment relationships are important, shape future development, and exert influences on well-being far beyond childhood.

To date, these investigations have focused primarily on psychosocial outcomes. Over the last three decades, there has been growing interest in linking early attachments to measures of physiology, with much of this work focused on activity of the hypothalamic–pituitary–adrenal axis and cortisol production in particular (for a review, see Hane & Fox, 2016). More recently, we and others have written about the emerging literature linking attachment experiences to the immune system and inflammatory processes (Ehrlich, 2019; Ehrlich, Miller, Jones, & Cassidy, 2016; Pietromonaco & Beck, 2019; Pietromonaco, DeVito, Ge, & Lembke, 2015), which is of particular interest given inflammation's direct role in the progression of some of the most common chronic diseases of aging. We refer readers to these reviews for in-depth discussions about why attachment-related experiences may be linked to biological systems, and how disruptions to some of these systems may give rise to differences in physical health across the lifespan. We have argued that attachment orientations and daily interactions with attachment figures each shape the ways in which individuals perceive, manage, and mitigate stress, all of which serve as important processes that could influence "wear and tear" on the body. Similarly, secure individuals, who have developed mental representations of themselves as lovable and worthy of care, may be more likely than insecure individuals to engage in health-promotive behaviors, manage their chronic diseases responsibly, and seek help when symptoms arise (e.g., Ciechanowski et al., 2004; Ehrlich et al., 2019). Collectively, these strategies play an important role in maximizing years of healthy living and slowing the progression of chronic disease.

In this chapter, we contemplate two questions that we hope will generate new lines of inquiry into the study of attachment and physical health. In so doing, we aim to provide concrete and testable hypotheses about the conditions under which one might expect and not expect to find a link between attachment and health.

What Evidence Supports a Link between Early Attachment and Physical Health?

Several changes in the understanding of chronic diseases have been instrumental to advancing discussion about how social experiences early in life could be linked to later physical health. First, diseases that were once viewed as health problems that emerged only later in life (e.g., cardiovascular disease) are increasingly viewed as conditions that have roots in earlier stages of development. In fact, precursors to chronic disease (e.g., fatty streaks in the intima of large muscular arteries; insulin resistance) are sometimes evident by adolescence. In addition, researchers have identified a number of childhood risk factors, including low socioeconomic status and high levels of adverse childhood events, that forecast risk for chronic disease decades later (e.g., Kittleson et al., 2006). The most stringent tests of the role of early experience in later physical health have controlled for the most likely confounds (e.g., adult income, education, health behaviors), thereby strengthening claims about the privileged role of early life experiences for subsequent health (Chen, Brody, & Miller, 2017).

Much of the research to date linking early childhood social experiences to adult physical health has relied on retrospective reports of early life experience, a design that has some notable limitations. Of particular concern is the fact that retrospective and prospective reports have only modest correspondence (Reuben et al., 2016), even for experiences that, presumably, would have been memorable (e.g., family member incarceration). Thus, although studies that have utilized retrospective reports of early attachment-related experiences provide a first step toward understanding how early attachments shape later health, the ability to draw strong conclusions based on these retrospective reports is limited.

Only a handful of long-term longitudinal samples are available to examine prospective associations between attachment experiences measured in childhood and adult physical health. One such ongoing study is the impressive Minnesota Longitudinal Study of Risk and Adaptation (Sroufe, Egeland, Carlson, & Collins, 2005). In one analysis, Puig and colleagues found that infant attachment security, assessed using the Strange Situation Procedure, was associated with self-reports of physical health at age 32 (Puig, Englund, Simpson, & Collins, 2013). Notably, adults who had been classified as insecurely attached were more likely to report inflammation-based diseases (e.g., diabetes, coronary heart disease) relative to adults who had been classified as secure. Using the same sample, Farrell and colleagues (2019) extended this work by showing that observations of maternal sensitivity across the first 3 years of life predicted a composite indicator of cardiometabolic risk (blood pressure, body mass index [BMI], waist circumference, and a measure of low-grade inflammation) at age 37. These important papers are among the first to demonstrate how attachment-related measures captured in early life can be used to predict physical health over 30 years later.

Critics of this approach to leveraging existing longitudinal studies will point out the lack of baseline health controls in these ongoing projects. Indeed, when these longitudinal studies began several decades ago, they were designed to focus on children's psychosocial outcomes, not physical health, so the lack of baseline health-relevant data is understandable. We encourage investigators who are planning new longitudinal studies to keep this criticism in mind and to consider including assessments of risk factors known to be associated with later disease (e.g., birthweight, pregnancy complications, breastfeeding duration), *even if health outcomes are not central to the initial study.*

Although the focus of this chapter is on the extent to which early attachment may predict later physical health, we highlight some exciting new evidence that suggests that these connections may not take decades to unfold and are in fact observable much earlier in the life course. Work by Bernard and colleagues suggests that, among children receiving child protective services, securely attached children had steeper declines in BMI acrosss toddlerhood than insecure children (Bernard, Frost, Jelinek, & Dozier, 2019). Additionally, in the same sample, insecure-organized and disorganized children had higher levels of C-reactive protein (a marker of low-grade inflammation) in early childhood compared to securely attached children (Bernard, Hostinar, & Dozier, 2019). These findings provide some intriguing evidence to suggest that, at least among at-risk children, the links between attachment and health are already present in childhood.

What Are the Limits of the Association between Early Attachment and Physical Health?

Preliminary evidence suggests that early attachment experiences are associated with later markers of physical health, but we recognize that there will be limits to the extent to which we should expect to find this link. Much of the work to date has focused on indicators of health that have ties to low-grade inflammation—a logical starting point for two reasons: (1) inflammation is a contributor to many chronic diseases of aging and (2) psychosocial stressors and other close relationship experiences appear to be associated with inflammation, making it a biological marker that appears to be sensitive to fluctuations in psychosocial stress.

For diseases and chronic conditions that have clear ties to health behaviors, stress, and coping, we predict that attachment processes are likely to be associated with those conditions. Conversely, we expect that the role of early attachment for later health will be limited for diseases that have an exceptionally strong genetic basis (e.g., Huntington's disease, some cancers). Similarly, for conditions that arise because of an extremely toxic external factor (e.g., severe environmental exposures), we would not expect early attachment to have much influence. Conversely, even for chronic conditions that are shaped by both genetic and environmental factors, it is possible that attachment experiences could play an important part in disease morbidity. Take the case of coronary artery disease. Both genetic and behavioral factors shape this disease, but evidence suggests that incorporating a healthy diet, exercising, and not smoking substantially reduces risk for coronary events—even among individuals with high genetic risk (Khera et al., 2016). These findings suggest that genetic risk is not deterministic, and there are behavioral modifications that high-risk individuals can make that give individuals some control over their long-term health and well-being. Could early attachment-based interventions reduce risk for health problems later in life? Evidence from Bernard and colleagues (described earlier) suggests that these interventions may have short-term health benefits, at least for securely attached children. Whether these benefits extend into adulthood is an exciting question that awaits future study.

Another boundary question concerns the extent to which attachment experiences predict disease *onset* versus disease *progression*. Numerous factors (e.g., genetics) are tied to disease onset, and these factors may largely shape whether or not someone is likely to receive a disease diagnosis. However, once that disease is present, attachment may play a more significant role in disease management and morbidity. The role of attachment for disease progression could be mediated by more proximal health behaviors and disease management that shape how well the disease is controlled (e.g., diabetes management; see Ciechanowski et al., 2004). For example, in a sample of children with asthma, the extent to which children perceived their parent as a secure base was related to families' active monitoring of their child's asthma symptoms, appropriate medication use, and collaborative relationship with medical providers (Ehrlich et al., 2019). This study relied on cross-sectional data, so the issue of disease onset versus progression will be an important one to sort out as more prospective longitudinal data become available.

Conclusions and Future Directions

We are encouraged by the emerging attempts to understand the link between early attachment and physical health, and we hope that additional research in the coming years will help clarify the conditions under which attachment shapes physical health. One priority for this work will be to identify whether attachment is a correlate or causal agent in the progression of disease. To clarify this question, research utilizing randomized trials of attachment-based interventions will be especially helpful, as these experimental designs allow for stronger conclusions about whether changes to children's attachment map onto corresponding differences in physical health. In addition, ongoing longitudinal studies, with assessments of attachment in infancy and childhood, will prove to be useful in evaluating whether these early experiences can predict chronic disease several decades later. Ideally, longitudinal studies of this nature would also include possible mechanisms assessed in the intervening years (e.g., health behaviors, stress, biological mechanisms). These investigations represent an important next step in clarifying the strength of the connection between early attachment and physical health.

We are also interested in exploring the ways in which early attachment may be associated with clinically relevant markers of health prior to adulthood. This work has proven to be especially challenging, given that childhood and adolescence is typically a developmental period of particularly good health. However, studies of children with chronic disease offer opportunities to evaluate whether social experiences predict disease morbidity across childhood and into adulthood. In addition, the increasing prevalence of childhood obesity in recent decades raises concerns for physicians and public health advocates who are understandably worried about the substantial economic burden and quality of life difficulties awaiting these children in adulthood. We propose that researchers view this global public health crisis with an "attachment lens." That is, to what extent do early attachment experiences shape risk for rapid weight gain and obesity in childhood and adolescence? Are insensitive parents more likely than sensitive parents to use food as a soothing strategy, or as a demonstration of love? Are these parents also more likely to use coercion and shame in connection to feeding (Savage, Fisher, & Birch, 2007)? These emotional complexities tied to food and feeding may provide some explanation for the proposed connections between attachment insecurity and obesity.

In sum, the next decade of research on early predictors of later physical health has the potential to expand the scope of outcomes connected to early attachment. Carefully designed studies, with measurement of possible confounding factors, will be important for evaluating the unique role of early attachment for later physical health.

ACKNOWLEDGMENTS

Preparation of this chapter was supported by the National Institutes of Health Common Fund (DP2 MD013947) and the Jacobs Foundation (Early Career Research Fellowship 2018-1288-07).

REFERENCES

Bernard, K., Frost, A., Jelinek, C., & Dozier, M. (2019). Secure attachment predicts lower body mass index in young children with histories of child protective services involvement. *Pediatric Obesity, 14,* e12510.

Bernard, K., Hostinar, C. E., & Dozier, M. (2019). Longitudinal associations between attachment quality in infancy, C-reactive protein in early childhood, and BMI in middle childhood: Preliminary evidence from a CPS-referred sample. *Attachment and Human Development, 21,* 5–22.

Chen, E., Brody, G., & Miller, G. E. (2017). Childhood close family relationships and health. *American Psychologist, 72,* 555–566.

Ciechanowski, P., Russo, J., Katon, W., Von Korff, M., Ludman, E., Lin, E., . . . Bush, T. (2004). Influence of patient attachment style on self-care and outcomes in diabetes. *Psychosomatic Medicine, 66,* 720–728.

Ehrlich, K. B. (2019). Attachment and psychoneuroimmunology. *Current Opinion in Psychology, 25,* 96–100.

Ehrlich, K. B., Miller, G. E., Jones, J. D., & Cassidy, J. (2016). Attachment and psychoneuroimmunology. In J. Cassidy & P. R. Shaver (Eds.), *Handbook of attachment: Theory, research, and clinical applications* (3rd ed., pp. 180–201). New York: Guilford Press.

Ehrlich, K. B., Miller, G. E., Shalowitz, M., Story, R., Levine, C., Williams, D., . . . Chen, E. (2019). Secure base representations in children with asthma: Links with symptoms, family asthma management, and cytokine regulation. *Child Development, 90,* e718–e728.

Farrell, A. K., Waters, T. E. A., Young, E. S., Englund, M. M., Carlson, E. E., Roisman, G. I., & Simpson, J. A. (2019). Early maternal sensitivity, attachment security in young adulthood, and cardiometabolic risk at midlife. *Attachment and Human Development, 21,* 70–86.

Hane, A. A., & Fox, N. A. (2016). Studying the biology of human attachment. In J. Cassidy & P. R. Shaver (Eds.), *Handbook of attachment: Theory, research, and clinical applications* (3rd ed., pp. 223–241). New York: Guilford Press.

Khera, A. V., Emdin, C. A., Drake, I., Natarajan, P., Bick, A. G., Cook, N. R., . . . Kathiresan, S. (2016). Genetic risk, adherence to a healthy lifestyle, and coronary disease. *New England Journal of Medicine, 375,* 2349–2358.

Kittleson, M. M., Meoni, L. A., Wang, N. Y., Chu, A. Y., Ford, D. E., & Klag, M. J. (2006). Association of childhood socioeconomic status with subsequent coronary heart disease in physicians. *Archives of Internal Medicine, 166,* 2356–2361.

Pietromonaco, P. R., & Beck, L. A. (2019). Adult attachment and physical health. *Current Opinion in Psychology, 25,* 115–120.

Pietromonaco, P. R., DeVito, C. C., Ge, F., & Lembke, J. (2015). Health and attachment processes. In J. A. Simpson & W. S. Rholes (Eds.), *Attachment theory and research: New directions and emerging themes* (pp. 287–318). New York: Guilford Press.

Puig, J., Englund, M. M., Simpson, J. A., & Collins, W. A. (2013). Predicting adult physical illness from infant attachment: A prospective longitudinal study. *Health Psychology, 32,* 409–417.

Reuben, A., Moffitt, T. E., Caspi, A., Belsky, D. W., Harrington, H., Schroeder, F., . . . Danese, A. (2016). Lest we forget: Comparing retrospective and prospective assessments of adverse childhood experiences in the prediction of adult health. *Journal of Child Psychology and Psychiatry, 57,* 1103–1112.

Savage, J. S., Fisher, J. O., & Birch, L. L. (2007). Parental influence on eating behavior: Conception to adolescence. *Journal of Law, Medicine, and Ethics, 35,* 22–34.

Sroufe, L. A., Egeland, B., Carlson, E. A., & Collins, W. A. (2005). *The development of the person: The Minnesota Study of Risk and Adaptation from Birth to Adulthood.* New York: Guilford Press.

Thompson, R. A. (2016). Early attachment and later development: Reframing the questions. In J. Cassidy & P. R. Shaver (Eds.), *Handbook of attachment: Theory, research, and clinical applications* (3rd ed., pp. 330–349). New York: Guilford Press.

West, K. K., Mathews, B. L., & Kerns, K. A. (2013). Mother–child attachment and cognitive performance in middle childhood: An examination of mediating mechanisms. *Early Childhood Research Quarterly, 28,* 259–270.

CHAPTER 26

The Continuing Influence of Early Attachment Orientations Viewed from a Personality–Social Perspective on Adult Attachment

Mario Mikulincer
Phillip R. Shaver

In this chapter, we deal with the continuing influence of individual differences in the functioning of the attachment behavioral system (attachment working models and orientations) formed during early parent–child relationships on later cognition, affect, and behavior. Specifically, we focus on three life domains—close relationships; emotion regulation and mental health; and the functioning of other behavioral systems (e.g., exploration, caregiving, sex)—domains in which research has revealed continuing effects of attachment orientations. We also consider the boundary conditions of these effects. Our discussion is based on a personality and social-psychological perspective and is informed by a large body of social and personality research on attachment in adulthood (Mikulincer & Shaver, 2016).

Continuity of Attachment Patterns from Infancy to Adulthood

Although personality and social psychologists have not conducted many long-term longitudinal studies of attachment orientations from childhood to adulthood because they work primarily with adult research participants (e.g., college students, married couples) using self-report measures (e.g., the Experiences in Close Relationships measure [ECR]; Brennan,

Clark, & Shaver, 1998), there is evidence of early parenting predictors of later self-reported attachment anxiety and avoidance. For example, Zayas, Mischel, Shoda, and Aber (2011) followed up 36 participants from one of Mischel's early studies of delay of gratification in 18-month-olds. They administered a brief version of the ECR to these participants when they were 22 years old and found strong negative associations (r's of approximately $-.70$) between insecure patterns of attachment in a current romantic relationship and maternal sensitivity measured 20 years earlier. However, these findings should be taken with caution because of the small sample size.

In a much more extensive study, Fraley, Roisman, Booth-LaForce, Owen, and Holland (2013) used data from the large-scale National Institute of Child Health and Human Development (NICHD) Study of Early Child Care and Youth Development to examine predictors of ECR scores at age 15 from early parenting variables. Insecurities of both kinds (anxiety and avoidance) were predicted by early maternal depression, increases over time in maternal depression, father absence, decreases over time in child's teacher-rated social competence with peers, and self-rated poorer friendship quality. Avoidance scores were predicted, in addition, by lower maternal sensitivity and decreases in sensitivity over time. ECR scores were not significantly related to infant temperament or to the various candidate genes investigated, suggesting that they were attributable primarily to social experiences rather than inheritance.

In short, adolescent and young adult ECR scores do relate in theoretically meaningful ways to early parenting (as initially suggested by retrospective reports of experiences with parents in Hazan and Shaver's [1987] pioneering studies, which launched the study of romantic attachment), in addition to being fairly stable over periods ranging from weeks to years (see, e.g., Fraley & Dugan, Chapter 18, this volume). However, the developmental trajectory of attachment patterns from infancy to adulthood was never expected to be simply direct and linear. Nor was it assumed by Bowlby (1973) or other attachment theorists that attachment working models and behavior patterns would be exclusively determined by early experiences. Rather, attachment working models can be updated throughout life (including in psychotherapy) and are affected by a broad array of factors, including the relationship partners one becomes involved with and a variety of other impactful life events, which can moderate the effects of mental residues of early experiences (Fraley & Roisman, 2019).

According to Simpson, Collins, Salvatore, and Sung (2014), the continuity of attachment patterns from infancy to adulthood is dynamic and involves successive transactions between the person and the environment over periods of years. Infant attachment patterns are carried from one point in time to another by mental representations that are responsive to social-emotional experiences in a wide variety of settings (family, school, peer relationships) and to current relationship experiences, so that later attachment representations are reflections of early prototypes, accumulated subsequent experiences, and current conditions.

Adult Attachment Orientations and Close Relationships

During the past 40 years, hundreds of studies have documented the substantial contribution of adult attachment orientations to the formation, maintenance, and quality of romantic and marital relationships (see Mikulincer & Shaver, 2016, for a review). According to Bowlby (1973), a person enters new relationships with working models shaped by past interactions with attachment figures, which tend to be projected onto any relationship partner who can potentially serve as a provider of a safe haven and a secure base. As a result, existing attachment orientations affect the way one anticipates, attends to, interprets, and recalls a current partner's behavior, biasing one's pattern of relating to this figure and the quality of the evolving relationship.

The projection of established attachment working models onto new relationships can be explained in terms of the social-cognitive process that Andersen and colleagues, following Freud, call *transference* (e.g., Andersen & Chen, 2002). When a representation of a previous relationship partner is implicitly primed by contextual cues (e.g., places where one interacted with that partner) or activated by resemblance cues in a new relationship partner, this representation will affect the ways in which the perceiver responds to the new partner. Moreover, since representations of significant others are linked to self-representations within an associative semantic network (e.g., Andersen & Chen, 2002), priming a significant-other representation is likely also to activate the associated self-representation, which in turn will bias self-appraisals within the new relationship. This makes it likely that early working models will be transferred to other relationship partners later in life and then influence the quality of the new relationship. Brumbaugh and Fraley (2007) provided direct evidence of this transference process during the initial stages of romantic relationships.

This transference process is not simple, however; it can be altered by a partner's own pattern of relating. That is, although existing working models can be automatically projected onto a new relationship partner, which occurs mainly when this partner is similar to past attachment figures, a partner's actual relational behaviors can disrupt the transfer process and weaken the influence of a person's attachment style on relationship quality. For example, a sensitive and responsive relationship partner can counteract the projection of insecure attachment working models onto this partner and cause positive changes in this partner's relational cognitions and behavior, which in turn can enhance relationship quality (Simpson & Overall, 2014). Arriaga, Kumashiro, Simpson, and Overall (2018) described specific partner responses that can increase a person's attachment security and buffer the destructive influence of his or her past attachment insecurities on close relationships (see also Arriaga & Kumashiro, Chapter 22, this volume).

These relational processes are not confined to couple or romantic relationships but can occur in any relational context in which an actual or symbolic (mentally represented) partner seems able to provide a safe haven and a secure base. This figure can have a close emotional relationship with the person (e.g., parent, sibling, friend) or can occupy the formal role of a "stronger and wiser" care provider in a specific context (e.g., teacher, therapist, manager, army officer, coach, priest). Numerous studies have shown that attachment orientations affect the quality of one's relationship with friends, teachers, therapists, leaders, and supervisors (see Mikulincer & Shaver, 2016, for a review). In addition, there is evidence that the responsiveness of teachers, therapists, and leaders has beneficial effects on interpersonal functioning of people with insecure attachment orientations (e.g., Davidovitz, Mikulincer, Shaver, Ijzak, & Popper, 2007; Håvås, Svartberg, & Ulvenes, 2015). There is also evidence that an adult's attachment working models are projected onto symbolic figures who can act as imaginary sources of a safe haven and secure base, biasing his or her relationship with God, pets, and groups (for reviews, see Granqvist, 2020; Mikulincer & Shaver, 2016).

Adult Attachment Orientations, Emotion Regulation, and Mental Health

Researchers have consistently shown that adults' attachment orientations contribute to emotion regulation and mental health (see Mikulincer & Shaver, 2016, for a review). Attachment-system activation is an inborn regulatory strategy aimed at mitigating distress by seeking proximity to protective others. The smooth functioning of this system results in a sense of attachment security that is a fundamental building block of psychological resilience and mental health. In contrast, failure to restore the sense of attachment security during interactions with inconsistent, unreliable, or insensitive attachment figures reduces resilience in coping with stressful life events and predisposes a person to break down psychologically in times of crisis (Mikulincer & Shaver, 2016). Attachment insecurity can therefore be viewed as a *general* vulnerability to psychological disorders, with the particular symptomatology depending on genetic, developmental, and environmental factors.

Attachment insecurities do not necessarily result in dysfunctions in emotion regulation and psychological disorders, and in fact a large array of factors (e.g., genetically determined temperament, personal and socio-economic resources, and life history) can buffer these negative influences of insecure working models. Moreover, beyond disorders such as separation anxiety and pathological grief, in which attachment injuries are the main causes and themes, attachment insecurities per se are unlikely to be sufficient causes of psychological disorders. Other factors are likely to converge with or amplify the effects of insecure attachment on the way to psychopathology.

Consider, for example, the relation between attachment-related avoidance and psychological distress. Many studies of large community samples have found no association between avoidant attachment and self-report measures of global distress (see Mikulincer & Shaver, 2016, for a review). However, studies that focus on highly stressful experiences (e.g., giving birth to an infant with a life-endangering illness) have indicated that avoidance is related to greater distress and poorer long-term adjustment (e.g., Berant, Mikulincer, & Shaver, 2008). Life history factors are also important. For example, traumatic life events, poverty, physical health problems, and involvement in turbulent romantic relationships during adolescence strengthen the link between attachment insecurity and psychopathology (e.g., Davila, Steinberg, Kachadourian, Cobb, & Fincham, 2004).

The link between insecure attachment and psychopathology is also complicated by research findings showing that psychological problems can increase attachment insecurity. For example, Mikulincer, Ein-Dor, Solomon, and Shaver (2011) assessed attachment insecurities and post-traumatic stress disorder (PTSD) among Israeli ex-prisoners of war (along with a matched control group of veterans) 18, 30, and 35 years after their release from captivity. Attachment anxiety and avoidance increased over time among the ex-prisoners, and the increases were predicted by the severity of PTSD symptoms at the first wave of measurement. These findings might reflect the action of a self-amplifying cycle by which attachment insecurities prospectively contribute to psychological disorder and the disorder then further heightens attachment insecurities, which in turn sustain or even exacerbate the disorder over time.

Adult Attachment Orientations and Other Behavioral Systems

According to Bowlby (1969/1982), interactions with a security-enhancing attachment figure and the resulting sense of attachment security set the foundation for the smooth functioning of other behavioral systems because people who feel secure have greater courage and more conflict-free mental resources to engage in and enjoy exploration and learning, caregiving, sex, and assertion of power. In contrast, when people are frightened and insecure, they are focused mainly on managing their distress rather than on nonattachment activities. In support of this view, numerous studies of adolescents and adults have shown that attachment insecurities have a detrimental effect on exploration and learning, care provision and prosocial behavior, power/autonomy assertion, and sex (see Mikulincer & Shaver, 2016, for a review).

Bowlby (1973) portrayed attachment security as a "secure base for exploration," suggesting that the attachment system is primary, comes first in development, and forms either a solid or a shaky foundation for the functioning of other behavioral systems. However, changes in the functioning of the other systems (e.g., failure to learn new skills and hence doubting one's competence and value; volunteering to help others and becoming more self-confident as a result) can feed back to attachment security. Moreover, genetic, life history, and cultural factors that shape the functioning of each behavioral system can buffer or amplify the influence of attachment working models. For example, although attachment insecurities can interfere with calm and confident learning of new information, this influence might be less notable among highly intelligent people or among those possessing the temperamental quality of effortful control. Similarly, although attachment insecurities can inhibit or interfere with a person's compassionate responses to others' suffering, this influence might be weakened in cultures that cultivate compassion and emphasize benevolent values.

Conclusion

The adolescent and adult attachment patterns studied, with self-report and observational measures and in survey, laboratory, and field experiments, have their origins in childhood relationships with parents and other care providers. Once established, these patterns, styles, or orientations contribute to mental health, the quality of close relationships, and the functioning of other behavioral systems. However, one should take into account that this contribution can be moderated or even overridden by the relationship partners one becomes involved with and the impactful life events one experiences across the lifespan. Moreover, attachment patterns can be impacted by life experiences and the quality of close relationships. The details of this mutual influence are delineated in thousands of published studies, many of them reviewed by us at book length (Mikulincer & Shaver, 2016). At present, there is no end in sight to this river of research, which is now firmly embedded in a wide variety of fields beyond social psychology, including individual, couple, and group psychotherapy; health psychology; education; religion; sports; and leadership. One large task for the future is to clarify relations between attachment theory and other theories applied in these diverse fields.

REFERENCES

Andersen, S. M., & Chen, S. (2002). The relational self: An interpersonal social-cognitive theory. *Psychological Review, 109,* 619–645.

Arriaga, X. B., Kumashiro, M., Simpson, J. A., & Overall, N. C. (2018). Revising working models across time: Relationship situations that enhance attachment security. *Personality and Social Psychology Review, 22,* 71–96.

Berant, E., Mikulincer, M., & Shaver, P. R. (2008). Mothers' attachment style, their mental health, and their children's emotional vulnerabilities: A seven-year study of children with congenital heart disease. *Journal of Personality, 76,* 31–66.

Bowlby, J. (1973). *Attachment and loss: Vol. 2. Separation.* New York: Basic Books.

Bowlby, J. (1982). *Attachment and loss: Vol. 1. Attachment* (2nd ed.). New York: Basic Books. (Original work published 1969)

Brennan, K. A., Clark, C. L., & Shaver, P. R. (1998). Self-report measurement of adult attachment: An integrative overview. In J. A. Simpson & W. S. Rholes (Eds.), *Attachment theory and close relationships* (pp. 46–76). New York: Guilford Press.

Brumbaugh, C. C., & Fraley, R. C. (2007). Transference of attachment patterns: How important relationships influence feelings toward novel people. *Personal Relationships, 14,* 513–530.

Davidovitz, R., Mikulincer, M., Shaver, P. R., Ijzak, R., & Popper, M. (2007). Leaders as attachment figures: Their attachment orientations predict leadership-related mental representations and followers' performance and mental health. *Journal of Personality and Social Psychology, 93,* 632–650.

Davila, J., Steinberg, S. J., Kachadourian, L., Cobb, R., & Fincham, F. (2004). Romantic involvement and depressive symptoms in early and late adolescence: The role of a preoccupied relational style. *Personal Relationships, 11,* 161–178.

Fraley, R. C., & Roisman, G. I. (2019). The development of adult attachment styles: Four lessons. *Current Opinion in Psychology, 25,* 26–30.

Fraley, R. C., Roisman, G. I., Booth-LaForce, C., Owen, M. T., & Holland, A. S. (2013). Interpersonal and genetic origins of adult attachment styles: A longitudinal study from infancy to early adulthood. *Journal of Personality and Social Psychology, 104,* 817–838.

Granqvist, P. (2020). *Attachment in religion and spirituality: A wider view.* New York: Guilford Press.

Håvås, E., Svartberg, M., & Ulvenes, P. (2015). Attuning to the unspoken: The relationship between therapist nonverbal attunement and attachment security in adult psychotherapy. *Psychoanalytic Psychology, 32,* 235–254.

Hazan, C., & Shaver, P. R. (1987). Romantic love conceptualized as an attachment process. *Journal of Personality and Social Psychology, 52,* 511–524.

Mikulincer, M., Ein-Dor, T., Solomon, Z., & Shaver, P. R. (2011). Trajectories of attachment insecurities over a 17-year period: A latent growth curve analysis of the impact of war captivity and posttraumatic stress disorder. *Journal of Social and Clinical Psychology, 30,* 960–984.

Mikulincer, M., & Shaver, P. R. (2016). *Attachment in adulthood: Structure, dynamics, and change* (2nd ed.). New York: Guilford Press.

Simpson, J. A., Collins, W. A., Salvatore, J. E., & Sung, S. (2014). The impact of early interpersonal experience on adult romantic relationship functioning. In M. Mikulincer & P. R. Shaver (Eds.), *Mechanisms of social connection: From brain to group* (pp. 221–234). Washington, DC: American Psychological Association.

Simpson, J. A., & Overall, N. C. (2014). Partner buffering of attachment insecurity. *Current Directions in Psychological Science, 23,* 54–59.

Zayas, V., Mischel, W., Shoda, Y., & Aber, J. L. (2011). Roots of adult attachment: Maternal caregiving at 18 months predicts adult peer and partner attachment. *Social Psychological and Personality Science, 2,* 289–297.

CHAPTER 27

Early Attachment from the Perspective of Life-History Theory

Ohad Szepsenwol
Jeffry A. Simpson

The attachment system is an innate motivational system that becomes activated in response to threatening or distressing stimuli and regulates proximity-seeking behaviors aimed at reestablishing felt security (Bowlby, 1969/1982; Sroufe & Waters, 1977). Human infants are defenseless and require the protection of stronger and wiser caregivers. Seeking proximity to a primary caregiver when threatened or distressed, therefore, is a behavioral strategy that presumably enhanced infants' reproductive fitness in our evolutionary past. The enduring effects of early attachment experiences on cognitive, emotional, and behavioral outcomes suggest that the attachment system may also serve evolutionary functions later in life. In this chapter, we suggest that both secure and insecure early attachment experiences and their representations act as mediators of important information about early environments that channel development toward evolutionarily adaptive trajectories. We draw on recent advances in life-history theory and attachment research to support this premise.

Life-History Theory

Life-history theory (LHT) outlines the trade-offs individuals make when investing their limited time, energy, and resources toward accomplishing important life tasks, such as growth and reproduction (Del Giudice, Gangestad, & Kaplan, 2016). For example, the number of children an individual has reflects a compromise between the reproductive advantages of having a large number of children in relation to the investments required to raise a healthy, competent child. Different types of strategies, known as life-history (LH) strategies, are associated with different physical, psychological, and demographic characteristics (phenotypes). One key insight of LHT is that the optimal LH strategy is contingent on several fundamental properties of the local environment to which individuals are "evolutionarily designed" to perceive and react.

Two principal parameters that calibrate LH strategies are the degree of harshness (morbidity and mortality) and unpredictability (random fluctuations) in the local environment (Ellis, Figueredo, Brumbach, & Schlomer, 2009). Environments that are harsh and/or unpredictable should motivate individuals to achieve as much as they can before a more probable early death. Hence, they promote a *fast* LH strategy, which entails a shorter growth period (e.g., early menarche and pubertal timing), early reproduction, and a greater number of children to offset higher child mortality rates. In contrast, environments that are safe and predictable, in which premature death is less likely, allow individuals to accrue embodied and material resources before reproducing and to invest more resources in their children to increase their competence and chances of survival. Such environments, therefore, promote a *slow* LH strategy, which entails an extended growth period (e.g., later menarche, delayed puberty), delayed reproduction, more stable pair bonds, and greater eventual parental investment.

Studies show that exposure to harshness and unpredictability during childhood have enduring effects on LH strategies (e.g., Simpson, Griskevicius, Kuo, Sung, & Collins, 2012). Presumably, this is because early environments signal to the developing child what future environments might be like, promoting the development of traits and capabilities that enhance fitness in such environments. These early-developing traits and capabilities form the basis for adult LH strategies (Simpson & Belsky, 2016).

Integrating LHT and Attachment Theory

The calibration of LH strategies to match environmental conditions occurs across development. For this process to occur, early local conditions (i.e., levels of harshness and unpredictability) must be detected and processed in a way that generates strategic physiological and psychological adjustments in the developing child. This is problematic because children are not directly aware of how safe and predictable their local environment is. They are, however, aware of the quality of parental care they receive, which tends to be better and more reliable in safe and predictable environments (Simpson & Belsky, 2016). Thus, through their caregiving behaviors, parents mediate the effects of local environments on their children.

The quality and reliability of interactions with caregivers affects and calibrates the child's attachment system. Through such repeated interactions, a child develops mental representations and expectations (internal working models [IWMs]) about the responsiveness and availability of caregivers (Bowlby, 1973; Main, Kaplan, & Cassidy, 1985). These IWMs shape the child's future behavior in similar situations. The attachment system, in other words, provides a mechanism through which information regarding the quality of the caregiving environment and, indirectly, the safety and predictability of the local environment, becomes internalized by the child, which can lead to phenotypic adjustments that enhance fitness. When the caregiving environment is harsh or unreliable (e.g., neglectful or inconsistent parenting), the child typically develops insecure attachment representations. Not being able to rely on the availability and responsiveness of the caregiver, the child often develops either a "hyperactivated" attachment system designed to force responsiveness from the caregiver (anxious-resistant attachment) or a "deactivated" system that suppresses proximity-seeking behaviors (avoidant-resistant attachment) (Main, 1981). In contrast, when the caregiving environment is reliably good (e.g., sensitive and responsive parenting), the child typically develops secure attachment representations, which include positive expectations about the availability and support of the caregiver and feeling safe and confident to explore the surrounding world.

How do early attachment representations help to shape LH strategies later in life? According to LH models (see Simpson & Belsky, 2016), secure attachment promotes the development of slow LH traits that should be more adaptive in safe, predictable environments, whereas insecure attachment promotes the development of fast LH traits that ought to be more adaptive in harsh and/or unpredictable environments (Szepsenwol & Simpson, 2019). Early attachment security should be a fundamental construct in this causal chain because it (1) sets the stage for attachment security throughout life (Fraley, 2002), (2) is important for the development of basic interpersonal and regulatory competencies that support a slow LH strategy (e.g., emotion regulation, social competence; Calkins & Leerkes, 2011; Groh et al., 2014), and (3) forecasts the emergence of personality traits that are more adaptive for a slow LH strategy (e.g., agreeableness, conscientiousness, emotional stability; Young, Simpson, Griskevicius, Huelsnitz, & Fleck, 2019). Early attachment security, therefore, may be an important mediator between sensitive, responsive parenting, rooted in safe and predictable early environments, and psychological traits that facilitate slow LH strategies. We now review evidence linking early attachment security with four of the main markers of a slow LH strategy.

Early Attachment Security Predicts Slow LH Traits

Mating Strategies

A main prediction of LHT is that growing up in a safe and predictable environment should forecast a long-term mating strategy characterized by stable, committed romantic relationships (Belsky, Steinberg, & Draper, 1991). Recent evidence from the Minnesota Longitudinal Study of Risk and Adaptation (MLSRA) reveals that this link is partially mediated by attachment representations. Individuals whose first 4 years of life were more predictable (based on the stability in parents' employment, cohabitation, and residence) were more likely to receive better early supportive parenting from their mothers, which predicted more secure attachment representations at age 19. Attachment security, in turn, predicted greater engagement or desire to engage in long-term romantic relationships at age 23 (Szepsenwol et al., 2017).

Direct evidence linking early attachment security with mating strategies is more limited. Several longitudinal studies, however, have found that early attachment security prospectively predicts interpersonal behaviors known to promote more stable romantic relationships. For example, individuals categorized as secure in the Strange Situation at 12 months of age have more positive emotional experiences in their romantic relationships in early adulthood and display less negative affect during conflict resolution and collaboration tasks with their romantic partners (Simpson, Collins, Tran, & Haydon, 2007). Similarly, individuals categorized as secure at 12 and 18 months exhibit better conflict-recovery skills in adulthood following conflict discussions with their romantic partners (Salvatore, Kuo, Steele, Simpson, & Collins, 2011). These findings suggest that the interpersonal skills necessary to enact a long-term mating strategy successfully are rooted in early attachment security.

Parental Attitudes and Behavior

LHT and attachment theory share the premise that parental behaviors in adulthood are influenced by early rearing experiences. According to LHT, growing up in a safe, predictable environment should forecast greater parental investment, a hallmark of a slow LH strategy. This may be especially true for men, for whom there is a stronger trade-off between investing in existing children and having more children via additional mating (Geary, 2000). Indeed, recent findings from the MLSRA reveal that males whose first 4 years of life were more predictable had more positive attitudes about parenting at age 32 and displayed more supportive parenting behavior in videotaped interactions with their infant children. Moreover, the connection between early predictability and better adult parenting was serially mediated by the quality of early parenting they had received from their mothers and the resultant security of their attachment representations at ages 19 and 26 (Szepsenwol, Simpson, Griskevicius, & Raby, 2015). Although this research did not examine early attachment security directly, it highlights the important intermediary role of the early caregiving environment and subsequent attachment representations in the link between early environments and adult parenting.

Pubertal Timing

Another key insight of LH models is that psychological development and physiological development should be interwoven and calibrated by the same early environmental cues (Belsky et al., 1991). For girls, this means that growing up in a safe, predictable environment should delay the onset of puberty, given that such environments favor somatic growth over early reproduction. Some evidence supports this idea and points to the involvement of early attachment in this process. For example, in findings from the National Institute of Child Health and Human Development Study of Early Child Care and Youth Development (SECCYD), girls who grew up in relatively poor families (lower income-to-needs ratio) but were classified as secure in the Strange Situation at 15 months experienced later menarche than lower income girls classified as insecure (Sung et al., 2016).

Physical Health

An additional important prediction of LHT is that individuals who grow up in a safe, predictable environment should experience better adult physical health and greater longevity compared to individuals who grow up in a harsh and/or unpredictable environment (Ellis et al., 2009). The reason for this is that safe and predictable environments have fewer uncontrollable sources of morbidity and mortality, which should promote a prolonged period of somatic growth and greater somatic maintenance at the expense of earlier reproduction. Evidence from the MLSRA indicates that the attachment system plays a key role in this process. Individuals who were classified as secure during infancy (at both age 12 months and age 18 months) were less likely to report having a diagnosed physical illness at age 32 (Puig, Englund, Simpson, & Collins, 2013; see also Ehrlich & Cassidy, Chapter 25, this volume).

Boundary Conditions

Our discussion thus far has focused on how early attachment security is prospectively related to slow LH traits. We do not mean to imply, however, that the enduring effects of early attachment on behaviors, cognitions, and emotions can be fully understood within an LHT framework. LHT is concerned with variables governing the pace of growth, reproduction, and aging. The purview of attachment theory, of course, extends well beyond this. For example, unlike attachment theory, LHT does not make predictions regarding the quality of one's living experience (e.g., life satisfaction), primarily because it has little significance for evolutionary fitness. Another example is religiosity. While some scholars have proposed a link between the attachment system and religious thoughts and behaviors (e.g., Kirkpatrick, 1998), it is unlikely that such links reflect an LH process. Although religiosity is associated with some LH outcomes in modern times (e.g., reproductive decisions), it is unlikely that religiosity mediated the pace of growth, reproduction, and aging during our ancestral past. Researchers, therefore, should be cautious when applying LH logic to attachment processes, ensuring that the predicted traits or behaviors were connected in theoretically meaningful ways to patterns of growth, reproduction, and aging in our ancestral past.

Future Directions

It is important to understand *how* early attachment representations are prospectively related to different LH strategies. Mediating mechanisms could have psychological, physiological, and/or behavioral components. One possibility involving all three components is that early attachment has an enduring impact on stress reactivity and both emotion regulation and expression, which in turn shapes interpersonal functioning throughout life (see Ehrlich & Cassidy, Chapter 25, this volume). Individuals who were securely attached as infants do show an early advantage in buffered hypothalamus–pituitary–adrenal axis reactivity (Gunnar, Broderson, Nachmias, Buss, & Rigatuso, 1996) and tend to express their emotions in more well-regulated ways (Calkins & Leerkes, 2011). This allows them to maintain better relationships, parent more effectively, and manage stress in a healthier way. In contrast, individuals who were insecurely attached as infants are typically more reactive to stress and express their emotions in poorly regulated ways (e.g., excessive anger, intensified distress), which may expedite the achievement of certain short-term goals (such as fending off rivals or gaining attention), but often is maladaptive in the long run. Thus, patterns of stress reactivity and emotion regulation and expression may mediate the relation between early attachment representations and adult LH strategies.

Conclusions

Early attachment representations serve an evolutionary function by mediating the effects of early environments on adult LH strategies. Early attachment security, which is rooted in supportive caregiving experiences that occurred in safe, predictable rearing environments, forecasts the development of a slow LH strategy characterized by delayed puberty, a long-term mating strategy, high parental investment, and a longer, healthier life. In the future, the productive integration of attachment theory and LHT will be facilitated by a better understanding of the mechanisms that link early attachment and LH strategies.

REFERENCES

Belsky, J., Steinberg, L., & Draper, P. (1991). Childhood experience, interpersonal development, and reproductive strategy: An evolutionary theory of socialization. *Child Development, 62,* 647–670.

Bowlby, J. (1973). *Attachment and loss: Vol. 2. Separation.* New York: Basic Books.

Bowlby, J. (1982). *Attachment and loss: Vol. 1. Attachment* (2nd ed.). New York: Basic Books. (Original work published 1969)

Calkins, S. D., & Leerkes, E. M. (2011). Early attachment processes and the development of emotional self-regulation. In K. D. Vohs & R. F. Baumeister (Eds.), *Handbook of self-regulation: Research, theory, and applications* (2nd ed., pp. 355–373). New York: Guilford Press.

Del Giudice, M., Gangestad, S. W., & Kaplan, H. S. (2016). LH theory and evolutionary psychology. In D. M. Buss (Ed.), *The handbook of evolutionary psychology* (2nd ed., Vol. 1, pp. 88–114). Hoboken, NJ: Wiley.

Ellis, B. J., Figueredo, A. J., Brumbach, B., & Schlomer, G. (2009). Fundamental dimensions of environmental risk: The impact of harsh versus unpredictable environments on the evolution and development of LH strategies. *Human Nature, 20,* 204–268.

Fraley, R. C. (2002). Attachment stability from infancy to adulthood: Meta-analysis and dynamic modeling of developmental mechanisms. *Personality and Social Psychology Review, 6,* 123–151.

Geary, D. C. (2000). Evolution and proximate expression of human paternal investment. *Psychological Bulletin, 126,* 55–77.

Groh, A. M., Fearon, R. P., Bakermans-Kranenburg, M. J., van IJzendoorn, M. H., Steele, R. D., & Roisman, G. I. (2014). The significance of attachment security for children's social competence with peers: A meta-analytic study. *Attachment and Human Development, 16,* 103–136.

Gunnar, M. R., Brodersen, L., Nachmias, M., Buss, K., & Rigatuso, J. (1996). Stress reactivity and attachment security. *Developmental Psychobiology, 29,* 191–204.

Kirkpatrick, L. A. (1998). God as a substitute attachment figure: A longitudinal study of adult attachment style and religious change in college students. *Personality and Social Psychology Bulletin, 24,* 961–973.

Main, M. (1981). Avoidance in the service of attachment: A working paper. In K. Immelmann, G. Barlow, M. Main, & L. Petrinovich (Eds.), *Behavioral development: The Bielefeld Interdisciplinary Project* (pp. 651–693). New York: Cambridge University Press.

Main, M., Kaplan, N., & Cassidy, J. (1985). Security in infancy, childhood, and adulthood: A move to the level of representation. In I. Bretherton & E. Waters (Eds.), Growing points of attachment theory and research. *Monographs of the Society for Research in Child Development, 50*(1–2, Serial No. 209), 66–104.

Puig, J., Englund, M. M., Simpson, J. A., & Collins, W. A. (2013). Predicting adult physical illness from infant attachment: A prospective longitudinal study. *Health Psychology, 32,* 409–417.

Salvatore, J. E., Kuo, S. I. C., Steele, R. D., Simpson, J. A., & Collins, W. A. (2011). Recovering from conflict in romantic relationships: A developmental perspective. *Psychological Science, 22,* 376–383.

Simpson, J. A., & Belsky, J. (2016). Attachment theory within a modern evolutionary framework. In J. Cassidy & P. R. Shaver (Eds.), *Handbook of attachment: Theory, research, and clinical applications* (3rd ed., pp. 91–116). New York: Guilford Press.

Simpson, J. A., Collins, W. A., Tran, S., & Haydon, K. C. (2007). Attachment and the experience and expression of emotions in romantic relationships: A developmental perspective. *Journal of Personality and Social Psychology, 92,* 355–367.

Simpson, J. A., Griskevicius, V., Kuo, S. I. C., Sung, S., & Collins, W. A. (2012). Evolution, stress, and sensitive periods: The influence of unpredictability in early versus late childhood on sex and risky behavior. *Developmental Psychology, 48,* 674–686.

Sroufe, L. A., & Waters, E. (1977). Attachment as an organizational construct. *Child Development, 48,* 1184–1199.

Sung, S., Simpson, J. A., Griskevicius, V., Kuo, S. I. C., Schlomer, G. L., & Belsky, J. (2016). Secure infant–mother attachment buffers the effect of early-life stress on age of menarche. *Psychological Science, 27,* 667–674.

Szepsenwol, O., Griskevicius, V., Simpson, J. A., Young, E. S., Fleck, C., & Jones, R. E. (2017). The effect of predictable early childhood environments on sociosexuality in early adulthood. *Evolutionary Behavioral Sciences, 11,* 131–145.

Szepsenwol, O., & Simpson, J. A. (2019). Attachment within LH theory: An evolutionary perspective on individual differences in attachment. *Current Opinion in Psychology, 25,* 65–70.

Szepsenwol, O., Simpson, J. A., Griskevicius, V., & Raby, K. L. (2015). The effect of unpredictable early childhood environments on parenting in adulthood. *Journal of Personality and Social Psychology, 109,* 1045–1067.

Young, E. S., Simpson, J. A., Griskevicius, V., Huelsnitz, C. O., & Fleck, C. (2019). Childhood attachment and adult personality: A life history perspective. *Self and Identity, 18,* 22–38.

TOPIC 6

CULTURE AND ATTACHMENT

- How are attachment processes manifested in different cultures?

- How does culture manifest itself in attachment processes?

CHAPTER 28

Attachment Theory
Fact or Fancy?

Heidi Keller

After initial resistance, attachment theory has become the leading theory of social-emotional development since its first formulation during the 1960s–1970s. It proposes that during ancestral times selective pressures resulted in children developing an emotional bond with one or a few caregivers during the first year of life in order to promote protective security. The quality of the attachment relationship is regarded as dependent upon parenting quality, specifically sensitive responsiveness to an infant's signals. In addition, this relationship organizes the child's further psychological development (Bowlby, 1969). Attachment is regarded as universal in its meaning, its developmental sequence, the conditions of its emergence, its qualities, and its predictive power for developmental consequences.

The majority of attachment researchers continue to claim validity of the original formulations 50 years later (e.g., Cassidy, 2016). Recently, some attachment scholars have argued that 21st-century attachment theory has developed from its origins and is substantially different from the original (Duschinsky, van IJzendoorn, Foster, Reijman, & Lionetti, 2020; Thompson, 2017). However, they mainly refer to topical extensions, such as from a focus on the infant–caregiver relationship to relationships and development in general, including psychopathology, and to diverse fields of application (for an overview, see Cassidy & Shaver, 2016). Attachment theory thus serves as an umbrella for attachment mini theories. Yet, attachment researchers also acknowledge that the theory was flawed from the beginning, with fuzzy definitions of core conceptions. Ross Thompson, who argues for the relevance and applicability of attachment theory as it is now conceptualized, acknowledged its shortcomings when he said that on some issues, "it is difficult to indicate definitively what attachment theory currently claims" (2017, p. 303). This conclusion is shared by critics of attachment theory in general and its change over the last 50 years in particular, such as Marga Vicedo, who asks, "And, what *is* attachment theory today?" (2020, p. 153).

In the following paragraphs I briefly summarize the major problems of attachment theory with respect to three theses:

1. The basic assumptions are mainly ambiguous and fuzzy or wrong.
2. Attachment theory is a purely monocultural theory that cannot claim universality.
3. Attachment theory does not meet the criteria for a good theory.

I will conclude that the description, explanation, and prediction of children's development in terms of attachment theory are not appropriate for many children on this planet and, therefore, not only are they unscientific but also ethical implications have to be taken into consideration (e.g., Rosabal-Coto et al., 2017).

The Basic Assumptions Are Mainly Ambiguous and Fuzzy or Wrong

The problematic aspects of attachment theory start with its definition. What is attachment as an emotional bond? Is it a relational strategy between a child and a particular caregiver? Is it a trait or a characteristic of the child that gives rise to predictions for further development (competence assumption)? Also problematic are ill-defined conceptions of sensitive parenting important to the quality of attachment relationships and the mechanisms by which this relationship becomes important to a child's development. Parental sensitivity is based on implicit assumptions about a particular cultural model of development and, related to this, favorable developmental outcomes. These implicit assumptions are tied to a particular conception of the person in a particular cultural historical time. Internal working models of relationships (are they a cognitive schema? an emotional bias?) are assumed to derive from children's attachment relationships, but there is little consensus among attachment researchers about how these models develop and how they function, as attachment researchers themselves have pointed out (Thompson, 2017).

It is stated that attachment evolved as an adaptation during the evolution of humankind and is therefore universal. Attachment theory—as it is understood and applied—is about children's well-being; evolutionary theory, however, is about reproductive success. Evolution does not pursue particular goals, such as security of attachment, and adaptation does not imply universality. Moreover, rhesus monkeys, with an extensive mother–child caregiving system, are taken as the primate model for human attachment development. But rhesus monkeys are just one primate species among many and therefore not representative of human development in different social ecological contexts (Vicedo, 2017). Moreover, variability is the human condition, so one model can never apply to all.

Another bias in the formulation of attachment theory is that Bowlby was informed and impressed by clinical cases of postwar traumatized children and conceptualized children's normal development from a deficit perspective. Thus, developmental resources and resilience are underestimated.

Attachment Theory Is a Purely Monocultural Theory That Cannot Claim Universality

The emergence of attachment theory must be understood in the historical context of the postwar Western world, as Marga Vicedo (2017) has convincingly argued. Several implicit assumptions are inherently part of this socioecological context and this historical epoch. The most important of these implicit assumptions starts with the credo that adults need to be the caretakers of small children. This assumption is tied to the prevalent family model in this context, specifically the two-generation nuclear family with a small number of children. These adults need to have time and resources to care for a baby in a particular way, including to be exclusively available and attentive to the baby and responsive to all the— even subtlest—signals. The preferred communication channel is face to face, which necessitates a dyadic mode of interaction, following a dialogical structure with the infant having the lead (e.g., German middle-class mothers react to the increased wakefulness around age 2 months with increased face-to-face contact and smiling; see Kärtner, Keller, & Yovsi, 2010; Wörmann, Holodynski, Kärtner, & Keller, 2012). Verbalization and mentalization of the infant's inner world (feelings, cognitions, intentions, preferences, wishes) lead to emphasizing particular dimensions of development, especially the development of a separate sense of self and an autobiographical embodiment of the self. Emotion expression, especially maintaining positive emotionality, is considered as crucial for children's healthy development. This socialization strategy is based in higher formal education and is associated with an inward turn, specifically reflecting about one's inner world and mental states (Eksen, 2010). The intensive dyadic social encounters are complemented by an equally important focus on infants learning to rely on themselves. Therefore, infants are referred to objects rather than to people because many people are regarded as overstimulating to an infant and distract the infant from him- or herself. This socialization strategy is aimed at reaching early psychological auton-omy in terms of a self-sufficient, self-contained, and separate self. Secure attachment would enable the child to become such an independent agent pursuing his or her own interests and intentions (Keller, 2007; Keller & Kärtner, 2013).

This socialization strategy contrasts sharply with the ideas and prac-tices that families value in many other parts of the world. However, there is not a single other strategy, but substantial cultural psychological and anthropological evidence to infer many different parenting strategies in different social ecologies (e.g., Lancy, 2005). A variety of family mod-els exists, with variations in composition with related and non-related members, different structures, and different functions. Different family systems necessitate different caregiving arrangements compared to the nuclear family that provided the context used by attachment theorists. Rural subsistence-based farming community households (which comprise four to six times the number of people in Western middle-class house-holds) have especially clear boundaries between children's and adults' worlds (see, e.g., Madagascan villagers in Scheidecker, 2017). In these small-scale farming communities, primary caregivers of small children are mainly other children, and there is not one or two main caregivers but a caregiving network. The biological mother may be an important part in this network, but she may also be one of several caregivers with equal responsibilities, or she may have a circumscribed role only (e.g., only breastfeeding). Children experience substantial amounts of body con-tact and motor stimulation, which emphasize different socialization goals than the Western middle-class philosophy. In many contexts, children are expected to suppress emotions in the presence of adults (but maybe not in children's groups), so that stranger anxiety does not appear in the behavioral repertoire (for an extensive discussion of cultural conceptions and differences in parenting strategies, see Keller & Chaudhary, 2017). Instead of an early differentiation between the self and others (such as the development of a categorical self), children are supposed to grow into a relational network with a conception of the self as a part of a social unit. It is within this socially symbiotic unit that, together with an emphasis on motor development, children become self-reliant and responsible mem-bers of the household at an early age. This parenting strategy is built not on children taking the lead but on caregivers structuring and leading.

Knowledge about socialization strategies from other contexts than the Western middle-class world is still restricted. There is some system-atic research from subsistence-based farmers (e.g., Gottlieb, 2004; Keller,

2007; Otto & Keller, 2014; Quinn & Mageo, 2013), which has been briefly summarized before. There are singular studies from hunter-and-gatherer and pastoral societies (e.g., Morelli, Henry, & Spielvogel, 2019). Much more culturally informed research is needed to derive a more comprehensive picture of children's development globally. In any case it can be concluded that the socialization goals and strategies that attachment theory claims are universally valid apply, if at all, only to a small part of the world's population. As discussed before, many children are raised in relational networks that are differently organized and structured compared to relationships in small nuclear families.

Attachment Theory Does Not Meet the Criteria for a Good Theory

A good theory consists of clearly defined interrelated theoretical assumptions that can be tested and accepted or rejected. One of the problems of attachment theory is that many of its core concepts are not clearly defined and, therefore, are subject to multiple interpretations. Attachment researchers appear more interested in confirming the theory than in testing it (see Mesman, Chapter 30, this volume). Researchers with results that do not fit their assumptions do not question those assumptions and possibly modify their theory but instead explain them post hoc in cultural or contextual terms. In a study by Agrawal and Gulati (2005) with an Indian urban middle-class sample, 100% of the children were classified as securely attached in the Strange Situation Procedure. The results were explained post hoc as expressing close proximity of Indian babies with their mothers during day and night. The influence of continuous body contact on the development of attachment security, however, was not tested. Another explanation that is offered to dismiss results that don't fit the theory concerns methodology. For example, Mesman, van IJzendoorn, and Sagi-Schwartz (2016, p. 871) concluded "that in many cases the coding is done by researchers who have not been formally trained by experts, which makes the quality of the classifications unclear." The experts are Western attachment researchers. The cultural knowledge of local coders, which may have influenced their coding, is regarded as disturbing.

Moreover, attachment researchers only accept research evidence that has been assessed with methods that have been developed by attachment researchers themselves and that are recognized by them, like the Strange Situation Procedure and the Attachment Q-Sort. This implies the confound of theory and method (see, e.g., Lamb, Thompson, Gardner, Charnov, & Estes, 1984). It also means that cultural evidence about local conceptions and practices of childrearing is ignored intentionally.

Conclusion

Children grow up in different learning environments and develop within the cultural scripts of their caregivers. Concomitant to their early experiences, pathways of development are constructed and co-constructed that differ from each other with respect to the timing, the structure, and the results of developmental achievements (Keller & Kärtner, 2013). The logical consequence is that attachment as defined in the Western middle-class culture cannot be regarded as a universal phenomenon. Nevertheless, health care services, parenting support programs, and interventions, as well as the educational systems in multicultural Western societies and their outreach in other parts of the world, rely on attachment theory as the gold standard for children's well-being and education. Yet, evaluating one system with the standards of another system leads to invalid results. For example, caregiving arrangements with relational networks of other children and very restricted contact with the mother and adults in general (cf. Scheidecker, 2017), cannot be evaluated as a deficit *per se* and corrected with intervention programs focusing on the mother and positive parenting derived from attachment theory (for scientific and ethical problems involved, see Morelli et al., 2017; Rosabal-Coto et al., 2017; Serpell & Nsamenang, 2014).

The formulation of attachment theory was an important paradigmatic shift in Western developmental sciences and will continue to represent a historical scientific landmark. However, 50 years later attachment theorists and researchers should not only acknowledge cultural differences in raising children and ideas about children's healthy development, but also take these differences seriously. Moreover, the conceptual and theoretical flaws of attachment theory that are widely recognized should be remedied. Researchers as well as practitioners should accept the ethical responsibilities that are an inherent part of their professions.

ACKNOWLEDGMENT

I am extremely grateful to Gilda Morelli and Marga Vicedo for many constructive comments to drafts of this chapter.

REFERENCES

Agrawal, P., & Gulati, J. (2005). The patterns of infant mother attachment as a function of home environment. *Journal of Human Ecology, 18*(4), 287–293.

Bowlby, J. (1969). *Attachment and loss: Vol. 1. Attachment*. New York: Basic Books.

Cassidy, J. (2016). The nature of the child's ties. In J. Cassidy & P. R. Shaver (Eds.), *Handbook of attachment: Theory, research, and clinical applications* (3rd ed., pp. 3–22). New York: Guilford Press.

Cassidy, J., & Shaver, P. R. (Eds.). (2016). *Handbook of attachment: Theory, research, and clinical applications* (3rd ed.). New York: Guilford Press.

Duschinsky, R., van IJzendoorn, M., Foster, S., Reijman, S., & Lionetti, F. (2020). Attachment histories and futures: Reply to Vicedo's "Putting attachment in its place." *European Journal of Developmental Psychology, 17*(1), 138–146.

Eksen, K. (2010). "Inward turn" and the Augustinian self. *Diametros, 25,* 132–145.

Gottlieb, A. (2004). *The afterlife is where we come from: The culture of infancy in West Africa.* Chicago: University of Chicago Press.

Kärtner, J., Keller, H., & Yovsi, R. D. (2010). Mother–infant interaction during the first three months: The emergence of culture-specific contingency patterns. *Child Development, 81*(2), 540–554.

Keller, H. (2007). *Cultures of infancy.* Mahwah, NJ: Erlbaum.

Keller, H., & Chaudhary, N. (2017). Is the mother essential for attachment?: Models of care in different cultures. In H. Keller & K. A. Bard (Eds.), *Contextualizing attachment: The cultural nature of attachment* (pp. 109–138). Cambridge MA: MIT Press.

Keller, H., & Kärtner, J. (2013). Development: The culture-specific solution of universal developmental tasks. In M. L. Gelfand, C.-Y. Chiu, & Y. Y. Hong (Eds.), *Advances in culture and psychology* (Vol. 3, pp. 63–116). Oxford, UK: Oxford University Press.

Lamb, M. E., Thompson, R. A., Gardner, W., Charnov, E. L., & Estes, D. (1984). Security of infantile attachment as assessed in the Strange Situation: Its study and biological interpretation. *Behavioral and Brain Sciences, 7,* 127–147.

Lancy, D. F. (2005). *The anthropology of childhood* (2nd ed.). Cambridge, UK: Cambridge University Press.

Mesman, J., van IJzendoorn, M. H., & Sagi-Schwartz, A. (2016). Cross-cultural patterns of attachment: Universals and contextual dimensions. In J. Cassidy & P. R. Shaver (Eds.), *Handbook of attachment: Theory, research, and clinical applications* (3rd ed., pp. 790–815). New York: Guilford Press.

Morelli, G., Henry, P. I., & Spielvogel, B. (2019). Learning prosociality: Insights from young forager and subsistence farmer children's food sharing with mothers and others. *Behavioral Ecology and Sociobiology, 73*(6), 1–20.

Morelli, G., Quinn, N., Chaudhary, N., Vicedo, M., Rosabal-Coto, M., Murray, M., . . . Takada, A. (2017). Ethical challenges of parenting intervention in low- to middle-income countries. *Journal of Cross Cultural Psychology, 49*(1), 5–24.

Otto, H., & Keller, H. (Eds.). (2014). *Different faces of attachment.* Cambridge, UK: Cambridge University Press.

Quinn, N., & Mageo, J. M. (Eds.). (2013). *Attachment reconsidered: Cultural perspectives on a Western theory.* New York: Palgrave Macmillan.

Rosabal-Coto, M., Quinn, N., Keller, H., Vicedo, M., Chaudhary, N., Gottlieb, A., & Morelli, G. A. (2017). Real world applications of attachment theory. In H. Keller & K. A. Bard (Eds.), *Contextualizing attachment: The cultural nature of attachment* (pp. 335–354). Cambridge, MA: MIT Press.

Scheidecker, G. (2017). *Kindheit, kultur und moralische emotionen: Zur sozialisation von furcht und wut im ländlichen Madagaskar.* Bielefeld, Germany: Transcript Verlag.

Serpell, R., & Nsamenang, A. B. (2014). *Locally relevant and quality ECCE programmes: Implications of research on indigenous African child development and socialization*. Paris: UNESCO.

Thompson, R. A. (2017). Twenty-first century attachment theory: Challenges and opportunities. In H. Keller & K. A. Bard (Eds.), *Contextualizing attachment: The cultural nature of attachment* (pp. 301–319). Cambridge, MA: MIT Press.

Vicedo, M. (2017). Putting attachment in its place: Disciplinary and cultural contexts. *European Journal of Developmental Psychology, 14*(6), 684–699.

Vicedo, M. (2020). On the history, present and future of attachment theory: Reply to Robbie Duschinsky, Marinus van IJzendoorn, Sarah Foster, Sophie Reijman & Francesca Lionetti "attachment histories and futures." *European Journal of Developmental Psychology, 17*(1), 147–155.

Wörmann, V., Holodynski, M., Kärtner, J., & Keller, H. (2012). A cross-cultural comparison of the development of the social smile: A longitudinal study of maternal and infant imitation in 6- and 12-week-old infants. *Infant Behavior and Development, 35*(3), 335–347.

CHAPTER 29

Pluralities and Commonalities in Children's Relationships
Care of Efe Forager Infants as a Case Study

Gilda Morelli
Linxi Lu

All children develop attachment relationships, except perhaps in the harshest circumstances. The ability to do so is part of our human legacy, representing a universal need to form meaningful, close ties with others (Baumeister & Leary, 1995). It is usual for children to form attachments with people they trust to meet their needs and to keep them safe in contexts of threat (Labile, Thompson, & Froimson, 2015), thereby distinguishing attachments from other types of social relationships. When safe from threats, children are better able to learn about and participate fully in their community. What it means for a child to feel threatened, to feel safe, and to trust are intimately tied to ecocultural aspects of community life. Thus, attachment relationships, and processes underpinning them, reflect and are responsive to local phenomena. We offer support for this thesis by considering basic relational features of biobehavioral synchrony and construals of self and other. We reflect on these features related to attachment relationships in contexts of infants' care in a small-scale foraging society.

Children's Care in Small-Scale Societies and Other-Regarding Relational Orientations[1]

Children's care has profound implications for their attachments, and the care of children varies in systematic ways across communities (Keller &

---

[1] The term *children* or *young children* refers to ~24-month-olds and younger; the term *infants* refers to ~15-month-olds and younger.

Kärtner, 2013). We have learned more about these associations by going beyond the families with Western middle-class lifestyles who are usually studied. In families with small-scale, subsistence lifestyles—the most prevalent lifestyles globally (e.g., Global Agriculture, n.d.)—it is common for children to grow up in extended or multigenerational households (versus nuclear), with many children (versus few), and more than a few child and adult caregivers (versus one or two adults). It is usual for these children to be near or in physical contact with caregivers and for caregivers to prefer proximal (e.g., tactile, kinesthetic) and other forms of care (e.g., anticipating children's needs). In such care contexts, children learn other-regarding relational orientations whereby they experience themselves as socially interdependent and obligated, and integrate others' needs and interests with their own (compared to self-regarding, to experience self as separate from others, to act on self-interests and needs) (e.g., Cohen, Hoshino-Browne, & Leung, 2007). Care intensifies social interconnections, increasing the likelihood that children will maintain them.

Diversity in children's care gives rise to a plurality of relational experiences and relationships. Alongside this plurality are relationship features common to all (Sutcliffe, Dunbar, Binder, & Arrow, 2012). One that stands out is biobehavioral synchrony.

Biobehavioral Synchrony

Synchrony refers to *temporally coordinated processes* between social partners that take place at the same time or close in time and are essential for affiliative relationships (Feldman, 2007). It can occur in different ways (e.g., in turn-taking or overlapping vocalizations), with different sensory modalities (e.g., gaze or touch), with one or several partners, and within and across biobehavioral systems. Experiences of synchrony between social partners fosters familiarity with each other's style and affective state and engenders shared experiences. Much of what we know about synchrony comes from studies of dyadic interactions, including parent–child, especially mother–child, interactions. With regular experiences of synchrony, over time, infants' and mothers' biobehavioral systems become mutually attuned so that they "accommodate the inclusion of the other" (Feldman, 2012, p. 43). As an example, mothers adapted their heart rhythms to that of their 3-month-olds, and vice versa, during gaze and vocal synchrony in face-to-face interactions (Feldman, Magori-Cohen, Galili, Singer, & Louzoun, 2011).

Synchrony takes place differently in mother–infant interactions related to community-based relational orientations. Cameroonian Nso mothers' (small-scale, subsistence farmers) contingent responsiveness to nondistressed vocalizations of their 3-month-olds was more physical than visual; German mothers' contingent responsiveness was more visual than physical (Kärtner, Keller, & Yovsi, 2010). Indian mothers and their 2-month-olds had more closely spaced vocal turns and more simultaneous vocalizations compared to French and U.S. mother–infant dyads (Gratier, 2003). Nso and Indian mothers' interactional styles, consistent with other-regarding relational orientations, arguably enhance infants' social interconnectedness. These styles may create infants' impression of *unity* with mother as they act together as *one in unison*. This is how Cowley and colleagues talk about chorusing between caregivers and infants in KwaZulu communities in South Africa (Cowley, Moodley, & Fiori-Cowley, 2004). A comparative style is alternating turn-taking synchronous interactions (e.g., face-to-face), characteristic of mother–infant interactions with self-regarding orientations, that creates infants' impression of a separated individual self.

Synchronous mother–child interactions associate with children's attachment relationships in families with Western lifestyles sensitized to self-regarding relational orientations. What of children's attachments in families with different lifestyles sensitized to other-regarding orientations? This orientation is particularly adaptive in small-scale societies where cooperation is crucial for survival. We turn to Efe foragers' care of infants to reflect on this question. We consider ecocultural correlates of infant care and how care safeguards infants from environmental threats and provides them with ample relational opportunities. In light of their care, we consider infants' experiences of synchrony with caregivers and the group as a whole, relational orientation, and attachments.

Efe Foragers and Care of Infants[2]

The Efe of the Democratic Republic of Congo, like other tropical foragers, subsist primarily by hunting and gathering forest foods. They reside in camps made up mostly of several extended families of brothers and their wives, children, parents, and unmarried sisters. Camps are nestled around open communal areas where most daily activities take place. The Efe move around camp at will, as do younger children who are also able to move in and out of the huts of kith and kin with few restrictions.

The Efe must deal with threats associated with nutritional and social uncertainty. There is high day-to-day and seasonal variability in access to food, and, on any one day, some Efe may have little to eat. Efe move camp in search of better opportunities for food, and when they do, residency

---

[2]The data reported on Efe care draw primarily from two published accounts: Morelli, Ivey Henry, and Foerster (2014) and Morelli, Henry, and Spielvogel (2019).

patterns typically change, sometimes significantly so. Several camps may merge when food is plentiful, and a camp may fracture into smaller groups when it is not. There are other reasons for changes in residential patterns. Efe often become ill and many die in the first decades of life. Others leave to visit families far away or in search of better prospects, with expectations of returning. What this means is that people on whom Efe depend may suddenly be gone and their return may be uncertain.

Efe deal with uncertainty by cooperating at extremely high levels, which reduces individual and shared risks. This pattern is obvious when it comes to the care of children. Mothers and fathers are not consistently able to supply enough food to keep themselves and their nutritionally dependent children healthy. They greatly rely on help from kin and non-kin to do both. The cooperative networks in which they participate are dynamic, favoring flexible social and economic associations based on repeated cooperation that nurture relationships. These reciprocal networks exist within broader relational networks that make it possible for mothers to respond rapidly to changing conditions. This means, at times, that mothers have to recalibrate their networks to include others they don't know well or at all.

Infants' Social Networks

Efe mothers' network of cooperative relationships largely determine the character of their infants' first social ties. But mothers alone do not determine the full extent of their infants' social life. As others seek out infants and vice versa, infants' social networks rapidly expand. In the first months of life, in *a 2-hour period,* Efe infants averaged nine social partners; by their first birthday, they averaged 14—and some infants had as many as 20 different social partners. It is unlikely for infants to have the same social partners over short periods of time. Only 30% of social partners, on average, were the same for infants as 4- to 6- and as 7- to 11-month-olds. Among them were mothers, fathers, and siblings.

Infants benefit from their network affiliations by the protection and care they receive. As more people care for infants, infants are more likely to obtain needed resources. Additionally, infants get practice adjusting to different interactional styles, which readies them to nimbly manage changing social scenes of multiple partners with diverse characteristics, permanency, and interests. In so doing, infants learn a complex set of behaviors for developing, sustaining, and renewing relationships. Regularly occurring changes in infants' social partners may support this learning. Such shifts occur with surprising frequency. Efe who were 4–6 months old, for example, experienced changes in social partners every 2–4 minutes on average, similar to younger and older infants. Despite this dynamic social landscape, most who care for Efe infants are familiar to them.

Early experiences with variable social environments should influence rapid development of neurobiological processes associated with attentional control systems. These systems ought to enhance infants' capacity to manage changing multisensory information across multiple social partners, and to change the focus of their attention and engagement quickly. The ability to develop flexible attentional systems is intricately linked to emotion regulatory processes (Swingler, Perry, & Calkins, 2015). In line with this thesis is the finding that Efe infants were rarely distressed by their quick-moving and varied social landscape. They were in good moods most times regardless of social partner. Infants seemed to enjoy their time with caregivers and their amiable moods made engaging them a pleasing experience (Sroufe, 2005). When Efe infants were less pleasing to be with (e.g., overly fussy), they spent more time with their mothers (Winn, Morelli, & Tronick, 1987).

As such socioemotional competences develop, infants become increasingly accomplished at social interactions. At the same time, caregivers are motivated to sustain contact with infants to enrich their cooperative partnerships with mothers. Such contacts provide means by which infants and caregivers learn about each other, commitment strengthens, and trust develops.

Caregiver Trustworthiness

One way Efe caregivers signal their trustworthiness is by responding quickly to infant distress, which most caregivers do. Furthermore, caregivers are exceptionally good at anticipating infant distress and acting to preempt it, which explains why distress rarely escalates. Another way is by giving infants what they ask for, which all caregivers did most times, and by offering infants unsolicited resources—notable food. Food sharing, one of the most prosocial acts of cooperation, is an expression of care and belonging.

Infants' trust in caregivers sets the groundwork for infants' attachment to them. But infants trust caregivers in different ways and to different degrees, so they may not form attachments to all trusted caregivers. Caregivers most involved in coregulating infant allostasis are likely to be among those infants trust a lot. Infant distress and hunger significantly disrupt biosocial regulatory processes; thus, caregivers who regularly safeguard infants from these threats are likely to be among the most trustworthy. As infants experience a good number of camp members as trustworthy caregivers, their trust of individual caregivers may generalize to the camp as a whole, making the camp a secure setting for infants.

Biobehavioral Synchrony

Efe infants should experience high levels of synchrony with many who care for them. Frequently, care involves regulating infant state and establishing infant internal rhythms—indicators of synchrony. Infants experience synchrony in other ways as they sit on the backs and hips of caregivers who are involved in rhythmically repetitive daily activities. Care is usually a multisensory experience with one caregiver—or several at the same time—singing to, patting, and rocking infants; and multisensory processing maximizes synchronous processes (Harris & Waug, 2002). Additionally, infants probably experience synchrony with people who are less directly involved with their care. This takes place in contexts of regularly occurring campwide activities characterized by rhythm and repetition such as storytelling, singing, drumming, and clapping (e.g., Ellamil, Berson, & Margulies, 2016).

Synchrony of tactile and kinesthetic interactions typifies a good proportion of infants' synchronous experience with caregivers, and a good many of these interactions overlap with infant signals. This is expected given their proximal style of care. Such synchrony creates for infant and caregiver a feeling of *acting as one in unison*. More intriguing, given that infants often interact with more than one partner at a time, infants and partners may perceive all of them as *many acting as one in unison*.

Attachment Relationships

Infants develop affiliative relationships with their network of caregivers with whom they've experienced different levels of synchrony and trustworthy experiences. These relationships are primed to be attachments. There is likely a core of caregivers—grandmothers, mothers, aunts, siblings—to whom infants form attachments. There are others with whom infants are emotionally ready to form attachments. Our current understanding of Efe infant attachments is as follows:

- Infants develop attachments with many in their caregiving networks.
- Infants are partial to some caregivers with whom they have developed attachments, but partiality can change rapidly.
- Infants are readily able to form attachments with others in their caregiving network. This is not meant to imply that infants shift attachments; only that those individuals are not always available.
- Infants experience attachments as an integrated system of relationships, not as a collection of single attachments.
- Infants' attachments are tied to safeguards against threats to health and social interdependencies.

Final Reflections

The safe, positive qualities of infants' diverse relationships, including with familiar partners who are experienced over and over again, enriches neural pathways underlying neurobiological and social plasticity. Such plasticity leaves many possibilities available for infants to develop attachment relationships, a thesis consistent with research on social experiences and adaptive neuroplasticity in early development (e.g., Guzzetta, 2019). What we are learning about biosocial opportunities related to infant care experiences should lead to a qualitative shift in theorizing on infant attachment relationships to accommodate the great diversity among communities in infants' care and relational orientations.

REFERENCES

Baumeister, R. F., & Leary, M. R. (1995). The need to belong: Desire for interpersonal attachments as a fundamental human motivation. *Psychological Bulletin, 117*(3), 497–529.

Cohen, D., Hoshino-Browne, E., & Leung, A. (2007). Culture and the structure of personal experience: Insider and outsider phenomenologies of the self and social world. In M. Zanna (Ed.), *Advances in experimental social psychology* (Vol. 39, pp. 1–67). Amsterdam: Elsevier.

Cowley, S. J., Moodley, S., & Fiori-Cowley, A. (2004). Grounding signs of culture: Primary intersubjectivity in social semiosis. *Mind, Culture, and Activity, 11*(2), 1–24.

Ellamil, M., Berson, J., & Margulies, D. S. (2016). Influences on and measures of unintentional group synchrony. *Frontiers in Psychology, 9*, 1–6.

Feldman, R. (2007). Parent–infant synchrony and the construction of shared timing: Physiological precursors, developmental outcomes, and risk conditions. *Journal of Child Psychology and Psychiatry, 48*(3–4), 329–354.

Feldman, R. (2012). Parent–infant synchrony: A biobehavioral modal of mutual influences in the formation of affiliative bonds. *Monographs of the Society for Research in Child Development, 77*(2), 42–51.

Feldman, R., Magori-Cohen, R., Galili, G., Singer, M., & Louzoun, Y. (2011). Mother and infant coordinate heart rhythms through episodes of interaction synchrony. *Infant Behavior and Development, 34*, 569–577.

Global Agriculture. (n.d.). Agriculture at a crossroads. Retrieved from *www.globalagriculture.org/report-topics/industrial-agriculture-and-small-scale-farming.html*.

Gratier, M. (2003). Expressive timing and interactional synchrony between mothers and infants: Cultural similarities, cultural differences, and the immigration experience. *Cognitive Development, 18*(4), 533–554.

Guzzetta, A. (Ed.). (2019). *Neural plasticity*. London: Hindawi.

Harris, A. W., & Waug, R. M. (2002). Dyadic synchrony: Its structure and function in children's development. *Developmental Review, 22*, 555–592.

Kärtner, J., Keller, H., & Yovsi, R. D. (2010). Mother–infant interaction during the first 3 months: The emergence of culture-specific contingency patterns. *Child Development, 81*(2), 540–554.

Keller, H., & Kärtner, J. (2013). The cultural solution of universal developmental tasks. In M. J. Gelfand, C.-y. Chiu, & Y.-y. Hong (Eds.), *Advances in culture and psychology* (Vol. 3, pp. 63–116). Oxford, UK: Oxford University Press.

Labile, D., Thompson, R. A., & Froimson, J. (2015). Early socialization: The influences of close relationships. In J. E. Grusec & P. Hastings (Eds.), *Handbook of socialization* (2nd ed., pp. 35–59). New York: Guilford Press.

Morelli, G., Henry, P. I., & Spielvogel, B. (2019). Learning prosociality: Insights from young forager and subsistence farmer children's food sharing with mothers and others. *Behavioral Ecology and Sociobiology, 73*(6), 86.

Morelli, G., Ivey Henry, P., & Foerster, S. (2014). Relationships and resource uncertainty: Cooperative development of Efe hunter-gatherer infants and toddlers. In D. S. Navarez, A. Fuentes, K. Valentino, & P. Grey (Eds.), *Ancestral landscapes in human evolution: Culture, childrearing and social well being.* (pp. 69–103). New York: Oxford University Press.

Sroufe, L. A. (2005). Attachment and development: A prospective, longitudinal study from birth to adulthood. *Attachment and Human Development, 7,* 349–367.

Sutcliffe, A., Dunbar, R., Binder, J., & Arrow, H. (2012). Relationships and the social brain: Integrating psychological and evolutionary perspectives. *British Journal of Psychology, 103*(2), 149–168.

Swingler, M. M., Perry, N. B., & Callkins, S. D. (2015). Neural plasticity and the development of attention: Intrinsic and extrinsic influences. *Development and Psychopathology, 27,* 443–457.

Winn, S., Morelli, G., & Tronick, E. (1987). The infant and the group: A look at Efe caretaking practices. In J. K. Nugent, B. M. Lester, & T. E. Brazelton (Eds.), *Cultural context of infancy* (pp. 87–109). Norwood, NJ: Ablex.

CHAPTER 30

Attachment Theory's Universality Claims
Asking Different Questions

Judi Mesman

The relationship between attachment theory and cultural approaches to the study of parenting and child development has been a rocky one. Even though John Bowlby firmly rooted attachment theory in explicitly evolutionary terms, using ethological research as a foundation for the theory's main elements (Bowlby, 1969/1982), critics have contended its claims of universality (e.g., Keller, 2018). Interestingly, criticism regarding cultural issues comes almost exclusively from those who do not identify as attachment researchers. Cultural criticism from within the ranks of attachment research has been virtually nonexistent. Self-criticism is surely less appealing than self-preservation, but it does constitute a vital aspect of reflective science that is motivated to move forward rather than stay put. If criticism only comes from the "outside," and is therefore more easily dismissed as invalid, important opportunities for growth may be missed.

Having been academically "raised" in one of the world's strongholds of attachment research, I was a firm believer of the universality assumptions of attachment theory and its methods. It wasn't until I started working with young scholars from the Global South, collecting video data of family life in over 20 countries, that I could not escape questioning the basis for some of these universality claims. This does not mean I have lost my admiration for the attachment framework, or my appreciation of the scientific rigor of attachment research and its many novel applications. I would like to argue that acknowledgment of the strengths of attachment research can coexist with the acknowledgment that somewhere along the

way, avenues of potential cultural enrichment have been trodden too nar-
rowly, and that uncomfortable questions need to be asked to make better
use of such avenues.

Summarizing the debate, attachment theory's proponents generally
support the notion that under nonextreme circumstances (i.e., in terms
of the availability of care and basic life resources), four hypotheses are
expected to be confirmed across cultures (Mesman, van IJzendoorn, &
Sagi-Schwartz, 2016):

1. According to the universality hypothesis, all children have the
   propensity to form attachments to one or more caregivers.
2. The normativity hypothesis states that the majority of children
   will form a secure attachment relationship, successfully balancing
   the need for care when in distress with the developmental need to
   explore.
3. The sensitivity hypothesis refers to the prediction that sensitive
   and responsive care predicts secure attachment in children.
4. The competence hypothesis states that a secure attachment relationship predicts adaptive child and adult functioning.

The research literatures relevant to these hypotheses has been critically interpreted by scholars within and outside attachment theory. The
general (evolutionary) notion of the importance of forging social relations and receiving consistent care by one or more caregivers for optimal
child development is rather uncontroversial. But when it comes to the
definitions and assessments of attachment and sensitivity, several scholars
have criticized what they see as a Western-centric and "etic" (perspective
from outside the social group) approach rather than "emic" (perspective
from inside the social group) approach to studying caregiver–child interactions (e.g., Keller, 2018; Otto & Keller, 2014). More specifically, critics
contend that relevant literatures on parenting and child development in
non-Western rural communities is ignored by attachment researchers,
and that promoting a single universalistic view of what constitutes good
parenting is not only inappropriate but even unethical. This is especially
relevant in the case of the competence hypothesis, where "positive" child
outcomes are often not defined according to local needs and opportunities. They argue that there are clearly too many variations in the concepts
and daily practices of caregiving across the globe to be able to claim universality of specific processes, let alone of standardized ways to assess the
quality of caregiver–child relationships.

A recent debate in *Child Development* shows the entrenchment of
the two positions on the universality of attachment-related constructs,
where an attempt to bridge the divide and a call for a "truce" (Mesman
et al., 2017) led to more criticism (Keller et al., 2018), followed by another

attempt that acknowledged the criticism, but arguably could have done more to question key assumptions in attachment theory (Mesman, 2018). Similarly, in a recent set of observational studies in non-Western contexts, including several rural ones, my coauthors and I advocated the importance of questioning Western formulations and assessments of the sensitivity construct, but we stayed within the confines of mainstream attachment theory rather than questioning the theory more directly (special issue of *Attachment and Human Development*: "Sensitivity Off the Beaten Track"). This illustrates a tension between a powerful theory that has engendered a large literature with an authoritative scientific approach to studying parenting and child development, and effort at acknowledging clear and salient cultural differences in caregiver–child interactions and seeking ways to integrate them into the existing attachment framework

The rigorous and highly standardized quantitative research approach of attachment theory is laudable, has led to numerous innovative avenues of research, and contributed to valuable insights on parenting and child development collected in highly informative volumes such as the *Handbook of Attachment* (Cassidy & Shaver, 2016). However, when it comes to cross-cultural questions, attachment research has been rather conservative, and may even have been prone to confirmation bias through an insistence on standardized measures that preclude different approaches that may yield different yet informative results. The reliance on overwhelmingly quantitative methods with gold standards of assessment (such as the Strange Situation Procedure [SSP]) increases the risk that relevant studies with different methods (such as the ethnographic methods that Ainsworth used in Uganda) and—more saliently—different conclusions will go unnoticed or unappreciated. In addition, larger publication traditions also seem to play a limiting role. Qualitative ethnographic studies conducted in nonurban non-Western regions are generally published in very different outlets than studies in mainstream attachment research, which results in separate literatures that rarely meet. This leads to limited opportunities for cross-fertilization and the discovery of new, sometimes uncomfortable questions about conclusions that have traditionally been regarded as confirmed. Especially in science, we must continue to ask these questions, or as James Baldwin (1955/1984) put it, "It is really quite impossible to be affirmative about anything which one refuses to question" (p. 131).

What are some of the questions that the field of attachment research needs to ask itself to move forward in understanding the role of culture in attachment processes? They should ideally be open-ended questions that provoke reflection and should not "answer" themselves simply by being posed. Below are four interrelated questions that seem most important for beginning an open-minded debate about the role of culture in attachment theory.

1. What exactly would attachment researchers consider evidence against the four hypotheses outlined above that hold universality claims? In other words, what type of findings could be "the black swan event" that would prove that not all swans are white? What findings might be so unexpected based on attachment theory that they would have a major impact on our understanding of attachment? It is good practice in science to formulate conditions under which a hypothesis should be rejected (Popper, 1959/2002), but scientists rarely do so explicitly or precisely. For example, it would be helpful to specify whether a finding that children with insecure attachment relations function better as they grow up in certain communities is a "deal breaker" for the competence hypothesis. Interestingly, many such specific cases of course already exist in many of our databases: The families that do not follow the average pattern and make our effect sizes for the expected associations medium-sized at best. This also touches upon a more far-reaching problem in many studies in the behavioral sciences: Average patterns dictate large-scale theories and rarely account for the many families for whom the pattern is absent or even reversed, that may sometimes even make up more than half of the sample. Do we do enough to account for those findings? This also means asking critical questions about how specific assessment methods, samples, and effect sizes play a role in this line of questioning, in favoring certain outcomes over others, and in deciding whether the findings are accepted within the attachment framework.

2. Why are there so few studies using the "gold standards" of attachment research in nonurban non-Western settings? As noted in the chapter on culture in the *Handbook of Attachment,* "the current cross-cultural database is almost absurdly small compared to the domain that should be covered" (Mesman et al., 2016, p. 809). With some minor adaptations, the SSP has, for example, been applied in rural Mali (True, Pisani, & Oumar, 2001) and rural Kenya (Kermoian & Leiderman, 1986), and both studies supported universality claims. However, these studies were conducted decades ago, and there seems to have been no attempt to continue such research using the gold-standard SSP with cultural modifications in communities off the beaten track. The few existing studies were conducted over 15 years ago (e.g., Kermoian & Leiderman, 1986; True et al., 2001) and all support universality claims. Why has this type of research not continued in more recent years, and therefore appears to lack urgency in this field? Will those few older studies be cited forever to assert universality without looking further because of practical constraints or because of a lack of curiosity? If the former, what can be done to overcome them, and if the latter, why are we not more curious about the usefulness of the SSP principles across settings?

3. Which literatures outside of mainstream attachment research could provide insights that might raise uncomfortable questions about the universality of attachment processes that may have been missed or dismissed rather than used to sharpen or even revise modern formulations of attachment theory? If we were to do our very best to find "black swans" in the scientific literature regardless of discipline or field, where would we find them and why have they not yet been used to inform attachment theory? An example is the application of principles from life-history theory (a branch from evolutionary theory) to explain unexpected findings from attachment research. In this line of work, a predominance of insecure attachment patterns in harsh contexts is interpreted as being adaptive to the challenging environment (Simpson & Belsky, 2016). In this case, another line of literature was used to strengthen attachment theory. But that is not the same as actively looking for theories and evidence-bases that raise questions about attachment theory. For example, what do we do with evidence from ethnographic work that shows that children in certain rural communities are cared for by more than 20 different people a day (Meehan & Hawks, 2013)? Reformulations of attachment theory have already allowed for multiple attachment figures, but 20? Are these children attached to the entire community? Can this still be described as "selective" or "preferential" attachment? And what about the omnipresence of juvenile caregivers in certain regions, some mere preschoolers themselves? Can they be attachment figures? In other words: It would be worth actively looking for literatures that provide very different pictures of caregiving from the ones we see in our Western labs and not just trying to squeeze their findings into attachment theory, but also using them to deepen our understanding of attachment, even if it means rejecting part of the original theory's claims.

4. How can the field of attachment research protect itself against potential confirmation bias when it comes to universality claims? Scholars strive for objectivity, but confirmation bias is a very powerful human tendency when it comes to processing information about deeply entrenched beliefs, including among scientists (Hergovich, Schott, & Burger, 2010). What can the field learn from scientific and practical insights into the mechanisms that foster entrenchment of ideas, and biased information processing? There is evidence that exposure to and continued engagement with a variety of disciplinary perspectives in higher education enhances critical thinking, and reduces the development of strong convictions regarding the "truth" about the world through more advanced epistemological skills (e.g., Ivanitskaya, Clark, Montgomery, & Primeau, 2002). The early specialization in a particular theoretical framework in a graduate program embedded in a research group that works exclusively

or primarily from that starting point may not be the best way to foster the development of new critical questions.

Attempting to answer these questions would likely open up many worthwhile avenues for discussion as well as innovative empirical and theoretical work that will inspire future generations of researchers interested in cultural processes in the formation of caregiver–child attachment bonds. Attachment research as a field can only grow if it is willing to entertain uncomfortable questions. We have seen growth in attachment theory through engagement with other fields, for example by acknowledging that the original theory was too mother-centric, that adaptation can be seen in a broader sense than just that of secure attachment, and that we simply do not yet know what processes are hidden in the transmission gap from caregiver attachment representation to child attachment quality. However, we must also allow future generations of researchers to answer such questions in ways that do not sit well with attachment theory. Answers that mean that attachment theory might need to be more modest about its claims and leave room for new generations to generate other theories to take over where the original framework simply does not deliver. Let us be their mentors who admit that our understanding of key issues in questions of universality versus culture-specificity of attachment is inadequate because the scope of our evidence base is incomplete and insufficient. Let us be brave enough to say to our students (paraphrasing Doris Lessing, 1962/1976): What you are being taught is the product of a particular subculture in which your teachers grew up, and that is likely to be an inherently self-perpetuating system. Because history shows us the impermanence of paradigms of thought, we encourage you to seek education outside of this subculture and develop your own judgment. In the same vein, although the conclusion of the chapter on culture in the *Handbook of Attachment* that "until further notice, attachment theory may . . . claim cross-cultural validity" (Mesman et al., 2016, p. 809) is attractive, it would be more elegant and productive to rephrase that to say, "Until further notice, we need to ask more critical questions before we can firmly claim cross-cultural validity of attachment theory."

REFERENCES

Baldwin, J. (1984). *Notes of a native son.* Boston: Beacon Press. (Original work published 1955)

Bowlby, J. (1982). *Attachment and loss: Vol. 1. Attachment* (2nd ed.). New York: Basic Books. (Original work published 1969)

Cassidy, J., & Shaver, P. R. (Eds). (2016). *Handbook of attachment: Theory, research, and clinical applications* (3rd ed., pp. 852–877). New York: Guilford Press.

Hergovich, A., Schott, R., & Burger, C. (2010). Biased evaluation of abstracts depending on topic and conclusion: Further evidence of a confirmation bias within scientific psychology. *Current Psychology, 29*(3), 188–209.

Ivanitskaya, L., Clark, D., Montgomery, G., & Primeau, R. (2002). Interdisciplinary learning: Process and outcomes. *Innovative Higher Education, 27*(2), 95–111.

Keller, H. (2018). Universality claim of attachment theory: Children's socioemotional development across cultures. *Proceedings of the National Academy of Sciences of the USA, 115,* 11414–11419.

Keller, H., Bard, K., Morelli, G., Chaudhary, N., Vicedo, M., Rosabal-Coto, M., . . . Gottlieb, A. (2018). The myth of universal sensitive responsiveness: Comment on Mesman et al. (2017). *Child Development, 89*(5), 1921–1928.

Kermoian, R., & Leiderman, P. H. (1986). Infant attachment to mother and child caretaker in an East African community. *International Journal of Behavioral Development, 9*(4).

Lessing, D. (1976). *The golden notebook.* St Albans, UK: Panther Books. (Original work published 1962)

Meehan, C. L., & Hawks, S. (2013). Cooperative breeding and attachment among the Aka foragers. In N. Quinn & J. M. Mageo (Eds.), *Attachment reconsidered: Cultural perspectives on a Western theory* (pp. 85–114). New York: Palgrave Macmillan.

Mesman, J. (2018). Sense and sensitivity: A response to the commentary by Keller et al. (2018). *Child Development, 89*(5), 1929–1931.

Mesman, J., Minter, T., Angnged, A., Cissé, I. A. H., Salali, G. D., & Migliano, A. B. (2017). Universality without uniformity: A culturally inclusive approach to sensitive responsiveness in infant caregiving. *Child Development, 89*(3), 837–850.

Mesman, J., van IJzendoorn, M. H., & Sagi-Schwartz, A. (2016). Cross-cultural patterns of attachment: Universal and contextual dimensions. In J. Cassidy & P. R. Shaver (Eds.), *Handbook of attachment: Theory, research, and clinical applications* (3rd ed., pp. 852–877). New York: Guilford Press.

Otto, H., & Keller, H. (Eds.). (2014). *Different faces of attachment: Cultural variations on a universal human need.* New York: Cambridge University Press.

Popper, K. (2002). *The logic of scientific discovery.* Abingdon-on-Thames, UK: Routledge. (Original work published 1959)

Simpson, J. A., & Belsky, J. (2016). Attachment theory within a modern evolutionary framework. In J. Cassidy & P. R. Shaver (Eds.), *Handbook of attachment: Theory, research, and clinical applications* (3rd ed., pp. 91–116). New York: Guilford Press.

True, M. M., Pisani, L., & Oumar, F. (2001). Infant–mother attachment among the Dogon of Mali. *Child Development, 72,* 1451–1466.

CHAPTER 31

Attachment and the Deep History of Culture

James S. Chisholm

Just after World War II, John Bowlby's "Psychology and Democracy" appeared in *The Political Quarterly*. I read it as a primitive model of the developmental origins of human cooperation and politics. Here I critique and expand on Bowlby's model according to current thinking in evolutionary-developmental biology and the recent "deep history" movement. I conclude that attachment processes both permeate and constrain culture. They permeate culture because they gave rise to it evolutionarily and give rise to it developmentally. And because they permeate culture, they also constrain it. No manifestation of culture could long exist that failed to meet infants' innate mammalian attachment needs. Moreover, attachment processes themselves have been highly canalized—naturally selected to entrain alternative reproductive strategies that can be evolutionarily adaptive in the risky and uncertain environments in which they develop (Belsky, Steinberg, & Draper 1991; Chisholm, 1996). What follows is an evolutionary-developmental account of how attachment processes might have become manifest in culture.

Bowlby's Model and "We-Ness"

Distressed by the war's brutality, Bowlby was concerned with "the psychological problem of ensuring persistent co-operative behaviour" (1946, p. 61) in groups of any kind. He believed the answer lay in the capacity of infants, first, to "libidinize" (emotionally value) mother, then others, groups of others, group leaders, and what he called the group's "policy" (he focused on political groups). The common denominator, he felt, was the ineffable feeling of "We'ness" (1946, p. 74)—the secure feeling of belonging to a valued group. Everyone's first experience of identity and cooperation/politics is in their first group, self-with-mother. I hope to show that Bowlby's early insight was prescient.

Bowlby's developmental model anticipates the first principle of evolutionary-developmental biology—"phenotype first"—which follows from the fact that selection operates on phenotypes, not genotypes. Bowlby locates the origin of human cooperation squarely in the infant's phenotype—in "the child's feelings for his mother" (1946, p. 64). In contrast, evolutionary models of human cooperation ignore or downplay development and attribute the fitness benefits of cooperation to adults. But how did adults learn to cooperate? What made them want to? The problem is that while evolution provides organisms with their genotypes (information about their environments of evolutionary adaptedness), selection can't "see" this (immaterial) information until it has been (materially) embodied during development. Selection can only work with what it already has—individual phenotypic differences. And what our ancestral mothers and infants already had were degrees of "goodness of fit" between their individual phenotypes, that is, in their attachment *relationships,* their capacity for "we-ness" and group identity.

I view a group's "policy" as its culture, in the specific sense of cultural identity. Its members identify with their group, their leaders, their shared beliefs and values and symbols thereof, and thereby make common cause to achieve their shared intentions. All politics is local identity politics. Everyone's first experience of identity and cooperation/politics is in their first group, self-with-mother. Everyone's first group is also an emotional descent group. With zero exceptions, each of our direct ancestors inherited not only half their mothers' DNA, but also the nongenetic (and potential epigenetic) effects of her behavior on their experience of attachment. I venture that attachment processes drove the evolution of our capacity for culture—the feeling of "we-ness," of hearts, minds, and political action.

Critique of Bowlby's Model

Bowlby's model of the development of human cooperation treats mother–infant cooperation as a given, however, and says nothing about its adaptive function or how it evolved. He also jumps straight from mother–infant groups to national political groups. In particular, he says nothing about male–female friendship and cooperation (e.g., Smuts, 1985), adult attachment, or conjugal groups. Nor, therefore, does he mention *kin* groups or the role of the father in kinship systems, which, from our deep hunter-gatherer past to the present, have so determined who cooperates with whom, for what, when, and how. The "deep history" movement suggests ways to build on Bowlby's model.

Deep History

"Deep history" (Shryock & Smail, 2011; Smail, 2008) is concerned with our evolutionary history from our last common ancestor with the chimpanzee and bonobo (6 million years ago) to the origin of writing ("shallow" history; 4,000 years ago). It differs from most traditional prehistory in its explicit focus on emotions and feelings (e.g., kinship, religion, exchange relations), which both express and entrain feelings of "we-ness." Smail argues that our deep history was driven by our basic great ape social emotions. Deep historical approaches are attentive to the expanding circles of group identity that characterize our past, from families, clans, bands, tribes, to states, but don't explain what motivated this increasing complexity.

The feeling of "we-ness" inspires kinship systems and motivates kinship behavior. "Deep kinship" attempts to trace the evolution of human kinship and social organization from their nonhuman primate origins (Trautman, Feeley-Harnik, & Mitani, 2011). The leading model is Chapais's *Primeval Kinship* (2008), which makes a strong case for the pivotal role of adult pair-bonding in the origin of human kinship. Of all the differences between chimp/bonobo and human social organization, the one that made a difference for us was the pair bond—Bowlby's missing conjugal group. On the other hand, Chapais treats pair-bonding as an evolutionary given and says nothing about how it evolved. The two models thus complement each other. Bowlby's model provides the explanans (attachment) but not the explanandum we want (the conjugal group). Chapais's model provides the explanandum (pair bonds), but no explanans ("bonding" is given). But in combination—with Bowlby's attachment as the process and Chapais's pair bond as its product—Bowlby's model of the development of our capacity for "we-ness" also works as a model of its evolution.

An Evolutionary–Developmental Rationale for Bowlby's Model

As I've argued elsewhere (Chisholm, 2003, 2017), Trivers's (1974) theory of parent–offspring conflict explains in principle how our capacity for "we-ness" may have evolved. At the beginning of hominin evolution all mothers were single mothers. Male parental investment didn't appear until adult males and females had evolved the capacity to form at least "proto-conjugal" groups. Trivers showed that parent–offspring conflict is inevitable because while mothers share 50% of their genes with each offspring, each offspring also shares 50% of its genes with its biological father. It would therefore have been in our ancestral infants' evolutionary interest to continually seek more resources from mother—continuing to nurse being paramount—in order to replicate *both* parents' genes. By the same token, it would also have been in mothers' evolutionary interest to replicate at least *two* copies of their genes, even if it means ceasing to nurse and investing in another child, existing or in the future. For Trivers, then, "socialization is a process by which parents attempt to mold each offspring . . . while each offspring [is expected] to resist . . . and to attempt to mold the behavior of its parents" (1974, p. 260).

Our ancestral mothers and infants had good reason to cooperate, however, because the evolution of our prolonged infant helplessness escalated our existing chimp/bonobo level of parent–offspring conflict into an early human mother–infant "arms race" (Kilner & Hinde, 2012). Infants would have exerted selection on mothers to continue nursing and mothers would have been selected to resist—but giving in more often to (thereby selecting for) infants with the ability to "mold" them into continuing to nurse. The effect would have been positive intergenerational feedback. Game theory shows that to avoid an increasingly expensive arms race the optimal strategy is for the conflicted parties to cooperate by each settling for less than they would like. As Shimon Peres advised, "In politics, as in family life, be careful not to win too much, because you may win the point and lose the game" (quoted in Remnick, 2002, p. 63). The short-term cost to both mother and infant of "giving in" to the other is balanced by the short-term benefit to each of reduced conflict. In the long term this is good for the infant—but giving in to her infant's short-term demands to continue nursing is not good for the mother's long-term fitness because it delays the birth of her next child. Parent–offspring conflict can thus lead to parent–offspring co-adaptation because "as offspring, individuals are under selection to adapt to . . . their parents' care, and as parents they are under selection to adapt to . . . their offspring's traits [attempts to 'mold' them]" (Kölliker, Royle, & Smiseth, 2012, p. 287). In other words, tolerating *not* winning too much from mother is practice for not winning too much from offspring—or anyone.

Solving one adaptive problem, however, often leads to another. Giving in to infant demands for prolonged nursing would increase birth intervals, slowing mothers' reproductive rates and increasing the risk of lineage extinction. But as Hrdy (2009, p. 101) noted, "Humans, who of all apes produce the largest, slowest maturing, and most costly babies, also breed the fastest." She made the case that this was possible only because our ancestral mothers got help with child care, turning us into "cooperative breeders." Among primates (except the callitrichids, the only other cooperatively breeding primate), only human mothers can have a child before the preceding one is independent; only human mothers ever have to decide which of their offspring gets what, when, or how; and only human mothers are known sometimes to neglect, reject, and even kill their offspring (Hrdy, 2009). Under conditions of risk and uncertainty, with high or unpredictable mortality rates, it can be evolutionarily rational for a mother to neglect, reject, or kill one child and invest instead in another with better prospects, either existing or in the future (Hrdy, 2009). Understanding mothers' potentially infanticidal intentions would have helped infants make the best of their bad bargain by adopting an alternative attachment strategy in order to avoid losing too much to mothers' inability or unwillingness to invest (Chisholm, 1996).

But again, how did the cooperative breeders learn to cooperate? What made them want to? In Bowlby's model they would have learned to cooperate when they themselves were infants. From an evolutionary-developmental perspective, however, they were *able* to learn as infants because *their* earlier infant ancestors had been selected to learn how to adapt to conflict with mother, giving them practice for adapting to conflict with their own infants. Adapting to conflict with their own infants was thus an exaptation of their adaptation to conflict with their mothers. Our earliest ancestral mother–infant dyads would then have been selected for their capacity for co-adaptation—for a better "goodness of fit" between their individual social-emotional-cognitive phenotypes. And mothers' helpers would *want* to cooperate because it felt good to express their feeling of "we-ness" with their mothers.

Politics: Parental Investment beyond the Family

More cooperative mothers would tend to rear more cooperative infants, who in turn would tend to be more cooperative as adults with other adult cooperators—including adults of the opposite sex. This set the stage for assortative mating for cooperativeness, cooperatively breeding males, and the emergence of Bowlby's missing conjugal group and Chapais's pair bond—the family. From this not-so-simple beginning there emerged endless forms of "we" groups, in expanding circles of kinship and complexity from families to clans, bands, tribes, kingdoms, states, and all of their institutional support groups (religious, economic, legal, military, etc.). Robertson (1991) suggested that this increasing political-economic complexity was driven by increasing parental investment "beyond the family." Parents, he argued, are always looking for ways "to shift the costs of reproduction out from the compact household into the wider social domain" (p. 122). For example, "Factories, banks, land registries, livestock markets and computer dating services reduce the need for large family corporations" (p. 39). In this view, large parts of the "wider social domain" are culturally constructed institutions for cooperative breeding. Unfortunately, as Marris (1996) notes, politics has a long history of shifting the cost of reproduction from those with political power to those without. For Marris, attachment processes permeate culture in the realm of politics and the costs of reproduction are fundamentally social-emotional. Chronic poverty and inequality make for risky and uncertain environments, subjecting the have-nots to chronic anxiety and insecurity about their uncertain futures. These are precisely the conditions in which insecure attachment styles can be evolutionarily adaptive—even if they are also bad for health and longevity and increase the risk for the inter-generational inheritance of insecurity. When parents' optimal reproductive strategy is to avoid lineage extinction by reproducing early and/or often, their offspring's optimal developmental strategy is to prepare for doing the same by adapting to—giving in to and making the best of—their parents' inability or unwillingness to invest. Attachment processes are thus manifest in the perpetuation—or not—of the "culture of poverty" (Leacock, 1971; Raikes & Thompson, 2005).

Conclusion

Bowlby's model of the developmental origin of human cooperation is worth exploring further because it also works as a model of its evolution. From the perspective of evolutionary-developmental biology it shows how and why attachment processes permeate culture—because they gave rise to it. The essence of culture is shared thinking—shared beliefs, values, and symbols thereof. And as Hobson put it, "The foundations of thinking were laid at the point when ancestral primates began to connect with each other emotionally in the same ways that human babies connect with their caregivers" (2004, p. 2).

ACKNOWLEDGMENTS

My thanks to the editors, Bernard Chapais, Daniel Smail, and Cyril Grueter, for their comments on an earlier version of this chapter.

REFERENCES

Belsky, J., Steinberg, L., & Draper, P. (1991). Childhood experience, interpersonal development, and reproductive strategy: An evolutionary theory of socialization. *Child Development, 62,* 647–670.

Bowlby, J. (1946). Psychology and democracy. *The Political Quarterly, 17,* 61–75.

Chapais, B. (2008). *Primeval kinship: How pair-bonding gave birth to human society.* Cambridge, MA: Harvard University Press.

Chisholm, J. S. (1996). The evolutionary ecology of attachment organization. *Human Nature, 7*(1), 1–37.

Chisholm, J. S. (2003). Uncertainty, contingency and attachment: A life history theory of theory of mind. In K. Sterelny & J. Fitness (Eds.) *From mating to mentality: Evaluating evolutionary psychology.* Hove, UK: Psychology Press.

Chisholm, J. S. (2017). How attachment gave rise to culture. In K. Bard & H. Keller (Eds.), *Contextualizing attachment: The cultural context of attachment.* Cambridge, MA: MIT Press.

Hobson, P. (2004). *The cradle of thought: Exploring the origins of thinking.* Oxford, UK: Oxford University Press.

Hrdy, S. B. (2009). *Mothers and others: The evolutionary origins of mutual understanding.* Cambridge, MA: Harvard University Press.

Kilner, R. M., & Hinde, C. M. (2012). Parent–offspring conflict. In N. J. Royle, P. T. Smiseth, & M. Kölliker (Eds.), *The evolution of parental care.* Oxford, UK: Oxford University Press.

Kölliker, M., Royle, N. J., & Smiseth, P. T. (2012). Parent–offspring co-adaptation. In N. J. Royle, P. T. Smiseth, & M. Kölliker (Eds.), *The evolution of parental care.* Oxford, UK: Oxford University Press.

Leacock, E. B. (Ed.). (1971). *The culture of poverty: A critique.* New York: Simon & Schuster.

Marris, P. (1996). *The politics of uncertainty: Attachment in private and public life.* London: Routledge.

Raikes, H. A., & Thompson, R. A. (2005). Links between risk and attachment security: Models of influence. *Applied Developmental Psychology, 26,* 440–455.

Remnick, D. (2002, January 7). The dreamer. *The New Yorker.*

Robertson, A. F. (1991). *Beyond the family: The social organization of human reproduction.* Berkeley: University of California Press.

Shryock, A., & Smail, D. L. (Eds.). (2011). *Deep history: The architecture of past and present.* Berkeley: University of California Press.

Smail, D. L. (2008). *On deep history and the brain.* Berkeley: University of California Press.

Smuts, B. (1985). *Sex and friendship in baboons.* Piscataway, NJ: Transaction.

Trautmann, T. R., Feeley-Harnik, G., & Mitani, J. C. (2011). Deep kinship. In A. Shryock & D. L. Smail (Eds.), *Deep history: The architecture of past and present.* Berkeley: University of California Press.

Trivers, R. L. (1974). Parent–offspring conflict. *American Zoologist, 14,* 249–264.

TOPIC 7

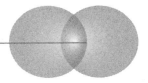

SEPARATION AND LOSS

- How do people respond to the loss of an attachment figure?

- What are the key processes and mechanisms involved?

CHAPTER 32

Losing a Parent in Early Childhood
The Impact of Disrupted Attachment

Ann Chu
Alicia F. Lieberman

Do infants and young children experience grief and mourning? What is the psychological meaning of their observable distress during lengthy separations from their primary attachment figures? Does their distress have long-term negative effects on their mental health? These questions guided early observations of infants separated from their mothers. The questions became more nuanced in the ensuing decades in response to accumulating knowledge about early childhood development and the role of environmental factors in shaping emotional experience and behavior. A return to attachment theory in an effort to integrate new research may contribute to our understanding of how the impact of prolonged separation compares to parental death.

Young children may respond with intense grief to both death and prolonged separation because, in both situations, the concrete manifestations and emotional effect of the caregiver's absence is immediate and severe. We use the term *loss* to encompass both death and prolonged separation but specify when each of these two experiences is involved. Because of diverse caregiving constellations that are becoming increasingly common, we use the term *caregiver* to refer to an attachment figure who plays a central role in the child's daily life and emotional organization.

Responses to Loss

Losing an attachment figure in the first 5 years of life is psychologically disorganizing because young children experience the violation of the developmentally appropriate expectation that their attachment figure will be available as a predictable protector (Bowlby, 1973, 1980; Lieberman, Compton, Van Horn, & Ghosh Ippen, 2003). Rupture of the foundational expectation of safety causes injury to the young child's emerging sense of self, manifested in distress behaviors that include inconsolable crying, sadness, lethargy, withdrawal, anger, searching for the caregiver, sensitivity to reminders of the caregiver, refusal of substitute caregivers, lack of interest in age-appropriate activities, changes in biological rhythms, and regression in developmental milestones (Zero to Three, 2016).

Early observations of young children separated from their caregivers buttressed the premise that caregiver loss is damaging to children with detailed filmed and written records of moment-to-moment child behaviors in response to separation (e.g., Bowlby, 1958; Bowlby & Robertson, 1953; Freud & Burlingham, 1944; Robertson, 1952; Spitz, 1946). Bowlby (1960, 1969) described a recurrent pattern in the temporal unfolding of the child's responses to prolonged separation, characterized by three phases—labeled *protest, despair,* and *detachment*—that can overlap and alternate with each other. In the initial *protest,* the infant shows distress through loud crying that may last intermittently for a week or more, interspersed with expressions of anger and refusing care from others as well as search behaviors that include looking for the caregiver or holding on to objects associated with the caregiver. *Despair* sets in when active demands for the caregiver diminish and the young child becomes increasingly apathetic and withdrawn, with low-keyed intermittent crying, sad facial expressions, and withdrawal from engagement with people and objects. *Detachment* is marked by an apparent return to interest in people and surroundings and acceptance of surrogate care, but also includes "selective forgetting" of the caregiver characterized by a striking lack of interest or ambivalence toward the returning caregiver and the absence of age-appropriate reunion behavior. This is a crucial stage in the child's emotional experience because detachment can be adopted as a habitual defense against emotional closeness. When this happens, avoidance of intimacy becomes the template for a working model of attachment grounded in the expectation that affectional bonds will be disrupted, often resulting in feelings of love triggering an anticipatory fear of loss and generating emotions of anxiety, sadness, and anger (see also Shaver & Mikulincer, Chapter 33, and Maccallum, Chapter 36, this volume).

Understanding of Loss

While early theorists agreed on young children's behavioral responses following the loss of a parent, they disagreed on whether young children have the cognitive and emotional maturity to experience an actual mourning process, including the prolonged and painful psychological restructuring that accompanies redirecting affectional bonds from the lost caregiver to a new object of affection. Bowlby believed that children might experience mourning as early as 6 months of age whenever their attachment behavior is activated, and their attachment figure is consistently absent. Anna Freud (1960), on the other hand, spoke for many leading psychoanalysts when she claimed that mourning presupposes mental capacities such as object constancy, which young infants do not attain in a stable manner until 3 years of age. Though this theoretical debate has not been empirically resolved, the distinction between external behaviors and the child's inner experience is important to keep in mind when trying to understand similarities in how infants and young children respond to caregiver death or prolonged separations from a primary caregiver.

Infants and toddlers are in the early processes of developing stable internal working models of attachment relationships. When this is disrupted by the loss of the caregiver, the child is confronted with the dilemma of how to give meaning to a developmentally incomprehensible event. Physical and mental representations of the caregiver coexist in painful contrast with the cessation of the daily routines upon which those representations are based and with longing for those pleasurable, safe expectations. During prolonged separation, this inner split may define the child's perceptions of the attachment figure and become the dominant structure in the working models of the self and, by extension, of the self in relation to attachment issues. The self-experience of the child becomes that of someone who cannot trust that one can love and be loved with the expectation that love will be safe and lasting.

Prolonged separation and death are differentiated by the continued existence versus the demise of the caregiver. As children mature, the finality of death becomes an increasingly central factor in organizing their mourning process. Piaget (1960) posited that young children have egocentric and preoperational thought processes that lead them to construe their thoughts and actions as causing the events that are important to them. Young children routinely believe that their parent left because of something they did ("Mommy left me because I yelled") and that the loss is a reversible state that can be remedied through the child's behavior ("Mommy will come back if I stop yelling"). As children develop their capacities and learn new facts about the loss from direct explanations or from overhearing others, their questions and hypotheses about the reasons for the loss also evolve. Their experience of loss needs to be readdressed and reintegrated in the course of development in a dynamic process that promotes factual understanding and internal acceptance.

Psychobiological Impact

Studies have consistently demonstrated the impact of elevated levels of stress hormones on brain structures such as the amygdala, hippocampus, and prefrontal cortex and on brain functions including learning, memory, and executive functioning. Disruptions in these biological systems in early childhood as a result of adverse childhood experiences have been linked to a broad range of deleterious physical and mental health outcomes (see Shonkoff & Garner, 2012). The integration of multiple research perspectives is converging into a "neuroscience of attachment" that conceives of attachment as a neural construct organized around detection and response to threat and safety cues (Coan, 2008). The National Scientific Council on the Developing Child summarized the research findings using a conceptual taxonomy comprising three types of stress responses: positive, tolerable, and toxic. A positive stress response is brief, mild-to-moderate in intensity, and occurs in the context of a responsive caregiver who helps the child cope. A tolerable response is associated with non-normative experiences that pose a significant level of threat or danger. When these adverse events are experienced in the context of a protective caregiving relationship, the level of stress response remains tolerable. The toxic stress response is characterized by strong, frequent, or prolonged activation of the stress response system in the absence of a protective caregiving relationship. Because young children's caregivers play a key role in the development of self-regulation, caregiver loss can result in chronic activation of the stress response system and lead to changes in brain structure and function as the substrates of changes in observable behavior and internal working models of attachment. Boyce and Ellis (2005) used evidence that biological sensitivity to context results in differential adaptations to the environment to highlight the importance of a multilevel approach to understanding the impact of adversity and trauma on children's stress responses and developmental trajectories.

Environmental Context and Intervention Strategies

The grieving process is often idiosyncratic and particularly unpredictable in early childhood because young children's responses are deeply affected by the quality of their relationships with the lost caregiver and with the new surrogate caregivers, the changing circumstances of the family, and environmental features. The quality of subsequent parental care (e.g., acceptance, degree of warmth and empathy, promoting autonomy in the child) is one of the most significant predictors of resilience (Norris-Shortle, Young, & Williams, 1993). In cases of parental death, the psychological functioning of the surviving parent is the most significant predictor of later outcomes (Wolchik, Tein, Sandler, & Ayers, 2006). The role of preexisting quality of attachment in predicting children's response to caregiver loss is not systematically documented. Rigorous research is inherently fraught with methodological problems for many reasons, including the impossibility of assessing quality of attachment retrospectively in the aftermath of the loss.

Young children's expressions of loss are distinctly different from adults' mourning behaviors. The frequent lack of a sustained sadness in young children may prevent adults from appreciating the depth and intensity of the child's reaction to the loss. It is often difficult for adults, coping with loss themselves, to notice, understand, and respond appropriately to young children's grief. Toddlers express their grief through play, fantasy, and drawings more clearly than through language. Preschool children may engage in questioning and watching adults in order to understand the loss. Adults may want to alleviate the child's pain by offering evasive or misleading explanations, including that the person is on a long trip or vacation, at work, or sleeping peacefully.

If adults deny or attempt to cover up the caregiver loss, young children may become aware that this is a taboo subject and repress their emotional reactions (Bowlby, 1979). The resulting incongruence between what the child knows and what adults allow the child to show can lead to chronic cognitive confusion and an inability to identify emotional experience. Young children may downplay or suppress their grief reactions to comply with an adult's wishful belief that recovery will proceed faster if the child "forgets" the loss. With no acceptable emotional outlet open to them, children's fears and confusion can evolve into maladaptive thoughts and behaviors in an effort to cope.

Young children need to maintain a mental connection with the absent caregiver and integrate that caregiver into their ongoing sense of self. Horowitz (1997) described the importance for grieving adults of continuously confronting their changed reality until the loss of the loved one is fully represented in memory and integrated into updated working models of the self. This process is particularly daunting for young children, who must undertake it in the context of their immaturity in memory formation, object permanence, logical thinking and understanding of cause and effect, emotional regulation, coping strategies, and dependence on others for the experience of safety and the search for meaning. Helping young children to retain or regain a healthy developmental trajectory in the aftermath of caregiver loss must involve a two-generation approach where the substitute caregivers receive the help they need in supporting the child (Lieberman et al., 2003).

Interventions should support the child's emotional connections with the new attachment figure, create a safe and consistent environment, identify and respond to traumatic reminders of the loss, and promote adjustment to changes in daily routines (Lieberman et al., 2003). In cases of parental death, adults can include young children in death rituals and in playing out what happened. Children require concrete descriptions of what happens to people when they die, including an explanation of the loss of functions, the permanence of death, and the sadness and other emotions that the survivors typically feel after a death. Children coping with prolonged separation from caregivers need reassurance that they will continue to be loved and protected during the separation. If the separation is prolonged but temporary, the child can anticipate the caregiver's return with concrete reminders such as photos, calendars where the days until reunion (if known) are marked, and, whenever feasible, telephone calls, cards, or other means of bridging the physical distance. If the separation is final but the caregiver is alive, the child needs age-appropriate explanations aligned with the facts, along with strategies to help integrate the loss and form a new substitute attachment relationship.

Conclusion

Attachment theory and empirical evidence point to the devastating impact of losing a parent—to death or prolonged separation—during the first 5 years of life. This potent form of early life stress disrupts the developing foundation of neurophysiological, emotional, social, and cognitive functioning in very young children. Understanding how children respond to, understand, and cope with the loss of a parent provides guidance for how to establish better intervention strategies and treatment guidelines as well as institutional and public health policies that promote young children's healthy attachment relationships and mental health.

REFERENCES

Bowlby, J. (1958). The nature of the child's tie to his mother. *International Journal of Psych-Analysis, 39,* 350–373.

Bowlby, J. (1960). Grief and mourning in infancy and early childhood. *Psychoanalytic Study of the Child, 15*(1), 9–52.

Bowlby, J. (1969). *Attachment and loss: Vol. 1. Attachment.* New York: Basic Books.

Bowlby, J. (1973). *Attachment and loss: Vol. 2. Separation.* New York: Basic Books.

Bowlby, J. (1979). On knowing what you are not supposed to know and feeling what you are not supposed to feel. *Canadian Journal of Psychiatry, 24*(5), 403–408.

Bowlby, J. (1980). *Attachment and loss: Vol. 3. Loss, sadness and depression.* New York: Basic Books.

Bowlby, J., & Robertson, J. (1953). A two-year-old goes to hospital. *Journal of the Royal Society of Medicine, 46*(6), 425–427.

Boyce, W. T., & Ellis, B. J. (2005). Biological sensitivity to context: I. An evolutionary-developmental theory of the origins and functions of stress reactivity. *Development and Psychopathology, 17*, 271–301.

Coan, J. A. (2008). Toward a neuroscience of attachment. In J. Cassidy & P. R. Shaver (Eds.), *Handbook of attachment: Theory, research, and clinical applications* (2nd ed., pp. 241–268). New York: Guilford Press.

Freud, A. (1960). Discussion of Dr. John Bowlby's paper. *Psychoanalytic Study of the Child, 15*(1), 53–62.

Freud, A., & Burlingham, D. T. (1944). *War and children.* New York: International University Press.

Horowitz, M. (1997). *Stress response syndromes* (3rd ed.). Northvale, NJ: Jason Aronson.

Lieberman, A. F., Compton, N., Van Horn, P., & Ghosh Ippen, C. (2003). *Losing a parent to death in the early years: Guidelines for the treatment of traumatic bereavement in infancy and early childhood.* Washington, DC: ZERO TO THREE Press.

Norris-Shortle, C., Young, P. A., & Williams, M. A. (1993). Understanding death and grief for children three and younger. *Social Work, 38*(6), 736–742.

Piaget, J. (1960). *The child's concept of the world.* Paterson, NJ: Littlefield, Adams.

Robertson, J. (1952). A two year old goes to hospital [Video file]. Retrieved from *www.youtube.com/watch?v=s14Q-_Bxc_U.*

Shonkoff, J. P., & Garner, A. S. (2012). The lifelong effects of early childhood adversity and toxic stress. *Pediatrics, 129*, 232–246.

Spitz, R. (1946). Grief, a peril in infancy [Video file]. Retrieved from *https://collections.nlm.nih.gov/catalog/nlm:nlmuid-9505470-vid.*

Spitz, R. (1947). Grief, a peril in infancy [Video file]. Retrieved from *https://collections.nlm.nih.gov/catalog/nlm:nlmuid-9505470-vid 9/24/2019.*

Wolchik, S. A., Tein, J., Sandler, I. R., & Ayers, T. S. (2006). Stressors, quality of the child–caregiver relationship, and children's mental health problems after parental death: The mediating role of self-system beliefs. *Journal of Abnormal Child Psychology, 34*, 212–229.

ZERO TO THREE. (2016). *DC:0-5: Diagnostic classification of mental health and developmental disorders of infancy and early childhood.* Washington, DC: Author.

CHAPTER 33

Attachment, Loss, and Grief Viewed from a Personality–Social Perspective on Adult Attachment

Phillip R. Shaver
Mario Mikulincer

Bowlby (1980) provided pioneering ideas concerning functional and dysfunctional emotional responses to the loss of an attachment figure. In this chapter, we extend Bowlby's ideas concerning grief responses and consider some of the psychological mechanisms underlying disordered grief processes and successful grief resolution, including how they relate to adult attachment security/insecurity. Our discussion is based on a personality–social psychological perspective and is informed by a large body of social and personality research on attachment in adulthood (see Mikulincer & Shaver, 2016).

Emotional Responses to the Loss of an Attachment Figure

Based on ethological observations of infants separated from their mothers, Bowlby (1980) argued that temporary separation from, or loss of, an attachment figure is one of the most distressing of all human experiences. An infant separated from a primary caregiver cries, thrashes, attempts to reestablish contact with the absent figure by calling and searching, and resists other people's soothing efforts. If the separation is prolonged, the infant grieves disconsolately, and anxiety and anger gradually give way to despair (Bowlby, 1980).

These negative emotional reactions are also observed in adolescence and adulthood following the unwanted breakup or loss of a romantic relationship. Such breakups can be devastating, and the resulting emotional reactions can be so intense that they erode a person's mental and physical health. Numerous studies have shown that unwanted breakups are associated with heightened physiological arousal and increased risk for emotional problems, physical illnesses, and even mortality (see Sbarra, 2012; Sbarra & Manvelian, Chapter 34, this volume). The most dramatic emotional reactions occur following the death of a primary attachment figure (Stroebe, Hansson, Schut, & Stroebe, 2008). This kind of loss is likely to bring forth an overwhelming and paralyzing torrent of negative affect that can disrupt psychological functioning for months. Despite variations in mourning rituals and expressions of grief across cultures, the death of an attachment figure evokes pain and despair everywhere in the world and has done so during all periods of recorded history (Rosenblatt, 2008).

According to Bowlby (1980), grief reactions are due to the attachment system's loss of a primary pillar of security, which causes an upsurge in hopelessness while searching for the lost attachment figure and the terror that accompanies the loss of a reliable source of protection, sympathy, and support. In line with this analysis, more intense grief is observed among adults who describe having a strong attachment to the person they have lost (e.g., Jerga, Shaver, & Wilkinson, 2011).

Coping with Loss: The Adaptive and Maladaptive Nature of Secondary Attachment Strategies

The loss of an attachment figure is not only a source of distress and despair; it is also a sign that the primary attachment strategy—proximity seeking—is not workable with respect to the lost figure and that one needs to adopt what Cassidy and Kobak (1988) called secondary attachment strategies—anxious hyperactivation of the attachment system, avoidant deactivation of the system, or a disorganized combination of both—to deal with the overwhelming pain of loss. Although these secondary strategies can be adopted even in response to short-term rejection or brief separations, Bowlby (1980) paid special attention to the use of these strategies during bereavement because the primary attachment strategy (seeking proximity and care) does not suffice following the death of an attachment figure.

Disordered Mourning

Bowlby (1980) suggested that secondary attachment strategies are involved in two major forms of disordered mourning: "chronic mourning" and "prolonged absence of conscious grieving" (p. 138). Chronic mourning (or *complicated grief*) is characterized by overwhelming anxiety and despair, prolonged problems in reestablishing normal life, ruminative thoughts and worries about the missing partner, and maintenance of an intense, active attachment to the deceased (as if this person is still alive) even years after the loss (see Chu & Lieberman, Chapter 32, this volume). An apparent absence of grief (or *delayed grief, inhibited mourning,* or *absent mourning*) is characterized by the lack of overt expressions of sadness or sorrow, emotional detachment from the missing partner, and a rapid return to normal life without major disruptions. According to Bowlby (1980), chronic mourning reflects a pervasive anxious hyperactivation of the attachment system, whereas absence of grief results from an avoidant deactivation, defensive shutdown, or suppression of attachment-related thoughts, feelings, and actions.

Anxious hyperactivation of the attachment system intensifies expressions of distress, neediness, and vulnerability and heightens attachment-related fears and worries that interfere with effective engagement in other activities (Cassidy & Kobak, 1988). Following the loss of an attachment figure, this hyperactivating strategy becomes more intense, rendering a person vulnerable to chronic mourning and depression (Mikulincer & Shaver, 2012). In contrast, avoidant deactivation of the attachment system involves dismissal of attachment needs, suppression of attachment-related thoughts and emotions, inhibition of proximity-seeking bids, and efforts to remain self-reliant and independent (Cassidy & Kobak, 1988). Following the loss of an attachment figure, these avoidant defenses can cause a person to suppress painful loss-related thoughts and feelings, avoid engaging in the mental labor required for grief resolution, and dismiss the importance of the lost relationship. These defenses direct attention away from painful memories and feelings (*defensive exclusion*) to such an extent that these mental representations may become mentally segregated or dissociated. However, these suppressed mental representations may continue to influence a person's responses without his or her being aware of it (Bowlby, 1980).

Bowlby (1980) claimed that prolonged absence of grieving could produce emotional problems and physical disorders if the bereaved person was strongly attached to the deceased. In such cases, defensive exclusion proves difficult because even subtle reminders of the deceased can reactivate suppressed or defensively excluded memories and feelings. Moreover, if the mourner shared many everyday activities and places with the deceased, these activities and places can become painful reminders of the loss, which in turn may have negative effects on mental and physical health.

It is important to note that bereaved individuals who rarely sought proximity to and comfort from a mate when he or she was alive and remained emotionally detached from the mate may be less likely to experience intense distress and pain, develop segregated or dissociated memories and emotions, or be overwhelmed by the intrusion of unwanted memories and feelings when reminded of the deceased's passing (Jerga et al., 2011). In such cases, absence of grieving may reflect a true absence of distress rather a defensive reaction against the psychological pain caused by the loss of an important attachment figure. Compatible with this possibility, many people who exhibit few signs of grief shortly after the loss of a partner do not display signs of distress, maladjustment, or poor health months or years later (see Bonanno, Boerner, & Wortman, 2008). In fact, avoidant people, who tend to remain emotionally detached even when involved in long-term relationships including marriage, often do not show strong signs of distress or pain following the death of a partner (e.g., Jerga et al., 2011).

Healthy Mourning: Attachment Reorganization and Grief Resolution

Some degree of hyperactivation and deactivation is also involved in the two major psychological tasks thought to be required for healthy grief resolution (Mikulincer & Shaver, 2012). One task involves accepting the death of the loved other, returning to everyday activities, and rearranging or "editing" one's hierarchy of attachment figures by forming new emotional bonds or upgrading existing ones. The other task involves maintaining a symbolic attachment to the deceased and integrating the lost relationship into one's personal identity and self-narrative. These two tasks are part of what Bowlby (1980) called "attachment reorganization"—the rearrangement of representations of the deceased attachment figure and the self in relation to this figure and the "editing" of the hierarchy of attachment figures (Fraley & Shaver, 2016). Attachment reorganization, like other developmental transitions, requires a gradual transfer of attachment functions (proximity seeking, safe haven, secure base) from the deceased to other security providers so that security needs can be met by these alternative figures. Moreover, just as adolescents must transfer attachment functions from parents to peers but continue to use their parents as attachment figures "in reserve," mourners can transform the deceased into an internal, symbolic source of security. In this way, the symbolic bond with the deceased as well as new or renewed attachments with living figures can sustain a bereaved person's sense of security.

How might anxious hyperactivation and avoidant deactivation contribute to attachment reorganization? Hyperactivation, by motivating a mourner to experience and express the deep pain of loss, reactivate memories of the deceased, and yearn for this person's proximity and love, can help the mourner explore the meaning and importance of the lost relationship and find new ways to maintain a symbolic bond with the deceased. When hyperactivation is regulated properly, a mourner can incorporate the past into the present without splitting off important elements of his or her self and identity tied to the lost attachment figure. Avoidant deactivation can also contribute to the reorganization process by enabling momentary detachment from the deceased and blocking the intrusion of painful thoughts and feelings. With this assistance, the bereaved individual can explore the new reality, return to mundane activities, and realize that life presents new and attractive opportunities following a loss. If this deactivation targets only the relationship with the deceased rather than all close relationships, it can even facilitate the formation of new attachment bonds and the adaptive transfer of attachment functions.

Without at least some periods of attachment-system hyperactivation, a mourner is not fully capable of integrating the lost figure into his or her identity. And without some degree of deactivation, the mourner may remain stuck in grief, unable to form emotional bonds with new relationship partners. Attachment reorganization requires both kinds of secondary strategies, operating in a dynamic balance or a graceful "oscillation" (see Stroebe, Schut, & Stroebe, 2005). With the passage of time and the successful transfer of attachment functions to other partners, this oscillation is gradually reduced and the mourner moves ahead with new attachments as well as a continuing symbolic bond with the deceased.

What are the factors that favor a successful oscillation between hyperactivation and deactivation? Although this oscillation process has not yet been systematically examined, we believe that it might depend on the extent to which (1) the deceased was a major source of security and (2) new relationship partners provide a source of security and comfort. If the lost figure was cold and rejecting while alive, hyperactivation may entrap the bereaved person in a welter of distress, confusion, and ambivalence (like a child returning to an abusive parent). Forming new relationships with emotionally distant and unresponsive partners can also prevent the transfer of attachment functions and a return to normal life. In both cases, reorganization may fail. Moreover, deactivation can be overgeneralized, leading to undifferentiated inhibition of attachment needs and problems in forming close relationships. Of course, these tentative ideas need to be tested in prospective studies examining patterns of attachment hyperactivation and deactivation throughout the grief process.

Bowlby (1980) also thought that attachment insecurities (anxiety, avoidance) can jeopardize attachment reorganization and complicate the grief process. Attachment-anxious individuals are unable to deactivate loss-related thoughts and feelings and return to ordinary life; avoidant individuals are unable to maintain comforting symbolic bonds with the deceased. In both cases, attachment insecurities can interfere with adaptive hyperactivation-deactivation oscillation, cause a person to rely more on one secondary strategy than the other, and suffer from either chronic mourning (in the case of attachment-anxious individuals) or prolonged absence of grief (in the case of attachment-avoidant individuals). In contrast, dispositional attachment security allows a person to steer clear of disordered mourning. Secure individuals can recall and think about a lost partner and discuss the loss more coherently (e.g., Hesse, 2016; Shaver & Tancredy, 2001). Moreover, their constructive coping strategies allow them to experience and express distress without suffering a disruption of normal functioning (e.g., Stroebe et al., 2005). In addition, their positive models of the lost partner allow them to continue to create or use a symbolic bond with the deceased, and their positive models of self allow them to cope with the loss and begin to form new relationships (Shaver & Tancredy, 2001). Indeed, there is extensive evidence showing that chronic attachment insecurities (anxiety, avoidance) are associated with disordered patterns of mourning (see Fraley & Shaver, 2016; Mikulincer & Shaver, 2012).

Concluding Remarks

Reactions to separation from and loss of an attachment figure are primary issues in Bowlby's theory. The intensity of loss reactions—often taking adults by surprise and seeming to be shockingly irrational (e.g., Didion, 2007)—provides some of the strongest evidence for the deep significance of attachment relationships and processes. If attachment were simply an attitude or a set of habitual expectations based on familiarity with a particular caregiver or romantic partner, its disruption would not cause the extreme misery that Bowlby and others noted in young children forcibly separated from parents, and that grief researchers observe in people who have lost an adult attachment figure to death. These predictable reactions are among the most important clues concerning the nature of attachment and the various ways of coping with attachment insecurity.

REFERENCES

Bonanno, G., Boerner, K., & Wortman, C. (2008). Trajectories of grieving. In M. S. Stroebe, R. O. Hansson, H. Schut, & W. Stroebe (Eds.), *Handbook of bereavement research and practice: Advances in theory and intervention* (pp. 287–307). Washington, DC: American Psychological Association.

Bowlby, J. (1980). *Attachment and loss: Vol. 3. Loss, sadness and depression.* New York: Basic Books.

Cassidy, J., & Kobak, R. R. (1988). Avoidance and its relationship with other defensive processes. In J. Belsky & T. Nezworski (Eds.), *Clinical implications of attachment* (pp. 300–323). Hillsdale, NJ: Erlbaum.

Didion, J. (2007). *The year of magical thinking*. New York: Vintage.

Fraley, R. C., & Shaver, P. R. (2016). Attachment, loss, and grief: Bowlby's views, new developments, and current controversies. In J. Cassidy & P. R. Shaver (Eds.), *Handbook of attachment: Theory, research, and clinical applications* (3rd ed., pp. 40–62). New York: Guilford Press.

Hesse, E. (2016). The Adult Attachment Interview: Protocol, method of analysis, and selected empirical studies: 1985–2015. In J. Cassidy & P. R. Shaver (Eds.), *Handbook of attachment: Theory, research, and clinical applications* (3rd ed., pp. 553–557). New York: Guilford Press.

Jerga, C., Shaver, P. R., & Wilkinson, R. B. (2011). Attachment insecurities and identification of at-risk individuals following the death of a loved one. *Journal of Social and Personal Relationships, 28,* 891–914.

Mikulincer, M., & Shaver, P. R. (2012). Attachment insecurities and disordered patterns of grief. In M. Stroebe, H. Schut, P. Boelen, & J. van den Bout (Eds.), *Complicated grief: Scientific foundations for health care professionals* (pp. 190–203). New York: Routledge.

Mikulincer, M., & Shaver, P. R. (2016). *Attachment in adulthood: Structure, dynamics, and change* (2nd ed.). New York: Guilford Press.

Rosenblatt, P. C. (2008). Grief across cultures: A review and research agenda. In M. S. Stroebe, R. O. Hansson, H. Schut, & W. Stroebe (Eds.), *Handbook of bereavement research and practice: Advances in theory and intervention* (pp. 207–222). Washington, DC: American Psychological Association.

Sbarra, D. A. (2012). Marital dissolution and physical health outcomes: A review of mechanisms. In L. Campbell, J. La Guardia, J. Olson, & M. Zanna (Eds.), *The Ontario Symposium: Vol. 12. The science of the couple* (pp. 205–227). Florence, KY: Psychology Press.

Shaver, P. R., & Tancredy, C. M. (2001). Emotion, attachment, and bereavement: A conceptual commentary. In M. S. Stroebe, W. Stroebe, R. O. Hansson, & H. Schut (Eds.), *Handbook of bereavement research: Consequences, coping, and care* (pp. 63–88). Washington, DC: American Psychological Association.

Stroebe, M., Hansson, R. O., Schut, H., & Stroebe, W. (Eds.). (2008). *Handbook of bereavement research and practice: Advances in theory and intervention*. Washington, DC: American Psychological Association.

Stroebe, M., Schut, H., & Stroebe, W. (2005). Attachment in coping with bereavement: A theoretical integration. *Review of General Psychology, 9,* 48–66.

CHAPTER 34

The Psychological and Biological Correlates of Separation and Loss

David A. Sbarra
Atina Manvelian

> True friendship is like sound health; the value of it
> is seldom known until it is lost.
> —attributed to CHARLES CALEB COLTON

This chapter considers two major themes, both of which center on adaptation to loss. In the latter half, we focus on the general experience of loss in adulthood, which is relevant for the study of bereavement as well as for nonmarital breakups and divorce. Before discussing relationship dissolution, however, we wish to shine a light on intact relationships. A deep understanding of the biopsychosocial correlates of loss, we believe, hinges on a deep understanding of the adult attachment bond itself. *What does it mean to say we are attached to another person?*

Building on the existing animal literature, Sbarra and Hazan (2008) argued that coregulation—an interdependence of biological systems within the pair bond around a homeostatic set point—is an emergent property of an attachment bond. In this definition, the word *emergent* is key. When two people fall in love and become attached, they often move from a point of relative physical and psychological distance to a place of extreme physical and psychological closeness. What emerges from this closeness—especially the intimate physical and sexual activity that often leads people to fall in love—is a pair bond (Zeifman & Hazan, 2016; see also Aviles & Zeifman, Chapter 7, this volume), and this pair bond is subserved by coregulation.

In Sbarra and Hazan's (2008) writing about coregulation, much of the focus was on physiological interdependence. However, ample literature now suggests that attachment relationships both shape and are shaped by psychological interdependence as well. For example, it appears that the brain represents threats to *close* others—but not threats to strangers—in similar neural regions as when representing threats to the self (Beckes, Coan, & Hasselmo, 2013). Similarly, if becoming attached involves the merging of the self with the other, a phenomenon that is well documented in psychological literature (e.g., Aron, Paris, & Aron, 1995), then responses to loss may be best understood and studied as a reorganization of mental representations of the self and the other.

Bowlby (1980) discussed this process of loss at length in the third volume of his trilogy. Perhaps most germane to the present analysis was Bowlby's idea that the key to healthy mourning was, "in some degree at least, a withdrawal of emotional investment in the lost person and that they may prepare for making a relationship with a new one" (p. 25). One of the reasons loss experiences create so much psychological distress is that people experience difficulties cleaving themselves from their former partner, reporting that they feel as if they are actually "losing a part of themselves" (Manvelian, Bourassa, Lawrence, Mehl, & Sbarra, 2018). We believe that this type of language is not simply metaphorical. If we take seriously the literature on coregulation (see LeRoy, Knee, Derrick, & Fagundes, 2019), this expression is probably closer to being literal than metaphorical.

When we experience loss, we lose the benefit conferred by our attachment figures—the homeostatic regulation around physiological *and* psychological set points. Accordingly, this experience portends not only emotional distress, but also autonomic hyperarousal, a loss of self, sleep difficulties, and many other challenges (Sbarra & Coan, 2017). In this sense, interpersonal loss is different from many other stressful experiences in that the pain of the loss is compounded by the fact that we are losing the person to whom we are accustomed to turning to in times of distress (see Bowlby, 1980).

How Do People Respond to the Loss of an Attachment Figure?

Normative Processes

We begin by thinking about normative responses to loss. The individual differences that shape adjustment to loss—that is, the behaviors, personality styles, or pathologies that give rise to or protect against risk for adverse outcomes following loss—do so, we argue, because they either exacerbate or help quell the normative challenge of loss: regulating a sense of felt security. Felt security within an attachment relationship is the sense that the world is predictable and safe, that we are loved, and that challenges are manageable because of the benefits afforded by the relationship; it is the emotional set point of the coregulatory processes operating within an attachment relationship (Mikulincer & Shaver, 2007; see also Mikulincer & Shaver, Chapter 26, this volume). For most people, separation and loss events disrupt this sense of felt security (Diamond, Hicks, & Otter-Henderson, 2008; Janoff-Bulman, 1992), but the extent to which this disruption is experienced as mild or severe, and the extent to which it is maintained over time, depends largely on individual differences.

Individual Differences

There are tremendous differences in how people respond to loss events. In our work on marital separation and divorce, for example, we have found that while there is an average-level increased risk for early death associated with the dissolution of marriage, this risk is actually limited to a subset of people, especially adults who have a tendency to become over-involved or to actively avoid their emotional experiences (Sbarra & Coan, 2017; see also Shaver & Mikulincer, Chapter 33, this volume). For example, although the majority of people are resilient in the face of attachment loss, the mortality risk associated with loss is particularly elevated among people who become depressed following the end of marriage (Malgaroli, Galatzer-Levy, & Bonanno, 2017), whereas *chronic* depression—which usually does not emerge after the end of marriage—does not confer an equivalent risk.

Relationship-Specific Factors

Responses to loss also vary depending on relationship-specific factors such as the level of commitment in the relationship, with longer relationship duration and greater closeness in the relationship being associated with higher levels of stress after a breakup (Frazier & Cook, 1993). The quality of the relationship can also moderate postbreakup distress, suggesting that some people may actually experience *positive* responses to the end of marriage. In a longitudinal, nationally representative sample of married adults, for example, women who ended low-quality marriages showed the highest levels of life satisfaction over a 10-year period (Bourassa, Sbarra, & Whisman, 2015). One key finding in this study was that these gains in life satisfaction were realized only among women in the lowest quality marriages—about 15% of the sample. The authors speculate that these substantial improvements in psychological well-being may be predicated on ending relationships characterized by extreme discord, abuse, or violence.

A small literature also suggests that the nature of the relational loss event itself can shape the degree of consequent distress. For example, life events that are characterized by humiliation or infidelity tend to be highly associated with the onset of major depressive disorder, with participants reporting higher levels of both depression and anxiety compared to those who did not experience such events (Cano & O'Leary, 2000). Romantic rejection and unrequited love are also characteristic of many breakups and highly associated with emotional pain and distress (Monroe, Rohde, Seeley, & Lewinsohn, 1999; Sbarra & Hazan, 2008). Still untested, however, is whether these events are so overpowering that they give rise to negative outcomes in general or whether some people (e.g., those with more secure attachment styles or states of mind) respond to even the most difficult breakups with transient distress, presumably because they have a generally positive representation of close others and see themselves as fundamentally lovable. This point highlights the way in which individual and relationship differences shape normative responses to loss (see Shaver & Mikulincer, Chapter 5, this volume).

What Are the Key Processes and Mechanisms Involved?

When considering the key processes and mechanisms that shape adaptation to loss, we again rely on the idea of felt security. The emotion regulation strategies that characterize anxious and avoidant dimensions of attachment insecurity (hyperactivation and deactivation, respectively) are behavioral strategies designed to maintain or restore one's sense of felt security (Mikulincer & Shaver, 2007). Loss events, however, pose an unusual demand on the attachment system because our partner is no longer available to help inhibit threats to felt security. People use emotion regulation scripts to manage threatening circumstances, with those high in anxiety relying on a *sentinel* script (amplifying the danger and notifying others about it) and with those high in avoidance using a *fight–flight* script (acting rapidly to escape without depending on others). Even though they have not been studied in the context of loss events, these scripts are likely to affect how people manage their emotions when relationships end. Maladaptation is observed most frequently when people rely on rigid emotion regulation scripts. We believe this is so because it limits emotion regulation flexibility (Bonanno & Burton, 2013), thereby keeping people stuck in perseverative loops of emotional overinvolvement (anxiety) or suppressive emotional states, where feelings related to the loss are pushed away (avoidance).

In contrast, attachment security is often defined in part by emotional equanimity, with people scoring high in attachment security being more mindful and accepting of present-moment experiences. We can compare maladaptive scripts to those that are more secure and express better emotional balance. Consider the following: "My wife is gone. This is so painful—I feel sadness everywhere. My heart is breaking. Breathe. Just breathe. It will be OK." Perhaps more than anything else, this statement is descriptive and experientially open—it acknowledges the awful pain of loss without becoming hyperfocused on it or avoiding it. In this way, people high in security have more access to and ease in dealing with their primary emotions, and when people allow primary emotions to be as they are, they gradually abate over time as people engage in the world around them. When people can engage in the world around them—see old friends, visit family, participate in new activities, meet new people— they are able to reorganize their sense of self and, in turn, become unattached from the person they have lost. However, when people are trapped in these experiences or energy is spent avoiding the pain of loss altogether, engagement with life experiences that can reorganize the attachment relationship in their minds along with their fundamental sense of self is inhibited.

Although not all of these ideas have been tested empirically in populations experiencing an attachment loss, a handful of studies designed to improve psychological distress support these basic contentions. For example, psychological treatments such as acceptance and commitment therapy (Hayes, Luoma, Bond, Masuda, & Lillis, 2006) or emotionally focused therapy (Johnson, 2019) advocate an open and curious stance toward emotional experiences—encouraging people to get in touch with their underlying emotions without attaching to them or avoiding them. Another behavioral target that is likely related to secure attachment and emotional equanimity is the capacity for self-compassion—the ability to take an emotionally equanimous and kind stance with respect to one's own experience. Self-compassion is associated with less emotional distress following a marital separation or divorce (Sbarra, Smith, & Mehl, 2012). Future research might empirically test if there is considerable overlap between those who rank high on self-compassion and those who experience attachment security, both of which are associated with better outcomes after loss (see Waters, Waters, & Waters, Chapter 14, this volume).

Conclusion

The authors of this volume were invited to answer a series of focused questions, and we would like to conclude our contribution with some questions of our own. First, we have speculated that social engagement is important for loss recovery, largely because it allows people to reorganize their attachment to a former partner and redefine their sense of self. This perspective, however, remains largely conjecture, and empirical studies on this topic would be a welcome addition to the literature. Second, we know little about how repeated loss events and the characteristics of these events shape how people enter into new relationships and experience losses in the future. If, for example, someone is rejected in a very hurtful way during a breakup, how does this shape the manner in which that person thinks, feels, and behaves in a new relationship and when that relationship ends? Third, can we induce or promote secure attachment to help people recover from breakups more effectively? If so, how? Especially in light of these new findings, we need more studies on coregulation. Can we assess coregulation with any degree of accuracy? What is it, and what is it not? How should "homeostatic set points" be assessed? In many ways, these questions bring us to our main conclusion: Any study of loss must draw upon the attachment literature and begin with a detailed understanding of the nature and function of attachment relationships.

REFERENCES

Aron, A., Paris, M., & Aron, E. N. (1995). Falling in love: Prospective studies of self-concept change. *Journal of Personality and Social Psychology, 69,* 1102.

Beckes, L., Coan, J. A., & Hasselmo, K. (2013). Familiarity promotes the blurring of self and other in the neural representation of threat. *Social Cognitive and Affective Neuroscience, 8,* 670–677.

Bonanno, G. A., & Burton, C. L. (2013). Regulatory flexibility: An individual differences perspective on coping and emotion regulation. *Perspectives on Psychological Science, 8,* 591–612.

Bourassa, K. J., Sbarra, D. A., & Whisman, M. A. (2015). Women in very low quality marriages gain life satisfaction following divorce. *Journal of Family Psychology, 29,* 490.

Bowlby, J. (1980). *Attachment and loss: Vol. 3. Loss, sadness and depression.* New York: Basic Books.

Cano, A., & O'Leary, K. D. (2000). Infidelity and separations precipitate major depressive episodes and symptoms of nonspecific depression and anxiety. *Journal of Consulting and Clinical Psychology, 68*(5), 774.

Diamond, L. M., Hicks, A. M., & Otter-Henderson, K. D. (2008). Every time you go away: Changes in affect, behavior, and physiology associated with travel-related separations from romantic partners. *Journal of Personality and Social Psychology, 95,* 385–403.

Frazier, P. A., & Cook, S. W. (1993). Correlates of distress following heterosexual relationship dissolution. *Journal of Social and Personal Relationships, 10,* 55–67.

Hayes, S. C., Luoma, J. B., Bond, F. W., Masuda, A., & Lillis, J. (2006). Acceptance and commitment therapy: Model, processes and outcomes. *Behaviour Research and Therapy, 44*(1), 1–25.

Janoff-Bulman, R. (1992). *Shattered assumptions: Towards a new psychology of trauma.* New York: Free Press.

Johnson, S. M. (2019). *Attachment theory in practice: Emotionally focused therapy (EFT) with individuals, couples, and families.* New York: Guilford Press.

LeRoy, A. S., Knee, C. R., Derrick, J. L., & Fagundes, C. P. (2019). Implications for reward processing in differential responses to loss: Impacts on attachment hierarchy reorganization. *Personality and Social Psychology Review, 23*(4), 391–405.

Malgaroli, M., Galatzer-Levy, I. R., & Bonanno, G. A. (2017). Heterogeneity in trajectories of depression in response to divorce is associated with differential risk for mortality. *Clinical Psychological Science, 5,* 843–850.

Manvelian, A., Bourassa, K. J., Lawrence, E., Mehl, M. R., & Sbarra, D. A. (2018). With or without you?: Loss of self following marital separation. *Journal of Social and Clinical Psychology, 37,* 297–324.

Mikulincer, M., & Shaver, P. R. (2007). *Attachment in adulthood: Structure, dynamics, and change.* New York: Guilford Press.

Monroe, S. M., Rohde, P., Seeley, J. R., & Lewinsohn, P. M. (1999). Life events and depression in adolescence: Relationship loss as a prospective risk factor for first onset of major depressive disorder. *Journal of Abnormal Psychology, 108*(4), 606.

Sbarra, D. A., & Coan, J. A. (2017). Divorce and health: Good data in need of better theory. *Current Opinion in Psychology, 13,* 91–95.

Sbarra, D. A., & Hazan, C. (2008). Coregulation, dysregulation, and self-regulation: An integrative analysis and empirical agenda for understanding attachment, separation, loss, and recovery. *Personality and Social Psychology Review,* 141–167.

Sbarra, D. A., Smith, H. L., & Mehl, M. R. (2012). When leaving your ex, love yourself: Observational ratings of self-compassion predict the course of emotional recovery following marital separation. *Psychological Science, 23*(3), 261–269.

Zeifman, D., & Hazan, C. (2016). Pair bonds as attachments: Mounting evidence in support of Bowlby's hypothesis. In J. Cassidy & P. R. Shaver (Eds.), *Handbook of attachment: Theory, research, and clinical applications* (3rd ed., pp. 416–434). New York: Guilford Press.

CHAPTER 35

Breaking the Marital Ties That Bind
Divorce from a Spousal Attachment Figure

Brooke C. Feeney
Joan K. Monin

One of the strongest attachment bonds formed in adulthood is the one formed with a spouse. According to attachment theory, neither love nor grief nor other forms of strong emotion are felt for just any person; instead, they are felt for particular individuals with whom one has established an attachment bond (Bowlby, 1969/1982, 1979). Once formed, an attachment bond tends to endure, and its disruption is strongly resisted. Because divorce involves the termination or reorganization of one of the strongest affectional bonds formed by adults, it is a highly significant life transition. This article describes an attachment perspective on responses to the loss of a spousal attachment figure, followed by a discussion of key processes and mechanisms underlying those responses, with a focus on the persistence of the attachment bond.

Response to the Loss of a Spousal Attachment Figure

In happy, well-functioning marriages, the attachment system works so that both partners feel safe and protected, each is able to depend on the other, and each is unafraid of the other's dependence. Attachment theory stipulates two important criteria for healthy functioning: First, to feel safe and protected, every individual (throughout the lifespan) requires the presence and availability of a trustworthy figure who is willing and able to provide a *safe haven* (comfort and support in times of need) and a *secure base* (from which to engage in exploration of the world and one's own capacities). Second, everyone must be able both to recognize when another person is a trustworthy attachment figure and to collaborate with him or her to maintain a mutually rewarding relationship (Bowlby, 1979). The absence of these important features of a marriage—for one or both partners—sets the stage for dysfunctional relations and separation and divorce (Feeney & Monin, 2016).

Attachment theory explains the many forms of emotional distress and personality disturbance (e.g., anxiety, anger, depression) to which separation and loss can give rise (Bowlby, 1979). Because attachment is an instinctive process that is elicited particularly during times of threat/ stress, the loss of a spousal attachment figure represents an ultimate threat that can provoke intense feelings of distress and have adverse effects on health and well-being, particularly if the bond is not broken for both couple members. Breaking attachment bonds is difficult and impactful even for those who wish to end their relationships because the presence and significance of an attachment bond is not always recognized until it is severed.

Studies on adjustment to divorce have shown that separated and divorced individuals have higher rates of physical and mental health disturbance than married individuals, and often higher rates even than widowed individuals (see Feeney & Monin, 2016, for a review). Separated and divorced individuals experience increased rates of acute and chronic physical illnesses, physical limitations, psychopathology, depression, suicide, homicide, violence, substance abuse, accidents and injuries, and disease-caused mortality (e.g., Bourassa, Ruiz, & Sbarra, 2019; Sbarra, 2015). Divorced individuals also report lower levels of happiness, life satisfaction, self-esteem, self-confidence, and competence (e.g., Gustavson, Røysamb, von Soest, Helland, & Mathiesen, 2012).

However, if divorced people are compared with people in the most unhappy marriages, the divorced have higher morale, fewer physical problems, fewer depressive symptoms, and greater life satisfaction, self-esteem, and overall health (Hawkins & Booth, 2005). Thus, the more unhappiness and distress experienced in a marriage, the greater the relief and potential benefit that may follow divorce (Gustavson et al., 2012). Following a period of both emotional and physical upheaval, most adults cope successfully with divorce, and some report opportunities for growth, increased independence, and increased life satisfaction (Perrig-Chiello, Hutchison, & Morselli, 2015).

Key explanations for the psychological and physical health effects of divorce include (1) the protective effects of marriage (e.g., healthier lifestyle, more financial resources, stable social network); (2) a social selectivity or preexisting pathology model, indicating that people who divorce are less physically or psychologically fit for marriage; and (3) a crisis model, indicating that divorce is a traumatic event that induces psychological distress and health problems that lessen as a person adjusts (e.g., Solomon & Jackson, 2014). Attachment theory unifies these perspectives by postulating that although the biological function of attachment is protection, and separation anxiety/distress is a normative response to a severed bond, some people are predisposed by previous experiences to react more strongly to it (Sbarra & Coan, 2017).

Attachment theory predicts differential experiences of the divorce process based on attachment orientation (McNelis & Segrin, 2019). Divorce should be particularly taxing for individuals with troubled attachment histories (insecure attachment orientations) because (1) the separation confirms their worst fears and expectations, (2) the divorce is likely to reactivate earlier unresolved separations from attachment figures, and (3) insecure individuals lack the inner resources and coping strategies for adjusting to divorce (Feeney & Monin, 2016). Attachment anxiety and avoidance are associated with greater divorce-related distress and poorer coping. Specifically, separated adults high in attachment anxiety show poor adjustment to divorce, higher levels of hyperactivating coping strategies, and the highest levels of blood pressure during a divorce-specific task (Feeney & Monin, 2016; Lee, Sbarra, Mason, & Law, 2011). Among avoidant individuals, those who were able to self-regulate showed improvements in their self-concept over time, whereas those who were less able to self-regulate showed either no improvement or worsening of their self-concept (Sbarra & Borelli, 2013). The divorce-related distress experienced by secure individuals, however, is likely buffered by their social and personal resources that facilitate coping.

Bowlby (1979) noted that adults generally respond to separation and loss in a series of stages (numbness, yearning and searching, disorganization and despair, then reorganization), and he identified characteristics of loss situations that interfere with healthy adjustment: (1) the relationship provided considerable self-esteem and role identity, which is less sustainable without the lost partner; (2) having no close relationship with another person to whom the individual can transfer some aspects of the attachment bond; and (3) a marriage that was conflicted or ambivalent. Favorable outcomes are more likely if the person is able to express his or her feelings of yearning, anger, sadness, and fear of loneliness, and if he or she has the support of another trusted person.

Key Processes and Mechanisms: Persistence of the Attachment Bond

Although there are many stressors with which divorced individuals must cope (e.g., economic problems, social network changes), the loss of the marital relationship itself, combined with continuing contact and involvement with the ex-spouse, has been viewed as the most stressful part of the divorce experience. Separation from a spouse elicits conflicting emotions in both partners, including anger, contempt, regret, resentment, longing, affection, wish for reconciliation, guilt, anxiety, panic, sadness, and loneliness—regardless of what led to the divorce (Feeney & Monin, 2016). This mixture of positive and negative emotions can be confusing and is attributed to the persistence of the attachment bond when intimate relationships are disrupted.

Many people going through divorce continue to have feelings of attachment toward their ex-spouses (Bourassa, Hasselmo, & Sbarra, 2019). Although feelings of attachment are greatest when the divorce is recent and the spouse was the initiator, attachment does not seem to be influenced by the length of marriage, suggesting that attachment bonds may be established quickly but broken slowly and that the loss of an attachment bond is as difficult for those married a few years as for those married many years. Once partners have significantly bonded, attachment often persists and resists dissolution—even in the face of anger, hurt, and knowledge that the relationship should be terminated (Feeney & Monin, 2016).

Continued feelings of attachment have been considered to be a primary cause of the emotional and adjustment problems that follow separation (Madden-Derdich & Arditti, 1999; Sbarra & Borelli, 2019). Continuing attachment may be accounted for by the biological predisposition to use attachment figures as a safe haven and secure base. Losing an attachment figure eliminates these protective functions and creates both separation anxiety and attachment system activation. The many challenges associated with divorce are stressors that are likely to intensify activation of the attachment system and create a desire for proximity to one's attachment figure (who was the spouse prior to the divorce). The process of detachment and reorganization is likely to be more difficult than either spouse anticipates because attachment bonds may be partly unconscious and sometimes masked by feelings of dissatisfaction with the spouse. This may explain why many couples headed for divorce separate and then reconcile at least once before ending the relationship, why some ex-spouses have sex when they were intending only to transfer their children, and why a majority of remarried men regret having divorced their former wives (see Feeney & Monin, 2016, for a review).

Because of the difficulty of detaching, divorced individuals often experience a deep vulnerability to their former spouse, which they feel they must guard against with defensive strategies to prevent the pain of reevoked attachment feelings (Feeney & Monin, 2016). Regardless of who initiated the divorce, both couple members are likely to be vulnerable, and the process of detachment is likely to be slow and painful for both.

In fact, before detachment occurs, the attachment bond may be reactivated if the attachment figure reappears and invites renewed attachment. Attachment feelings and behaviors can be easily reactivated by drawing the former spouse back into old behavior patterns. Mikulincer and Florian (1996) proposed that adaptation to loss of an attachment figure involves a dialectical interplay of two opposing forces: the desire to maintain proximity to the lost person and the simultaneous desire to detach from the person to form new relationships.

Despite a large empirical literature on other aspects of the divorce experience, little is known about postdivorce relationships between ex-spouses. Clinical and empirical reports have shown that continued relations with a former spouse are often problematic and postdivorce harmony is rare (Buunk & Mutsaers, 1999). Few relationships offer as many opportunities for anger, blame, hatred, retaliation, desires for revenge, and violence as the ones between former spouses, particularly given that ex-spouses know each other's vulnerabilities. Remarriages may also contribute to poor postdivorce relations because a continuing relationship with a former spouse may be threatening to a new spouse and create conflict in the new marriage.

Attachment theory provides a basis for explaining some of the negative ways that former spouses behave toward each other. Bowlby (1969/1982) explained that behavior of an aggressive sort (protest, anger) often plays a role in maintaining affectional bonds. For example, when separation is perceived to be temporary, anger may hasten reunion and make it less likely that another separation will occur. This may explain why high levels of disagreement and conflict typically occur during the first year of marital separation; why many women continue to suffer physical and verbal abuse after separation and divorce, typically by men who do not want the relationship to end; and why many relationships without a history of violence often become violent at the time of separation (Feeney & Monin, 2016).

It is important to note, however, that a majority of divorced individuals report at least occasional contact with their ex-spouses, and that continuing attachment (presumably relatively secure attachment) might be associated with healthy development as well (Masheter, 1991). For example, research on children's continued contact with both parents has acknowledged the benefits of cooperative postdivorce relationships between ex-spouses (Gürmen, Huff, Brown, Orbuch, & Birditt, 2017). Cooperative postdivorce parenting can reduce role strain for custodial parents and the sense of estrangement and loss for noncustodial parents (Masheter, 1991). In fact, it has been argued that for couples who share custody of children, detachment can be only limited and some degree of attachment, if transferred effectively into constructive behavior, might be beneficial (Madden-Derdich & Arditti, 1999).

Given the strength of the attachment bond, divorced couples may need protection from each other during and after divorce in the form of agreed-upon rules of engagement and civility to set limits on dysfunctional behavior. The challenge is to redefine the relationship in a way that is mutually supportive, while minimizing behaviors that adversely affect adjustment (Madden-Derdich & Arditti, 1999; Sbarra & Borelli, 2019). Because the relationship between former spouses often determines the emotional climate in which families function after a divorce, this redefinition process has significant implications for the functioning of the family in its new form.

Both theoretical and empirical work on the redefinition process is needed (Sbarra & Borelli, 2019). Perhaps as postdivorce attachments are reorganized so that some of the earlier positive feelings and a new commitment to cooperative interdependence (e.g., in parenting) can be beneficial, the disappointment/animosity engendered by the failed marital relationship can fade into the background of memory. This redefinition process may involve a process of transition from an attachment bond to an affiliative bond, which, according to attachment theory, relies on a separate behavioral system. This redefinition process also involves the coordination and maintenance of joint caregiving responsibilities toward the children (perhaps motivated by recognition of the importance of the child's continuing secure attachment to both parents), while recognizing that other aspects of the prior marital relationship (attachment, sexuality, and caregiving toward the spouse) no longer apply. Positive relations between ex-spouses serve the interests of both spouses' caregiving systems, enhancing the children's well-being and the divorced parents' reproductive fitness. Attachment-based interventions may assist in the redefinition process.

REFERENCES

Bourassa, K. J., Hasselmo, K., & Sbarra, D. A. (2019). After the end: Linguistic predictors of psychological distress 4 years after marital separation. *Journal of Social and Personal Relationships, 36*(6), 1872–1891.

Bourassa, K. J., Ruiz, J. M., & Sbarra, D. A. (2019). Smoking and physical activity explain the increased mortality risk following marital separation and divorce: Evidence from the English Longitudinal Study of Ageing. *Annals of Behavioral Medicine, 53,* 255–266.

Bowlby, J. (1979). *The making and breaking of affectional bonds.* London: Tavistock.

Bowlby, J. (1982). *Attachment and loss, Vol. 1: Attachment* (2nd ed.). New York: Basic Books. (Original work published 1969)

Buunk, B. P., & Mutsaers, W. (1999). The nature of the relationship between remarried individuals and former spouses and its impact on marital satisfaction. *Journal of Family Psychology, 13,* 165–174.

Feeney, B. C., & Monin, J. K. (2016). Divorce through the lens of attachment theory. In J. Cassidy & P. R. Shaver (Eds.), *Handbook of attachment: Theory, research, and clinical applications* (3rd ed., pp. 941–965). New York: Guilford Press.

Gürmen, M. S., Huff, S. C., Brown, E., Orbuch, T. L., & Birditt, K. S. (2017). Divorced yet still together: Ongoing personal relationship and coparenting among divorced parents. *Journal of Divorce and Remarriage, 58,* 645–660.

Gustavson, K., Røysamb, E., von Soest, T., Helland, M. J., & Mathiesen, K. S. (2012). Longitudinal associations between relationship problems, divorce, and life satisfaction: Findings from a 15-year population-based study. *Journal of Positive Psychology, 7,* 188–197.

Hawkins, D. N., & Booth, A. (2005). Unhappily ever after: Effects of long-term, low-quality marriages on well-being. *Social Forces, 84,* 451–471.

Lee, L. A., Sbarra, D. A., Mason, A. E., & Law, R. W. (2011). Attachment anxiety, verbal immediacy, and blood pressure: Results from a laboratory analog study following marital separation. *Personal Relationships, 18,* 285–301.

Madden-Derdich, D. A., & Arditti, J. A. (1999). The ties that bind: Attachment between former spouses. *Family Relations, 48,* 243–249.

Masheter, C. (1991). Postdivorce relationships between ex-spouses: The roles of attachment and interpersonal conflict. *Journal of Marriage and the Family, 53,* 103–110.

McNelis, M., & Segrin, C. (2019). Insecure attachment predicts history of divorce, marriage, and current relationship status, *Journal of Divorce and Remarriage, 60,* 404–417.

Mikulincer, M., & Florian, V. (1996). Emotional reactions to interpersonal losses over the life span: An attachment theoretical perspective. In C. Magai & S. H. McFadden (Eds.), *Handbook of emotions, adult development, and aging* (pp. 269–285). San Diego, CA: Academic Press.

Perrig-Chiello, P., Hutchison, S., & Morselli, D. (2015). Patterns of psychological adaptation to divorce after a long-term marriage. *Journal of Social and Personal Relationships, 32,* 386–405.

Sbarra, D. A. (2015). Divorce and health: Current trends and future directions. *Psychosomatic Medicine, 77,* 227–236.

Sbarra, D. A., & Borelli, J. L. (2013). Heart rate variability moderates the association between avoidance and self-concept reorganization following marital separation. *International Journal of Psychophysiology, 88,* 253–260.

Sbarra, D. A., & Borelli, J. L. (2019). Attachment reorganization following divorce: Normative processes and individual differences. *Current Opinion in Psychology, 25,* 71–75.

Sbarra, D. A., & Coan, J. A. (2017). Divorce and health: Good data in need of better theory. *Current Opinion in Psychology, 13,* 91–95.

Solomon, B. C., & Jackson, J. J. (2014). Why do personality traits predict divorce?: Multiple pathways through satisfaction. *Journal of Personality and Social Psychology, 106,* 978–996.

CHAPTER 36

Normal and Pathological Mourning
Attachment Processes in the Development of Prolonged Grief

Fiona Maccallum

The death of a loved one can trigger a range of emotional, behavioral, and cognitive reactions we collectively label as grief. Individual reactions vary significantly in terms of intensity, frequency, and duration, but common experiences include yearning, distress, anger, numbness, a feeling that the loss is not real, a confused sense of self, and a loss of purpose and meaning in life. In recent years, increasing empirical attention has been directed toward understanding the heterogeneity observed in grief responses. It has been repeatedly found that although the majority of bereaved individuals appear to adapt to their loss, 7–10% experience an intense and debilitating grief response that can persist unabated for years, and is associated with significant impairment (Maciejewski, Maercker, Boelen, & Prigerson, 2016). Rigorous debate surrounds the optimal definition of this syndrome, which has been termed *prolonged grief disorder (PGD), complicated grief,* or *persistent complex bereavement disorder* (see Maciejewski et al., 2016; World Health Organization, 2018). In light of this debate, increasing attention has been directed toward understanding the mechanisms that facilitate or inhibit adaption in bereavement. Perhaps not surprisingly, attachment processes, long central to theoretical models of grief, have been strongly implicated in PGD (Maccallum & Bryant, 2013; Shear & Shair, 2005).

The separation distress typically observed during bereavement is a manifestation of disrupted attachment relationships. There is general consensus that symptoms largely resolve when the permanence of the loss is integrated into long-term memory and attachment representations are updated to reflect the reality of the death (Maccallum & Bryant, 2013; Mikulincer & Shaver, 2008). Contemporary adult attachment theories focus on two underlying dimensions that reflect the development of secure versus insecure attachments: attachment anxiety and attachment avoidance. Higher levels of either, or both, dimensions contribute to attachment insecurity. Attachment anxiety refers to a person's appraisals of the availability and responsiveness of attachment figures in times of stress. Attachment avoidance relates to a person's trust in the ability of others to provide comfort in times of stress (see Shaver & Mikulincer, Chapter 33, this volume). Those high in attachment anxiety doubt the responsiveness of their attachment figure and engage in frequent reassurance seeking. Conversely, higher avoidance is associated with deactivating strategies, such as withdrawing and minimizing emotional involvement (Mikulincer & Shaver, 2008).

Crucially, in the context of bereavement stress, the attachment system is activated but may also be significantly disrupted if an attachment figure has died. Theoretical models (e.g., Maccallum & Bryant, 2013; Mikulincer & Shaver, 2008) argue that high attachment anxiety should produce a hyperactivation of the attachment system. This can involve strong yearning and vigorous searching for the deceased in an attempt to achieve physical proximity and regulate emotional distress. The inevitable failure to achieve the goal of reunion perpetuates yearning and distress and can reinforce negative appraisals about one's ability to cope without the deceased. Furthermore, because attachment processes also facilitate exploratory behavior, anxious attachment should contribute to reduced willingness to explore new situations without the deceased, further reinforcing distress and low self-efficacy. High attachment avoidance, on the other hand, should promote disengagement from others and may generate negative thoughts and feelings toward the deceased to minimize the impact of the loss.

Many of the risk factors for poor bereavement outcomes involve threats to the development of secure attachment relationships (Lobb et al., 2010; Maccallum & Bryant, 2013). Most typical studies examining attachment in relation to bereavement have assessed the link between symptom severity and trait (chronic) measures of attachment anxiety and avoidance in adults and have focused on depression. Providing support for the role of attachment anxiety, higher levels of anxious attachment, with or without attachment avoidance, are associated with greater symptomatology, whereas higher levels of attachment avoidance in the absence of anxiety are associated with less symptomatology (Field & Sundin, 2001; Fraley & Bonanno, 2004). This suggests that in some circumstances attachment avoidance may represent a protective factor. More recent studies employing specific measures of PGD, however, suggest a complex picture for attachment avoidance. Much of this work has found that higher attachment avoidance is linked with more severe PGD symptomatology (Boelen & Klugkist, 2011; Wijngaards-de Meij et al., 2007; Yu, He, Xu, Wang, & Prigerson, 2016). Notably, however, the strength and direction of this relationship is moderated by factors including high versus low relationship satisfaction, and whether people are asked about their relationship-specific or general attachment style (see Maccallum & Bryant, 2013). Attachment avoidance may contribute to bereavement complications over the longer term by reducing the likelihood an individual will utilize available social supports or develop new attachments. However, it is also important to recognize that most studies examining attachment processes in PGD have not included pre-loss assessments. It is possible that the intense distress and trust disturbances associated with PGD reduce expectations that others can play an effective role in easing distress. That is, attachment style assessed post-loss may be influenced by symptoms of PGD or other bereavement experiences, and thus not reflect a pre-loss trait vulnerability. Further prospective and longitudinal work is needed to explore such possibilities.

Nonetheless, studies examining the linear associations between attachment style and symptom severity have identified different relationships between the attachment dimensions and depression and PGD, suggesting there may be some differences in the etiological pathways of these bereavement outcomes. However, bereaved individuals also typically experience symptoms from more than one diagnostic group (Simon et al., 2007). Accordingly, studies have begun to examine attachment and PGD using statistical methods that cluster individuals based on shared symptom presentations rather than diagnostic severity. Maccallum and Bryant (2018) used this technique with a community sample of bereaved individuals. Participants underwent a clinical assessment using standardized measures of PGD (Maciejewski et al., 2016) and major depression (Beck, Ward, Mendelson, Mock, & Erbaugh, 1961). Attachment style was measured using the Experiences in Close Relationships—Short Form (Wei, Russell, Mallinckrodt, & Vogel, 2007). This study identified three subgroups of participants that could be distinguished by level of attachment anxiety. One subgroup had a high probability of symptoms of both PGD and major depression, and high attachment anxiety; a second subgroup had primarily depressive symptoms and moderate attachment anxiety; and a third subgroup had few if any symptoms and low attachment anxiety. Higher attachment avoidance differentiated the two high-symptom groups (PGD/depression and depression) from the low-symptom group but did not differentiate between the PGD/depression and depression subgroups. This finding is consistent with the idea that attachment anxiety and avoidance may contribute differentially to chronic bereavement distress.

Another attachment process that has been the focus of study in bereavement is how an individual attempts to maintain a bond with the deceased person. "Continuing bonds" are typically divided into two categories: concrete (or physical) bonds, such as maintaining the deceased's possessions, and symbolic (or internalized) bonds, such as recalling cherished memories. A reliance on concrete bonds is thought to represent a failure to incorporate the reality of the loss (Field, 2008). However, the few studies that have examined such bonds in PGD have generated inconsistent findings (see Maccallum & Bryant, 2013). For example, Boelen, Stroebe, Schut, and Zijerveld (2006) found that the tendency to cherish possessions was predictive of later PGD only as a trend, whereas feeling calmed and supported by memories of the deceased was a relatively strong predictor over time. Stroebe, Schut, and Boerner (2010) propose that the degree to which any bond is adaptive or maladaptive must be considered in the context of the individual's attachment style. They suggest that secure individuals may be able to retain a wider range of bonds because they are not driven by a desire to physically reconnect with the deceased. However, for those high in attachment anxiety, both concrete *and* symbolic bonds may be motivated by a desire to regain physical proximity, and thus either could signal a failure to integrate the loss. That is, the adaptiveness of a bond is dependent on the individual's underlying attachment-related needs and motivations.

Maccallum and Bryant (2013) expanded these ideas into a theoretical model of PGD incorporating attachment. According to this model, attachment styles are a component of a person's self-identity that influences their bereavement responses by interacting with other aspects of self-identity. Of primary importance in this model is the degree to which the bereaved person's sense of self is constructed around the deceased person. Where a person's self-identify has become dominated by goals related to the deceased (e.g., caregiving, retirement plans, emotional/practical dependence), the reality of the loss represents a significant threat to their self-coherence. Accordingly, such individuals may seek to avoid specific information that reinforces the finality of the death but may be drawn to reminders of the person given the importance of that person for their self-identify (Maccallum & Bryant, 2019). However, memories of the deceased, even positive reminders, may serve to highlight the discrepancy between desired goals (e.g., reunion) and the current reality, and trigger yearning, rumination, and further distress. The experience of grief itself may also be a means of honoring and maintaining a bond with the deceased person. The combination of these factors is thought to impede integration of the reality of the loss, and hinder modification of the self to include meaningful goals and roles that reflect the physical absence of the deceased. Individuals who have a self-identity that includes a variety of personally meaningful goals and roles *independent* of the deceased can also experience acute distress but should experience less threat to their self-coherence. They should therefore be less motivated to avoid the reality of the loss and more likely to engage in emotional processing that leads to integration and modification of their now unachievable goals. This is not to say that the deceased was less important; rather, alternate aspects of their identity can be drawn on to provide respite or buffer them against the loss, making them less vulnerable to developing PGD.

Anxious and avoidant attachment styles are thought to interact with self-identify to produce different cognitive, emotional, and behavioral tendencies that impact the patterns of grief (see also Shear & Shair, 2005). There are many reasons why one's self-identity may become dominated by the deceased beyond attachment dynamics (e.g., prolonged period as a carer), however, an anxious attachment style will increase the likelihood that this happens and is considered a vulnerability factor. Attachment anxiety would also amplify separation distress and attempts to gain proximity to the deceased and facilitate the development of an idealized view of the lost partner/relationship (see Field & Sundin, 2001). Those with high attachment anxiety may also increase proximity seeking to alternate attachment figures (if available). In contrast, those high on attachment avoidance (only) are considered less likely to develop a self-identify dominated by the deceased, and so are considered less vulnerable to PGD; however, where present, attachment avoidance may be associated with avoidance of reminders and interfere with the development of new attachments and social connections, both of which may hinder processing of the loss and revision of the self. They would be less likely to demonstrate the separation distress observed with PGD and may experience more negative thoughts about the deceased. It is also possible PGD symptoms themselves may increase reported avoidant attachment tendencies (Maccallum & Bryant, 2013). More work is needed to understand the complex and inconsistent findings relating to attachment avoidance and PGD.

Effective cognitive behavioral treatments for PGD recognize the importance of attachment processes (Bryant et al., 2014). Treatments acknowledge the significance of the loss and incorporate therapeutic exposure to facilitate the emotional processing and revision of self-identity. Letter writing and "empty-chair" techniques facilitate direct communication with the deceased, and structured goal setting can be used to assist individuals to develop a meaningful alternate future. When possible, clients are encouraged to cultivate positive and supportive connections via reminders and memories of the deceased person. However, not all individuals with PGD benefit from this approach, and more work is needed to understand why treatment sometimes fails. It is possible the general perception that only attachment anxiety places clients "at risk" for PGD may lead some clinicians to overlook the potential impacts of attachment avoidance. Work may benefit from additional cognitive therapy and graded exposure techniques directed toward appraisals relating to vulnerability and trust in order to facilitate exploration and the development of flexible emotional coping strategies.

At the heart of PGD is the loss of a central attachment figure. Although most people are able to integrate their loss and find ways of living meaningfully without the deceased person, some become stuck in a state of acute, prolonged grief. Research on PGD is in its relative infancy. Most studies that have investigated adult attachment styles in relation to bereavement and PGD have focused on spousal loss. Any relationship that dominates a person's self-identity is likely to place that person at risk for developing PGD, but there may be aspects of certain relationships that amplify the likelihood of PGD (Maccallum & Bryant, 2013). Moreover, research has overwhelmingly focused on the loss of the attachment figure; little attention has been paid to the loss of an attachment-related role, such as occurs in parents when a child dies (see also Shaver & Mikulincer, Chapter 33, this volume). As the field matures, we will gain a deeper understanding of the complex interactions between attachment and the cognitive, behavioral, biological, and emotional factors that underlie chronic and debilitating grief reactions.

REFERENCES

Beck, A. T., Ward, C. H., Mendelson, M., Mock, J., & Erbaugh, J. (1961). An inventory for measuring depression. *Archives of General Psychiatry, 4,* 561–571.

Boelen, P. A., & Klugkist, I. (2011). Cognitive behavioral variables mediate the associations of neuroticism and attachment insecurity with prolonged grief disorder severity. *Anxiety, Stress and Coping: An International Journal, 24*(3), 291–307.

Boelen, P. A., Stroebe, M. S., Schut, H. A. W., & Zijerveld, A. M. (2006). Continuing bonds and grief: A prospective analysis. *Death Studies, 30,* 767–776.

Bryant, R. A., Kenny, L., Joscelyne, A., Rawson, N., Maccallum, F., Cahill, C., . . . Nickerson, A. (2014). Treating prolonged grief disorder: A randomized controlled trial. *JAMA Psychiatry, 71,* 1332–1339.

Field, N. P. (2008). Whether to relinquish or maintain a bond with the deceased. In M. S. Stroebe, R. O. Hansson, H. Schut, & W. Stroebe (Eds.), *Handbook of bereavement research and practice: Advances in theory and intervention* (pp. 113–132). Washington, DC: American Psychological Association.

Field, N. P., & Sundin, E. C. (2001). Attachment style in adjustment to conjugal bereavement. *Journal of Social and Personal Relationships, 18,* 347–361.

Fraley, R. C., & Bonanno, G. A. (2004). Attachment and loss: A test of three competing models on the association between attachment-related avoidance and adaptation to bereavement. *Personality and Social Psychology Bulletin, 30,* 878–890.

Lobb, E. A., Kristjanson, L. J., Aoun, S. M., Monterosso, L., Halkett, G. K. B., & Davies, A. (2010). Predictors of complicated grief: A systematic review of empirical studies. *Death Studies, 34,* 673–698.

Maccallum, F., & Bryant, R. A. (2013). A cognitive attachment model of prolonged grief: Integrating attachments, memory, and identity. *Clinical Psychology Review, 33,* 713.

Maccallum, F., & Bryant, R. A. (2018). Prolonged grief and attachment security: A latent class analysis. *Psychiatry Research, 268,* 297–302.

Maccallum, F., & Bryant, R. A. (2019). An investigation of approach behaviour in prolonged grief. *Behaviour Research and Therapy, 119,* 103405.

Maciejewski, P. K., Maercker, A., Boelen, P. A., & Prigerson, H. G. (2016). "Prolonged grief disorder" and "persistent complex bereavement disorder," but not "complicated grief," are one and the same diagnostic entity: An analysis of data from the Yale Bereavement Study. *World Psychiatry, 15,* 266–275.

Mikulincer, M., & Shaver, P. R. (2008). An attachment perspective on bereavement. In M. S. Stroebe, R. O. Hansson, H. Schut, & W. Stroebe (Eds.), *Handbook of bereavement research and practice: Advances in theory and intervention* (pp. 87–112). Washington, DC: American Psychological Association.

Shear, M. K., & Shair, H. (2005). Attachment, loss, and complicated grief. *Developmental Psychobiology, 47,* 253–267.

Simon, N. M., Shear, M. K., Thompson, E. H., Zalta, A. K., Perlman, C., Reynolds, C. F., . . . Silowash, R. (2007). The prevalence and correlates of psychiatric comorbidity in individuals with complicated grief. *Comprehensive Psychiatry, 48,* 395–399.

Stroebe, M. S., Schut, H., & Boerner, K. (2010). Continuing bonds in adaptation to bereavement: Toward theoretical integration. *Clinical Psychology Review, 30,* 259–268.

Wei, M., Russell, D. W., Mallinckrodt, B., & Vogel, D. L. (2007). The Experiences in Close Relationship scale (ECR)—Short Form: Reliability, validity, and factor structure. *jJournal of Personality Assessment, 88,* 187–204.

Wijngaards-de Meij, L., Stroebe, M., Schut, H., Stroebe, W., van den Bout, J., van der Heijden, P., & Dijkstra, H. (2007). Neuroticism and attachment insecurity as predictors of bereavement outcome. *Journal of Research in Personality, 41,* 498–505.

World Health Organization. (2018). *International classification of diseases for mortality and morbidity statistics* (11th rev.). Geneva, Switzerland: Author.

Yu, W., He, L., Xu, W., Wang, J., & Prigerson, H. G. (2016). How do attachment dimensions affect bereavement adjustment?: A mediation model of continuing bonds. *Psychiatry Research, 238,* 93–99.

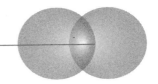

ATTACHMENT-BASED
INTERVENTIONS

- How do attachment-based interventions work?

- What are the key processes and mechanisms involved?

CHAPTER 37

Attachment-Based Interventions to Promote Secure Attachment in Children

Marian J. Bakermans-Kranenburg
Mirjam Oosterman

History and Overview

The history of documented attachment-based interventions is relatively short, spanning just over 30 years. The first published randomized intervention study with infant–parent attachment outcomes was conducted in Australia with highly anxious mothers who were offered support and anti-anxiety techniques, and were encouraged to show appropriate maternal behavior ($N = 80$; Barnett, Blignault, Holmes, Payne, & Parker, 1987), though without positive effects on infant attachment security. In spite of this first unsuccessful trial, the number of attachment-based intervention programs has increased hugely over the past decades, as evident from the comprehensive *Handbook of Attachment-Based Interventions* (Steele & Steele, 2018) presenting attachment-based interventions aimed at promoting security in infants and children, adolescents, and adults.

What is special about infant attachment interventions is that the "object" of the intervention is addressed only indirectly: Efforts to promote secure attachments are never directed to children, but rather to the caregiving environment. John Bowlby (1949) laid a firm basis for such an approach, arguing that the therapist should not focus on problems "inside" individuals, but instead should address stable patterns of interaction within close relationships (see Duschinsky, 2020). This implies that for the enhancement of attachment security in infants and children, caregivers and patterns of caregiver–child interaction should be the focus of attachment-based interventions. Consistent with this implication, attachment-based interventions focus on caregivers and patterns of caregiver–child interaction, in particular on caregiver sensitivity.

In the next sections we will discuss why and how parenting sensitivity has become the focus of interventions, and how effective such interventions have been in promoting parenting sensitivity and secure attachment. We briefly review two interventions that represent quite different approaches to promoting parenting sensitivity, and we elaborate on a shared feature, namely the use of video feedback. We try to explain what might make video feedback a working ingredient for enhancing parenting sensitivity and conclude with some outstanding issues. Understanding what works for whom will help us enhance the effectiveness of future intervention efforts.

Parenting Sensitivity as the Focus of Attachment-Based Interventions

Based on her work in Uganda and Baltimore, Mary Ainsworth concluded that secure attachment relationships resulted from the child's experience of sensitive parenting, that is, the child's signals and needs are accurately perceived and interpreted and responded to in an adequate and prompt way (Ainsworth, Blehar, Waters, & Wall, 1978). Indeed, empirical studies and meta-analyses have shown that sensitive parenting is a key determinant to promoting secure child–parent attachment relationships. Although the strength of this association is smaller than originally thought, caregiver sensitivity is the best documented predictor of secure attachment and virtually all attachment interventions have promoting sensitivity as a central aim (Bakermans-Kranenburg, van IJzendoorn, & Juffer, 2003).

Several approaches to improving parental sensitivity have been tried and tested. Broadly speaking, three approaches can be distinguished. The first approach centers on supporting the parent(s). Given the negative impact of stress on sensitivity, providing and enhancing parents' social and material support may result in lower parental stress levels, which in turn may lead to improved parenting sensitivity. Examples of this approach are a home-visiting program by volunteers to support adolescent mothers in Chile (Aracena et al., 2009) and the Mom2Mom program in Israel (Kaitz, 2018). The second approach aims to change parents' insecure mental representations of attachment or traumatic experiences that may hinder sensitive parenting behaviors. Through discussions about past and present attachment experiences and their influence on current thinking and parenting, "ghosts" from the past would be banished from the family theater (Fraiberg, Adelson, & Shapiro, 1975) and enable the parent to show more sensitive parenting. Contemporary examples of this approach include Minding the Baby (Slade et al., 2018) and Child–Parent Psychotherapy (Toth, Michl-Petzing, Guild, & Lieberman, 2018). In the third approach, the efforts are directed toward improving parental sensitivity at the behavioral level, without directly focusing on underlying factors on the representational or environmental levels that may hamper parenting sensitivity. Examples are the VIPP-SD program (Juffer, Bakermans-Kranenburg, & van IJzendoorn, 2017) and the Attachment and Biobehavioral Catch-up (ABC) intervention (Dozier & Bernard, 2017).

Somewhat unexpectedly, a meta-analysis showed that the third approach was the most effective in enhancing parenting sensitivity in randomized controlled trials, even in multiproblem samples (Bakermans-Kranenburg et al., 2003), with a combined effect size of Cohen's $d = 0.45$ for behavior-focused approaches versus $d = 0.27$ for all other approaches. Moreover, the behavioral approach was most effective in improving infant–parent attachment security ($d = 0.39$ for behavior-focused approaches versus $d = 0.06$ for all other approaches). A relevant observation here is that only interventions that were quite effective in improving parental sensitivity ($d > 0.40$) also showed positive effects on the infant–parent attachment relationship. This strongly suggests that effects on attachment security are indeed mediated by effects on parenting sensitivity, and it provides a further rationale for interventions to aim to enhance parenting sensitivity as a way to promote a secure child–parent attachment.

Two Examples

Given the documented effectiveness of interventions with a behavioral focus, one example of such an approach is presented here, along with an example of a broader intervention that is group-based rather than individual, and also includes attention to parental representations of past and present.

The Video-feedback Intervention to promote Positive Parenting (VIPP; Juffer, Bakermans-Kranenburg, & van IJzendoorn, 2008) program consists of four to six home-based sessions involving the intervener and the parent (sessions 5 and 6 with both parents if available), using personalized video feedback addressing themes such as distinguishing between the child's exploration versus attachment signals, verbalizing the child's behavior, and sensitivity chains that comprise a signal of the child (e.g., reaching for a toy), followed by a sensitive response of the parent (giving it to the child), and the child's reaction to that response (a happy smile to the parent). During each session, the videotaped parent–child interaction of the previous session is reviewed with the parent(s) to illustrate the themes of the intervention and to train the observation skills of the parent(s), for example by providing "subtitles" for the behavior of the child and encouraging the parent(s) to join by asking questions about the child's (sometimes subtle) signals. In the VIPP-SD program, sensitive discipline is an additional focus. Concepts from both attachment theory and coercion theory are used, stimulating parents to reinforce children's positive behaviors and set limits in an effective way. The program is implemented without the sensitive discipline component (VIPP) with parents of infants up to their first birthday, and with this additional component (VIPP-SD) when families with "terrible twos" and older children are targeted. The VIPP and VIPP-SD programs have been shown to be effective in various samples (see Juffer et al., 2017), with a combined effect size of $d = 0.47$ for enhanced caregiving sensitivity, based on 12 randomized controlled trials. The combined effect size for improved child outcomes was $d = 0.37$; for attachment it was $d = 0.36$, while a combined effect size of $d = 0.26$ was found for reduced child problem behavior.

Apart from sensitivity-focused, brief interventions, a variety of broad and more intensive attachment-based interventions have been developed and documented over the years, such as STEEP and Minding the Baby (see Steele & Steele, 2018). A recent addition to this family tree of intensive and broad interventions is the Group Attachment-Based Intervention (GABI; Steele, Murphy, Bonuck, Meissner, & Steele, 2019). GABI is a center-based intervention for parents with infants and toddlers identified as at risk of maltreatment. They visit the center up to three times weekly during a 26-week period. Each session lasts about 2 hours and consists of three parts. First, parents and children interact with one another, and these interactions are videotaped for later review. Second, the parents are separated from the children and meet as a group with the therapist, reviewing the videotape of a given parent interacting with his or her child as a basis for discussing current parenting issues as well as past experiences. In the third part, children and parents are reunited for a period of play before the session ends. The group-based approach has the benefit of providing mutual support and is assumed to be effective in engaging participants who perceive group treatments as less stigmatizing. The first randomized controlled trial tested the efficacy of GABI ($N = 78$; Steele et al., 2019) with families living in an impoverished urban area with high prevalence of domestic violence. The trial showed an increase in maternal sensitivity ($d = 0.71$) and a decrease in maternal hostility ($d = 0.45$). Dyadic reciprocity was also enhanced by the intervention ($d = 0.95$), although less so for mothers with the highest levels of adverse childhood experiences. The effects on attachment security will be available but are currently unknown. If such effects on attachment are established, GABI would provide a promising intervention format for parents in fragile circumstances at risk of maltreating their children.

How Does It Work?

An important similarity between these two interventions, shared with several other attachment-based interventions such as ABC, is the use of videotaped parent–child interactions. The meta-analyses (Bakermans-Kranenburg et al., 2003) showed that interventions with video feedback were more successful in improving parental sensitivity than interventions without the video-feedback component.

The persuasiveness of video footage had already been shown by the work of James and Joyce Robertson in the 1950s and 1960s. Their silent films in combination with verbal commentary on the child's behavior and affectional needs may be considered as a first example of the technique of "speaking for the child" (Juffer & Steele, 2014). This technique has become an important tool in attachment interventions and may be one of the explanations for the effectiveness of video feedback. Figure 37.1 provides an illustration of potentially active ingredients of video feedback. As shown in the figure, video fragments of the child's behavior, emotional expressions and body language in combination with the provision of "subtitles" as suggested and elicited by the intervener may stimulate parents to take the child's perspective and lead to a more accurate perception of the child's needs (Juffer, Struis, Werner, & Bakermans-Kranenburg, 2017). An additional

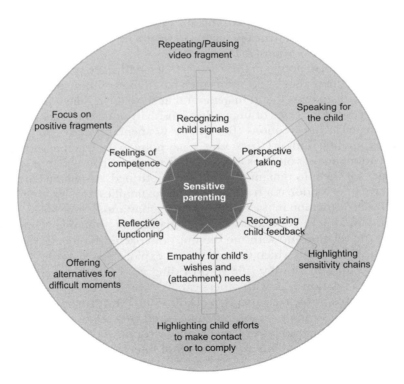

FIGURE 37.1. A model of potential active ingredients in Video-feedback Interventions to promote Positive Parenting and Sensitive Discipline (VIPP-SD). The outer circle contains strategies used during video-feedback intervention; the middle circle presents the aimed-for effects of these strategies in the parent, promoting enhanced sensitive parenting.

explanation for the effectiveness of video feedback refers to the possibility of focusing on video fragments of positive interactions in order to reinforce and encourage parents to show similarly sensitive behavior in daily interactions with their child (Juffer et al., 2008). Moreover, such a focus boosts feelings of parental competence. Highlighting child efforts to comply with difficult tasks or demands may stimulate parental empathy, paving the way for an understanding, sensitive response to a child who tries hard but only partly succeeds. Furthermore, watching and analyzing specific interaction patterns may help parents to reframe their thoughts and beliefs and recognize their own role in the interaction with their child (Juffer & Steele, 2014). Steele, Murphy, and Steele (2015) argued that this novel way of thinking may lay the foundation for changes in the general capacity to reflect on the emerging self and the other, defined as "reflective functioning" (Fonagy, Steele, Steele, Moran, & Higgitt, 1991). Reflective functioning may in turn pave the way for sensitive parenting because it comprises the capacity to see the child as a separate person motivated by internal mental states such as feelings, wishes, and desires. This may explain why parental reflective functioning is meta-analytically related to secure infant–parent attachment (Zeegers, Colonnesi, Stams, & Meins, 2017).

It is also worth noting in this context that GABI, at 26 weeks, is a longer-term commitment than short-term video-based interventions such as VIPP-SD. The meta-analysis found in general that short-term interventions were more successful in terms of improving sensitivity and attachment security than long-term interventions (Bakermans-Kranenburg et al., 2003). This perhaps puzzling finding (*"less is more"*) may point to the fact that short-term interventions are less onerous for the families and as a consequence it might be easier for them to remain involved and motivated. A specific barrier to long-term intervention is attrition, especially in families with multiple problems. Indeed, attrition in the GABI study was substantial, over 60%.

Finally, a more generic working mechanism of attachment interventions is the relationship with the therapist or coach, who ideally provides the secure base from which the parent can explore new parenting behaviors. According to Bowlby (1988), providing a secure therapeutic base, from which relationships with others can be explored, is an essential part of the therapist's role (see also Byng-Hall, 1999). Staff turnover can thus be detrimental to intervention outcomes, and this relational dimension of interventions should also be taken into account when considering the optimal number of sessions and duration of interventions.

Outstanding Issues

Most of our ideas about the active ingredients of interventions (see Figure 37.1) are speculative. Moreover, they may be differentially effective for different families, depending not only on the nature and level of the risk in a specific family but also on characteristics of both parent and child. The average effectiveness of an intervention is an underestimation for some families, and an overestimation for others. According to the *differential susceptibility* model, parents and children with specific genetic, neurobiological, or temperamental characteristics are not only more vulnerable to environmental stressors, but also benefit more from interventions changing the environment for the better. Supporting evidence for this model has accumulated in the past decade (see Bakermans-Kranenburg & van IJzendoorn, 2015). In the case of attachment interventions, differential susceptibility effects can play a role on two levels: First, some parents may be more susceptible to (specific elements of) the intervention program than others, with more pronounced changes in their parenting behavior as a result, and second, children may be more or less susceptible to (specific) changes in their caregiving environment, resulting in variation in change on the child and relationship level. Whether and to what extent parent and child susceptibility are associated, potentially multiplying the influence of differential susceptibility, is an important issue for future research.

ACKNOWLEDGMENT

The authors would like to thank Femmie Juffer for her helpful comments to the manuscript.

REFERENCES

Ainsworth, M. D. S., Blehar, M. C., Waters, E., & Wall, S. (1978). *Patterns of attachment: A psychological study of the Strange Situation*. Hillsdale, NJ: Erlbaum.

Aracena, M., Krause, M., Pérez, C., Méndez, M. J., Salvatierra, L., Soto, M., . . . Altimir, C. (2009). A cost-effectiveness evaluation of a home visit program for adolescent mothers. *Journal of Health Psychology, 14,* 878–887.

Bakermans-Kranenburg, M. J., & van IJzendoorn, M. H. (2015). The hidden efficacy of interventions: Gene × environment experiments from a differential susceptibility perspective. *Annual Review of Psychology, 66,* 381–409.

Bakermans-Kranenburg, M. J., van IJzendoorn, M. H., & Juffer, F. (2003). Less is more: Meta-analysis of sensitivity and attachment interventions in early childhood. *Psychological Bulletin, 129,* 195–215.

Barnett, B., Blignault, I., Holmes, S., Payne, A., & Parker, G. (1987). Quality of attachment in a sample of 1-year-old Australian children. *Journal of the American Academy of Child and Adolescent Psychiatry, 26,* 303–307.

Bowlby, J. (1949). The study and reduction of group tensions within the family. *Human Relations, 2,* 123–128.

Bowlby, J. (1988). *A secure base: Clinical applications of attachment therapy*. London: Routledge.

Byng-Hall, J. (1999). Family and couple therapy: Toward greater security. In J. Cassidy & P. R Shaver (Eds.), *Handbook of attachment: Theory, research, and clinical applications* (pp. 625–645). New York: Guilford Press.

Dozier, M., & Bernard, K. (2017). Attachment and biobehavioral catch-up: Addressing the needs of infants and toddlers exposed to inadequate or problematic caregiving. *Current Opinion in Psychology, 15,* 111–117.

Duschinsky, R. (2020). *The cornerstones of attachment research.* Oxford, UK: Oxford University Press.

Fonagy, P., Steele, M., Steele, H., Moran, G. S., & Higgitt, A. C. (1991). The capacity for understanding mental states: The reflective self in parent and child and its significance for security of attachment. *Infant Mental Health Journal, 12,* 201–218.

Fraiberg, S., Adelson, E., & Shapiro, V. (1975). Ghosts in the nursery: A psychoanalytic approach to the problems of impaired infant–mother relationships. *Journal of the American Academy of Child Psychiatry, 14,* 387–422.

Juffer, F., Bakermans-Kranenburg, M. J., & van IJzendoorn, M. H. (Eds.). (2008). *Promoting positive parenting: An attachment-based intervention.* New York: Taylor & Francis.

Juffer, F., Bakermans-Kranenburg, M. J., & van IJzendoorn, M. H. (2017). Pairing attachment theory and social learning theory in video-feedback intervention to promote positive parenting. *Current Opinion in Psychology, 15,* 189–194.

Juffer, F., & Steele, M. (2014). What words cannot say: The telling story of video in attachment-based interventions. *Attachment and Human Development, 16,* 307–314.

Juffer, F., Struis, E., Werner, C., & Bakermans-Kranenburg, M. J. (2017). Effective preventive interventions to support parents of young children: Illustrations from the Video-feedback Intervention to promote Positive Parenting and Sensitive Discipline (VIPP-SD). *Journal of Prevention and Intervention in the Community, 45,* 202–214.

Kaitz, M. (2018). Mom2Mom: An attachment-based home-visiting program for mothers of young infants. In H. Steele & M. Steele (Eds.), *Handbook of attachment-based interventions* (pp. 245–272). New York: Guilford Press.

Slade, A., Simpson, T. E., Webb, D., Albertsen, J. G., Close, N., & Sadler, L. (2018). Minding the Baby: Complex trauma and attachment-based home intervention. In H. Steele & M. Steele (Eds.), *Handbook of attachment-based interventions* (pp. 151–173). New York: Guilford Press.

Steele, H., Murphy, A., Bonuck, K., Meissner, P., & Steele, M. (2019). Randomized control trial report on the effectiveness of Group Attachment-Based Intervention (GABI©): Improvements in the parent–child relationship not seen in the control group. *Development and Psychopathology, 31*(1), 203–217.

Steele, H., & Steele, M. (Eds.). (2018). *Handbook of attachment-based interventions.* New York: Guilford Press.

Steele, M., Murphy, A., & Steele, H. (2015) The art and science of observation: Reflective functioning and therapeutic action. *Journal of Infant Child and Adolescent Psychotherapy, 14,* 216–231.

Toth, S. L., Michl-Petzing, L. C., Guild, D., & Lieberman, A. F. (2018). Child–parent psychotherapy: Theoretical bases, clinical applications, and empirical support. In H. Steele & M. Steele (Eds.), *Handbook of attachment-based interventions* (pp. 296–317). New York: Guilford Press.

Zeegers, M. A. J., Colonnesi, C., Stams, G.-J. J. M., & Meins, E. (2017). Mind matters: A meta-analysis on parental mentalization and sensitivity as predictors of infant–parent attachment. *Psychological Bulletin, 143,* 1245–1272.

CHAPTER 38

Mechanisms of Attachment-Based Intervention Effects on Child Outcomes

Mary Dozier
Kristin Bernard

Bowlby (1969/1982) considered societal interventions that increased the availability of attachment figures and individual interventions that enhanced parental sensitive responsiveness as central to the contribution attachment theory and research could make to society. A number of interventions have been developed in the last several decades that have the goal of enhancing children's attachment quality as well as having downstream effects on children's self-regulatory capabilities. These interventions typically conceptualize parent behavior and/or representations as the mechanism by which interventions have effects on attachment and on child self-regulation (see Figure 38.1 for conceptual model). In this chapter, we consider evidence regarding intervention effects on attachment and self-regulation outcomes, and evidence regarding the mechanism of the intervention's effects. Finally, we examine evidence that attachment quality serves as a mechanism for intervention effects on later child outcomes.

What Is the Evidence That Attachment-Based Interventions Affect Child Attachment and Child Self-Regulation?

Attachment and Biobehavioral Catch-up (ABC; Dozier & Bernard, 2019), Video-feedback Intervention to promote Positive Parenting and Sensitive Discipline (VIPP-SD; Juffer, Bakermans-Kranenburg, & van IJzendoorn, 2017), Child–Parent Psychotherapy (CPP; Lieberman, Weston, & Pawl,

1991; Toth, Michi-Petzing, Guild, & Lieberman, 2019), and Minding the Baby (MTB; Sadler et al., 2013; Slade et al., 2020) are among the attachment-based interventions with the strongest evidence base with regard to enhancing infant attachment and other more distal child outcomes.

ABC

ABC is a 10-session home-visiting intervention for parents of children between birth and 24 months of age that seeks to enhance parental nurturance in distress contexts and sensitivity in nondistress contexts, and to reduce intrusive/frightening behaviors (Dozier & Bernard, 2019). Parent coaches present manualized content that includes research evidence and videos. They also make "in-the-moment" comments at a high rate (approximately one comment per minute), which support parents' practice of intervention targets. Children of parents randomized to the ABC intervention show secure attachments at higher rates and disorganized attachments at lower rates than children of parents randomized to a control intervention of the same structure as ABC (Bernard et al., 2012). Positive effects of ABC are also seen across a range of developmental domains and include cognitive outcomes (e.g., better receptive vocabulary and executive functioning at preschool age), interpersonal outcomes (e.g., greater feelings of security in middle childhood), and physiological outcomes (e.g., more normative cortisol production in infancy, early childhood, and middle childhood) domains (see Dozier & Bernard, 2019).

VIPP-SD

VIPP-SD is implemented through seven in-home sessions that focus on enhancing parental empathy and sensitive discipline for parents of children between the ages of 1 and 5. Parents are video-recorded each session, with the video played back to highlight patterns of interaction that are consistent with themes related to sensitive parenting (e.g., comforting a child, supporting exploration) and sensitive discipline (e.g., positive reinforcement, sensitive time-out). Efficacy for VIPP-SD comes from an impressive set of 12 randomized clinical trials. Meta-analytic evidence across these studies demonstrates that VIPP-SD is efficacious in enhancing attachment security, reducing attachment disorganization, and reducing child behavior problems (Juffer et al., 2017).

CPP

CPP, developed by Alicia Lieberman and colleagues, targets parental representations and experiences of trauma as a way of enhancing parental responsiveness and child outcomes. CPP therapists aim to provide corrective attachment experiences to parents and children by fostering positive parent–child interactions during sessions, exploring parents' maladaptive perceptions about attachment relationships, and creating a trusting therapeutic alliance (Lieberman et al., 1991; Toth et al., 2019). CPP is implemented through about 50 sessions that can occur in office or home settings. CPP has shown effects on attachment in some samples (e.g., Toth, Rogosch, Manly, & Cicchetti, 2006), but not in others (e.g., Lieberman et al., 1991). The intervention has affected distal child outcomes, including reductions in children's angry behavior and behavior problems as reported by parents (Lieberman, Ghosh Ippen, & Van Horn, 2006), decreases in children's negative representations of self and parents (Toth, Maughan, Manly, Spagnola, & Cicchetti, 2002), and higher morning cortisol production (Cicchetti, Rogosch, Toth, & Sturge-Apple, 2011) relative to children who received a control intervention.

MTB

MTB (Sadler et al., 2013; Slade et al., 2020) is an integrated approach focusing on physical health and attachment needs of high-risk infants and their mothers. A team including a nurse practitioner and a clinical social worker work together to implement the intervention through alternating weekly sessions from the prenatal period (third trimester) through the first year of the child's life and biweekly thereafter. Slade, Sadler, and colleagues model their program after CPP as well as the Nurse–Family Partnership intervention (Donelan-McCall & Olds, 2019), a multifaceted home-visiting approach. In two separate randomized clinical trials, children assigned to MTB showed higher rates of secure attachment than children assigned to a control condition (Sadler et al., 2013; Slade et al., 2020). Parents who received MTB reported fewer externalizing behaviors among their children than were reported by parents in the control group (Ordway et al., 2014).

Taken together, evidence supports the efficacy of these and other attachment-based interventions on children's attachment quality and more distal effects on self-regulation. These more distal outcomes are not targeted specifically by the interventions, thus representing downstream effects.

What Are the Mechanisms for the Effects of Attachment-Based Interventions on Child Outcomes?

As exemplified in Figure 38.1, attachment-based interventions typically target either parental behaviors, such as responsive parenting (e.g., ABC

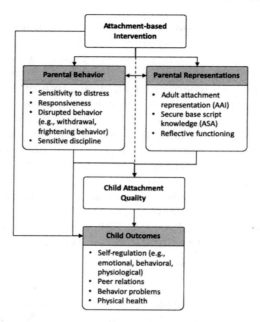

FIGURE 38.1. Conceptual model for mechanisms of attachment-based intervention effectiveness on child outcomes.

and VIPP-SD), or parental representations (e.g., CPP and MTB) as primary. Given the broader literature linking responsive parenting and parental representations to children's attachment security, we would expect that changes in these targets would mediate intervention effects on attachment security (as indicated by the dotted line in Figure 38.1) and other child outcomes. We consider the evidence that interventions effectively target parental behaviors or representations, and the evidence that behaviors or representations serve as mechanisms of intervention effects on child outcomes.

Intervention Effects on Parental Behavior

A primary intervention mechanism proposed for both ABC and VIPP-SD, and secondarily for CPP, is parental sensitive responsiveness. The ABC intervention leads to greater parental sensitivity than a control intervention among high-risk parents, foster parents, low-income Early Head Start parents, and adoptive parents, with effects seen immediately following the intervention and 3 years after the intervention has been implemented (Berlin, Martoccio, & Jones Harden, 2018; Dozier & Bernard, 2019); furthermore, parents who receive ABC show reduced parental withdrawal, a dimension of disrupted parenting behavior (Yarger, Bronfman, Carlson, & Dozier, 2020). For VIPP, intervention effects are also consistently seen on parental sensitivity across diverse samples of parents (e.g., low-income, adoptive, insecure), with a combined effect size in the medium range (Juffer et al., 2017).

Although relatively few studies have reported on mechanisms by which attachment-based interventions exert their effects on child outcomes, emerging evidence supports parental behavior as a key mediator. For example, changes in parental sensitivity mediate ABC's effects on language development (Raby, Freedman, Yarger, Lind, & Dozier, 2019), behavioral compliance (Lind, Bernard, Yarger, & Dozier, 2020), and stress-related cortisol production (Berlin, Martoccio, Bryce, & Jones Harden, 2019). Additionally, reductions in maternal withdrawal mediate ABC's effects on disorganized attachment (Yarger et al., 2020), a finding that is consistent with evidence supporting disrupted parenting behavior as a mediator of another attachment-based home-visiting intervention's effect on disorganized attachment (Tereno et al., 2017).

Intervention Effects on Parental Representations

Although changing parental representations is central to several interventions' theories of change, few studies have reported on intervention effects on parental representations. In one randomized trial, MTB enhanced mothers' level of reflective functioning (Slade et al., 2020), and in a second randomized trial, a subset of the most high-risk mothers showed enhanced reflective functioning (Sadler et al., 2013). Additionally, parents who received ABC demonstrated higher secure-base script knowledge, as assessed by the Attachment Script Assessment, than parents who received a control intervention (Raby, Waters, Tabachnick, Zajac, & Dozier, 2019). These studies offer preliminary evidence that attachment-based interventions may influence parents' own schemas about attachment relationships. Presumably, when targeting parental representations, effects on children are mediated by changes in parental behaviors that result from changes in parental representations. However, to our knowledge no studies have demonstrated that changes at the level of parental representation mediate effects on parenting behavior or child outcomes.

What Is the Evidence That Attachment Quality Mediates Intervention Effects on Downstream Child Outcomes?

Attachment security is a predictor of a host of child outcomes, such as psychopathology, peer relations, and physical health, and thus is often conceptualized as a key mechanism of change for intervention effects on distal child outcomes. However, to date, there is limited empirical evidence of attachment security as a mediator of intervention effects. In one study, Guild, Toth, Handley, Rogosch, and Cicchetti (2017) found that attachment security mediated the small, nonsignificant effect of CPP on teacher-reported peer relations at 9 years old. Similarly, Bernard, Frost, Jelinek, and Dozier (2019) found a significant indirect effect of ABC on children's obesity risk (i.e., body mass index [BMI]) via secure attachment, although direct effects of ABC on BMI were nonsignificant. Given that attachment quality is typically considered as a categorical variable, most studies are underpowered to detect effects when considering attachment in mediation models.

Conclusion

Relatively strong evidence exists to support claims that attachment-based interventions can engage purported intervention mechanisms (parental behavior in particular) and can enhance child outcomes. As we have discussed in this chapter, the evidence is especially strong regarding intervention effects on downstream child outcomes, which is of course critical. Evidence demonstrating that purported mechanisms actually mediate intervention effects on child outcomes is emerging in the literature, but does not constitute a strong evidence base. One reason for the limited evidence base is that the focus on intervention mechanisms is relatively recent. For example, the National Institute of Mental Health (NIMH) did not consider intervention mechanisms as a primary focus before 2010. In recent years, however, NIMH has pushed for study of intervention mechanisms, arguing that change would occur more rapidly if we understood the mechanism by which interventions work. Studying mechanisms has lagged behind study of outcomes, but work is progressing in this area. A second likely reason for the limited evidence is that many intervention studies are underpowered to detect mediation effects. Statistical power to detect mediation effects is often limited in intervention studies, especially when using categorical variables (Fritz & MacKinnon, 2007). Indeed, investigators may not have tested for such effects, knowing that their sample sizes did not allow adequate power to detect effects.

For the most part, what needs to change in order to affect critical developmental outcomes remains an open question. The evidence supporting parental sensitivity is the strongest at this point, but that may be because it is the easiest variable to measure. Many interventions target nurturance to distress in addition to sensitivity (with sensitivity usually operationalized as responsiveness during nondistress conditions); however, evidence of mechanisms does not yet extend to nurturance, at least partially because it represents a relatively low base-rate event. Nonetheless, nurturance is key to the models of change and could well serve as an important mechanism of change. Similarly, parental representations may serve as a key intervention mechanism, but the evidence supporting it as such is limited.

We suggest that investigators embrace the opportunity to study intervention effects at the level of intervention mechanism. Such studies will require investigators to address methodological limitations of previous research, such as sampling that achieves adequate power and assessing purported mechanisms at appropriate assessment points (i.e., pre- and postintervention). Identifying intervention mechanisms, especially those common across varied models, may offer insights that help refine and strengthen existing interventions. Furthermore, evidence of intervention mechanisms may inform theory, as experimental designs offer opportunities to test causal associations between key attachment variables (e.g., parental behavior, attachment security) and later developmental outcomes.

As we have described in this chapter, attachment-based interventions have been shown to have a host of effects on child outcomes soon after completion of the intervention, in domains ranging from attachment to cortisol production to language development (e.g., Bernard et al., 2012; Cicchetti et al., 2011; Toth et al., 2019). Some would argue that it is critical that such effects are sustained over time. Although many studies of attachment-based interventions are not designed or funded to study long-term effects, evidence from several randomized clinical trials support the long-term efficacy of some attachment-based interventions (e.g., Guild et al., 2017; Zajac, Raby, & Dozier, 2020). The short-term and long-term effects of attachment-based interventions on children and on their parents suggest the possibility that such interventions could have positive societal outcomes by enhancing perspective-taking, empathy, and self-regulation.

REFERENCES

Berlin, L. J., Martoccio, T. L., Bryce, C. I., & Jones Harden, B. (2019). Improving infants' stress-induced cortisol production through attachment-based intervention: A randomized clinical trial. *Psychoneuroendocrinology, 103*, 225–232.

Berlin, L. J., Martoccio, T. L., & Jones Harden, B. (2018). Improving Early Head Start's impacts on parenting through attachment-based intervention: A randomized clinical trial. *Developmental Psychology, 54*, 2316–2327.

Bernard, K., Dozier, M., Bick, J., Lewis-Morrarty, E., Lindhiem, O., & Carlson, E. (2012). Enhancing attachment organization among maltreated infants: Results of a randomized clinical trial. *Child Development, 83*, 623–636.

Bernard, K., Frost, A., Jelinek, C., & Dozier, M. (2019). Secure attachment predicts lower body mass index in young children with histories of child protective services involvement. *Pediatric Obesity, 14,* e12510.

Bowlby, J. (1982). *Attachment and loss: Vol. 1. Attachment.* New York: Basic Books. (Original work published 1969)

Cicchetti, D., Rogosch, F. A., Toth, S. L., & Sturge-Apple, M. L. (2011). Normalizing the development of cortisol regulation in maltreated infants through preventive interventions. *Development and Psychopathology, 23,* 789–800.

Donelan-McCall, N. S., & Olds, D. L. (2019). The Nurse–Family Partnership: Theoretical and empirical foundations. In H. Steele & M. Steele (Eds.), *Handbook of attachment-based interventions* (pp. 79–103). New York: Guilford Press.

Dozier, M., & Bernard, K. (2019). *Coaching parents of vulnerable infants: The Attachment and Biobehavioral Catch-up approach.* New York: Guilford Press.

Fritz, M. S., & MacKinnon, D. P. (2007). Required sample size to detect the mediated effect. *Psychological Science, 18,* 233–239.

Guild, D. J., Toth, S. L., Handley, E. D., Rogosch, F. A., & Cicchetti, D. (2017). Attachment security mediates the longitudinal association between Child–Parent Psychotherapy and peer relations for toddlers of depressed mothers. *Development and Psychopathology, 29,* 587–600.

Juffer, F., Bakermans-Kranenburg, M. J., & van IJzendoorn, M. H. (2017). Pairing attachment theory and social learning theory in video-feedback intervention to promote positive parenting. *Current Opinion in Psychology, 15,* 189–194.

Lieberman, A. F., Ghosh Ippen, C., & Van Horn, P. (2006). Child–Parent Psychotherapy: 6-month follow-up of a randomized clinical trial. *Journal of the American Academy of Child and Adolescent Psychiatry, 45,* 913–918.

Lieberman, A. F., Weston, D. R., & Pawl, J. H. (1991). Preventive interaction and outcome with anxiously attached dyads. *Child Development, 62,* 199–209.

Lind, T., Bernard, K., Yarger, H. A., & Dozier, M. (2020). Promoting compliance in children referred to Child Protective Services: A randomized clinical trial. *Child Development, 91,* 563–576.

Ordway, M. R., Sadler, L. S., Dixon, J., Close, N., Mayes, L., & Slade, A. (2014). Lasting effects of an interdisciplinary home visiting program on child behavior: Preliminary follow-up results of a randomized trial. *Journal of Pediatric Nursing, 29,* 3–13.

Raby, K. L., Freedman, E., Yarger, H. A., Lind, T., & Dozier, M. (2019). Enhancing the language development of toddlers in foster care by promoting foster parents' sensitivity: Results from a randomized control trial. *Developmental Science, 22,* e12753.

Raby, K. L., Waters, T. E. A., Tabachnick, A., Zajac, L., & Dozier, M. (2019). *ABC enhances secure base script knowledge among mothers with child welfare involvement.* Unpublished manuscript, University of Delaware, Newark, DE.

Sadler, L. S., Slade, A., Close, N., Webb, D. L., Simpson, T., Fennie, K., & Mayes, L. C. (2013). Minding the Baby®: Enhancing reflectiveness to improve early health and relationship outcomes in an interdisciplinary home visiting program. *Infant Mental Health Journal, 34,* 391–405.

Slade, A., Holland, M. L., Ordway, M. R., Carlson, E. A., Jeon, S., Close, N., . . . Sadler, L. S. (2020). Minding the Baby®: Enhancing parental reflective functioning and infant attachment in an attachment-based, interdisciplinary home visiting program. *Development and Psychopathology, 32*(1), 123–137.

Tereno, S., Madigan, S., Lyons-Ruth, K., Plamondon, A., Atkinson, L., Guedeney, N., . . . Guedeney, A. (2017). Assessing a change mechanism in a randomized home-visiting trial: Reducing disrupted maternal communication decreases infant disorganization. *Development and Psychopathology, 29,* 637–649.

Toth, S. L., Maughan, A., Manly, J. T., Spagnola, M., & Cicchetti, D. (2002). The relative efficacy of two interventions in altering maltreated preschool children's representational models: Implications for attachment theory. *Development and Psychopathology, 14,* 877–908.

Toth, S. L., Michi-Petzing, L., Guild, D., & Lieberman, A. F. (2019). Child–Parent Psychotherapy: Theoretical bases, clinical applications, and empirical support. In H. Steele & M. Steele (Eds.), *Handbook of attachment-based interventions* (pp. 296–317). New York: Guilford Press.

Toth, S. L., Rogosch, F. A., Manly, J. T., & Cicchetti, D. (2006). The efficacy of toddler–parent psychotherapy to reorganize attachment in the young offspring of mothers with major depressive disorder: A randomized preventive trial. *Journal of Consulting and Clinical Psychology, 74,* 1006–1016.

Yarger, H. A., Bronfman, E., Carlson, E., & Dozier, M. (2020). Intervening with Attachment and Biobehavioral Catch-up to decrease disrupted parenting behavior and attachment disorganization: The role of parental withdrawal. *Development and Psychopathology, 32*(3), 1139–1148.

Zajac, L., Raby, K. L., & Dozier, M. (2020). Sustained effects on attachment security in middle childhood: Results from a randomized clinical trial of the Attachment and Biobehavioral Catch-Up (ABC) intervention. *Journal of Child Psychology and Psychiatry, 61*(4), 417–424.

CHAPTER 39

Attachment-Based Intervention Processes in Disordered Parent–Child Relationships

Sheree L. Toth
Michelle E. Alto
Jennifer Warmingham

Attachment-Based Interventions and Disorganized Attachment

Disorganized attachment was first operationalized by Main and Solomon (1990) in the context of Ainsworth's Strange Situation (Ainsworth, Blehar, Waters, & Wall, 1978). In this paradigm, infants who display conflicted, disoriented, or fearful behaviors that disrupt typical organized attachment behaviors (e.g., avoidance, resistance, proximity seeking, and contact maintenance in relation to the caregiver) can be classified as having disorganized attachment (Main & Solomon, 1990). These disorganized behaviors are thought to result from a breakdown of the child's organized regulation strategies and a simultaneous activation of the child's fear system (Main & Solomon, 1990). For infants and children with disorganized attachment, the caregiver becomes a source of both protection and threat. As such, disorganized attachment during infancy and childhood is considered to be a manifestation of a disordered parent–child relationship.

Risk for disorganized attachment is higher in certain populations, including children exposed to maltreatment (Cyr, Euser, Bakermans-Kranenburg, & van IJzendoorn, 2010), high levels of marital discord (Owen & Cox, 1997), parental depression (Toth, Rogosch, Manly, & Cicchetti, 2006), parental substance abuse (Cyr et al., 2010), and parents with unresolved loss or trauma (van IJzendoorn, 1995). Although attachment disorganization is associated with certain risks and experiences within the caregiving environment, it is important to note that designation of disorganized attachment only characterizes the quality of a specific parent–child relationship and does not provide evidence of traumatic exposures (e.g., childhood maltreatment).

Both parent and child behaviors contribute to the quality of the attachment relationship and both are important to consider as targets for intervention. Frightened, frightening, or atypical parental behavior is often seen in dyads characterized by disorganized attachment relationships (Lyons-Ruth, Bronfman, & Parsons, 1999; Main & Hesse, 1998). More specifically, disorganized attachment is associated with higher levels of disrupted parenting behavior that includes affective communication errors, role/boundary confusion, fearful/disoriented behaviors, intrusiveness/negativity, and withdrawal (Yarger, Bronfman, Carlson, & Dozier, 2020). Infants or children with disorganized attachment struggle to consistently use their caregiver as a source of comfort in times of stress and may instead become disoriented or misdirect their bids for attention or comfort. This disorganized attachment behavior can be confusing, frustrating, or perceived as rejecting by a caregiver. Therefore, attachment disorganization can create daily challenges in the parenting environment and for child development. In fact, research has shown a small but significant association between disorganized attachment in childhood and later behavioral and mental health problems (Groh, Roisman, van IJzendoorn, Bakermans-Kranenburg, & Fearon, 2012).

A number of attachment-based interventions have been developed to prevent and address disorganized attachment in the context of the parent–child relationship. Attachment theory provides a framework for understanding the parental behaviors and dyadic interaction styles that serve as precursors to healthy parent–child relationships. Attachment-based interventions use a number of strategies to target these precursors as mechanisms of change in preventing disorganized attachment. For example, Child–Parent Psychotherapy (CPP; Lieberman, Ghosh Ippen, & Van Horn, 2015) targets parents' unresolved childhood experiences and attachment representations as a means of increasing their sensitivity when interacting with their children. Another intervention, Attachment and Biobehavioral Catch-up (ABC; Dozier & Bernard, 2019), uses explicit parent coaching and video feedback to enhance parents' nurturance, increase their ability to follow the child's lead, and reduce their frightening behavior. Other attachment interventions also have been developed with similar techniques and goals (see Toth, Gravener-Davis, & Guild, 2013).

Meta-analyses have examined whether attachment interventions are effective in reducing disorganized attachment in children (Bakermans-Kranenburg, van IJzendoorn, & Juffer, 2005; Facompré, Bernard, & Waters, 2017). Bakermans-Kranenburg and colleagues' (2005) initial meta-analysis found that overall, the interventions examined were not effective in changing disorganized attachment classifications. However, this meta-analysis highlighted the fact that those interventions that were found to be effective targeted samples at elevated risk for disorganized attachment and focused on key mechanisms of risk. Specifically, interventions were more effective in populations characterized by infant risk (i.e., adopted, irritable, or premature) than in populations characterized by parental risk (i.e., impoverished, socially isolated, insecure attachment representations). In addition, interventions that focused on parental sensitivity were most effective. Facompré and colleagues (2017) updated this meta-analysis with seven new studies published between 2005 and 2013. Contrary to Bakermans-Kranenburg and colleagues' study, they found that attachment-based interventions were in fact effective in increasing rates of organized attachment compared to control conditions. In addition, interventions were more effective in maltreated samples, further emphasizing the importance of providing attachment-based interventions for children who have experienced serious relational trauma typified by maltreatment.

In both meta-analyses described above, interventions primarily targeted one or more of three main foci: (1) parental sensitivity (e.g., by providing information on infant development, modeling appropriate infant touch and massage, providing video feedback intended to promote sensitive responsiveness); (2) providing support to parents (e.g., by providing supportive general counseling, social, financial, legal, health, or educational services); and/or (3) parental representations of attachment (e.g., by examining parents' internal working models of their caregiving role and their attachment histories). In both meta-analyses, interventions that targeted sensitivity were most effective in decreasing disorganization, although the greater effect of sensitivity-focused interventions over support- and representational-focused interventions was statistically significant in Bakermans-Kranenburg and colleagues' (2005) analyses only. The variable strength of sensitivity-focused interventions in changing disorganized attachment is consistent with research showing that although insensitivity has a significant but small role in the development of disorganized attachment (van IJzendoorn, Schuengel, & Bakermans-Kranenburg, 1999), it may not distinguish disorganized attachment from organized-insecure attachment the same way it distinguishes organized-secure from organized-insecure attachment. Instead, parental frightened, frightening, or atypical behavior may be more uniquely related to disorganized attachment (Madigan, Moran, & Pederson, 2006; Schuengel, Bakermans-Kranenburg, & van IJzendoorn, 1999). Frightening parental behavior can also include atypically disrupted affective communication between the parent and the infant (Lyons-Ruth et al., 1999). These behaviors have been uniquely linked to disorganized attachment (Lyons-Ruth et al., 1999; Madigan et al., 2006) and therefore are compelling potential targets of intervention for disordered parent–child relationships.

Attachment-Based Intervention Processes

Despite the strong theoretical underpinning and promising outcomes from interventions that target parental sensitivity, support, and parental representations in populations at risk for disordered parent–child relationships, the literature currently lacks substantive empirical evidence that these factors act as mediators, or change processes, of intervention effects on attachment disorganization. One recent study found that lower levels of maternal withdrawal mediated the effect of an attachment-based intervention (ABC) on disorganized attachment (Yarger et al., 2020; see also Dozier & Bernard, Chapter 38, this volume, for a related discussion of mechanisms of intervention effects on attachment and self-regulation outcomes). Although these findings are encouraging, there is a great need for growth in this area of the literature. Thus, assessing specific precursors to disorganized attachment as mediators will be essential as future studies that test intervention effects become more focused on understanding change processes.

Because there are often multiple theoretical mediators of attachment-based intervention effects depending on the clinical population, there are challenges to assessing all possible mediators in the context of intervention studies. As such, study design and thoughtful selection of mediators is often difficult to balance against participant burden. Furthermore, mediators should be closely tied to the theoretical change processes being targeted by the intervention. For example, employing a reliable interaction paradigm, coding system, and/or measure of parental behavior specific to disorganized attachment may be particularly important in samples of families at high risk for disorganized attachment, as change in these behaviors from baseline may help to explain intervention effects. Two behavioral coding systems have been specifically developed to assess parental behavior associated with disorganized attachment: Main and Hesse's (1998) FR (frightened or frightening) parental behavior scales, and Bronfman, Madigan, and Lyons-Ruth's (2007) Atypical Maternal Behavior Instrument and Classification (AMBIANCE) coding system for disrupted communication. FR behaviors includes threatening, frightened, dissociative, timid/deferential, spousal/romantic, and disorganized parental behavior. The AMBIANCE includes items from the FR coding system and adds dimensions observed among at-risk mothers that are theoretically related to infant fear and disorganized attachment. Specifically, the AMBIANCE assesses negative-intrusive behavior, role confusion, disorientation, affective communication errors, and withdrawal. Despite these coding systems' strong theoretical and empirical bases for detecting parental behaviors associated with disorganized attachment, few studies have capitalized on their utility for detecting change processes in attachment intervention studies. However, recent work by Yarger et al.

(2020), mentioned above, utilized the AMBIANCE system to code maternal behavior during the Strange Situation and found promising results linking dimensions of this coding system to changes in disorganized attachment in the context of an attachment-based intervention.

Measurement of theorized mechanisms of change that could promote decreases in disorganized attachment are often challenging to select and ascertain, as many measures include lab-based interaction paradigms that require time-intensive coding. Lotzin and colleagues (2015) provide an extensive review of observational coding methods that are used in parent–child research in the early years of child development. However, the time and cost associated with learning and coding interactive paradigms often limit their practicality for many intervention studies. More streamlined approaches to measuring mechanisms of change are warranted as greater importance is placed on identifying mechanisms of change and as research on therapeutic interventions moves into real-world settings for effectiveness trials (Lotzin et al., 2015).

Lotzin and colleagues (2015) also provide recommendations for intervention studies targeting parenting behavior and/or the parent–child relationship. Specifically, they suggest that selection of an instrument and paradigm assessing these mechanisms should include a thorough assessment of validity and sensitivity to change so that any true effects can be captured. Selection of a measure should also match the mechanisms of change proposed by the intervention and should be measured prior to the outcome measure in order to establish temporal precedence when testing mediation. Attention to measurement and thoughtful instrument selection are both important steps to identifying mechanisms of change for attachment-based interventions.

Although little research on attachment-based interventions has empirically examined processes that account for change in attachment classification, there is a growing body of work that has investigated processes that account for change in maternal behavior. Some preliminary findings indicate that clinician-related factors, such as quality of therapist or adherence to the intervention model, are important elements that could lead to positive change in maternal behavior (Caron et al., 2018; Suchman, Decoste, Rosenberger, & McMahon, 2012). In attachment-based interventions for parents of young children, clinicians often provide important *in vivo* feedback on parental interactions and statements about the child, which consequently helps promote sensitive maternal behaviors and decrease intrusive or frightening behaviors (Caron et al., 2018). As such, clinician adherence to the intervention model may be a process affecting maternal behavior change over the course of an intervention.

In addition to therapist adherence, maternal reflective functioning, parental representations of the child, and parental depression each were independent mediators of intervention effects on improvement in maternal caregiving behavior in the Mothers and Toddlers Program in a sample of substance-using mothers (Suchman et al., 2012). This finding is consistent with the idea that parenting behaviors are multiply determined, and further shows the importance of targeting and assessing multiple levels of parental functioning in attachment-based interventions. Furthermore, promotion of adaptive coping strategies to help manage symptoms of psychopathology for mothers presenting with mental disorders may be an important point of intervention that can aid in the promotion of adaptive parent–child relationships. These studies together show the potential for multiple mediators, including parental behaviors, psychopathology, representations, model adherence, and therapist-related factors, to play important roles in the processes by which evidence-based models can promote healthy parent–child interactions.

Conclusions

Parenting interventions aimed at healing disordered parent–child relationships show promising evidence across clinical populations. However, we have much more to learn about the processes that underlie intervention effects. Close attention to measure selection, study design, and assessment of possible mediators is essential to improving understanding of these interventions and the processes involved in the promotion of healthy parent–child relationships. Future work should focus on assessing both positive, supportive parental behaviors and insensitive and/or frightening parental behaviors. Families involved in services across clinical populations present with both challenges and strengths. Although a focus on disordered parent–child relationships calls greater attention to families' challenges, assessment and promotion of inherent family strengths is an important tenant of attachment-based interventions that should not be overlooked. Importantly, future research may help to reflect the shared and differential processes of change across clinical samples, which will help clinicians and researchers understand more about how to promote supportive parenting and healthy developmental trajectories for children.

REFERENCES

Ainsworth, M., Blehar, M., Waters, E., & Wall, S. (1978). *Patterns of attachment: A psychological study of the Strange Situation.* Hillsdale, NJ: Erlbaum.

Bakermans-Kranenburg, M. J., van IJzendoorn, M. H., & Juffer, F. (2005). Disorganized infant attachment and preventive interventions: A review and meta-analysis. *Infant Mental Health Journal, 26*(3), 191–216.

Bronfman, E., Madigan, S., & Lyons-Ruth, K. (2007). *Atypical maternal behavior instrument for assessment and classification (AMBIANCE): Manual for coding disrupted affective communication: Version 2.0.* Unpublished manual, Harvard University Medical School.

Caron, E. B., Bernard, K., Dozier, M., Caron, E. B., Bernard, K., Dozier, M., . . . Dozier, M. (2018). *In vivo* feedback predicts parent behavior change in the Attachment and Biobehavioral Catch-up intervention. *Journal of Clinical Child and Adolescent Psychology, 47*(1), 35–46.

Cyr, C., Euser, E. M., Bakermans-Kranenburg, M. J., & van IJzendoorn, M. H. (2010). Attachment security and disorganization in maltreating and high-risk families: A series of meta-analyses. *Development and Psychopathology, 22*(1), 87–108.

Dozier, M., & Bernard, K. (2019). *Coaching parents of vulnerable infants: The Attachment and Biobehavioral Catch-up approach.* New York: Guilford Press.

Facompré, C. R., Bernard, K., & Waters, T. E. A. (2017). Effectiveness of interventions in preventing disorganized attachment: A meta-analysis. *Development and Psychopathology, 30*(1), 1–11.

Groh, A. M., Roisman, G. I., van IJzendoorn, M. H., Bakermans-Kranenburg, M. J., & Fearon, R. P. (2012). The significance of insecure and disorganized attachment for children's internalizing symptoms: A meta-analytic study. *Child Development, 83*(2), 591–610.

Lieberman, A. F., Ghosh Ippen, C., & Van Horn, P. J. (2015). *Don't hit my mommy: A manual for Child–Parent Psychotherapy with young witnesses of family violence* (2nd ed.). Washington, DC: ZERO TO THREE Press.

Lotzin, A., Lu, X., Kriston, L., Schiborr, J., Musal, T., Romer, G., & Ramsauer, B. (2015). Observational tools for measuring parent–infant interaction: A systematic review. *Clinical Child and Family Psychology Review, 18*(2), 99–132.

Lyons-Ruth, K., Bronfman, E., & Parsons, E. (1999). Maternal frightened, frightening, or atypical behavior and disorganized infant attachment patterns. *Monographs of the Society for Research in Child Development, 64*(3), 67–96.

Madigan, S., Moran, G., & Pederson, D. R. (2006). Unresolved states of mind, disorganized attachment relationships, and disrupted interactions of adolescent mothers and their infants. *Developmental Psychology, 42*(2), 293–304.

Main, M., & Hesse, E. (1998). *Frightening, threatening, dissociative, timid-deferential, sexualized and disorganized parental behavior: A coding system for frightened/frightening (FR) parent–infant interactions.* Unpublished manual, University of California at Berkeley.

Main, M., & Solomon, J. (1990). Procedures for identifying infants as disorganized/disoriented during the Ainsworth Strange Situation. In M. T. Greenberg, D. Cicchetti, & E. M. Cummings (Eds.), *Attachment in the preschool years: Theory, research, and intervention* (pp. 121–160). Chicago: University of Chicago Press.

Owen, M. T., & Cox, M. J. (1997). Marital conflict and the development of infant–parent attachment relationships. *Journal of Family Psychology, 11*(2), 152–164.

Schuengel, C., Bakermans-Kranenburg, M. J., & van IJzendoorn, M. H. (1999). Frightening maternal behavior linking unresolved loss and disorganized infant attachment. *Journal of Consulting and Clinical Psychology, 67*(1), 54–63.

Suchman, N. E., Decoste, C., Rosenberger, P., & McMahon, T. J. (2012).

Attachment-based intervention for substance-using mothers: A preliminary test of the proposed mechanisms of change. *Infant Mental Health Journal, 33*(4), 360–371.

Toth, S., Gravener-Davis, J., & Guild, D. (2013). Relational interventions for child maltreatment: Past, present, and future perspectives. *Development and Psychopathology, 25*(4, Pt. 2), 1601–1617.

Toth, S. L., Rogosch, F. A., Manly, J. T., & Cicchetti, D. (2006). The efficacy of toddler–parent psychotherapy to reorganize attachment in the young offspring of mothers with major depressive disorder: A randomized preventive trial. *Journal of Consulting and Clinical Psychology, 74*(6), 1006–1016.

van IJzendoorn, M. H. (1995). Adult attachment representations, parental responsiveness, and infant attachment: A meta-analysis on the predictive validity of the Adult Attachment Interview. *Psychological Bulletin, 117*(3), 387–403.

van IJzendoorn, M. H., Schuengel, C., & Bakermans-Kranenburg, M. J. (1999). Disorganized attachment in early childhood: Meta-analysis of precursors, concomitants, and sequelae. *Development and Psychopathology, 11*(2), 225–249.

Yarger, H. A., Bronfman, E., Carlson, E., & Dozier, M. (2020). Intervening with Attachment and Biobehavioral Catch-up to decrease disrupted parenting behavior and attachment disorganization: The role of parental withdrawal. *Development and Psychopathology, 32*(3), 1139–1148.

CHAPTER 40

Therapeutic Mechanisms in Attachment-Informed Psychotherapy with Adults

Alessandro Talia
Jeremy Holmes

Attachment-informed psychotherapy (AIP; Holmes & Slade 2017) is an interpersonal model that uses developmental and relational perspectives to view psychopathologies and therapeutic interventions. In this model, psychological disorders are seen as associated with fundamental disruptions in people's capacity to trust others and themselves. Some patients have experienced their caregivers as unreliable, inconsistent, or repeatedly disconfirming of their perceptions and sense of self. Others report histories of active threat or abuse. Some patients have been abandoned, either by forced separations or death. Arising out of these and other developmental difficulties and traumata, attachment theory views psychological disorders as self-protective strategies, adaptive in their developmental context, which now constrain people's affective lives and limit their ability to learn from experience. In the context of a secure therapeutic relationship, AIP aims to reactivate patients' trust, so that such suboptimal strategies can be softened or relinquished entirely.

In our brief contribution, we outline a number of attachment-informed therapeutic processes, drawing on Bowlby's writing, contemporary psychotherapy research, and our own clinical experience. We see AIP as a meta-model; its "mechanisms" are "common factors" that are applicable across a variety of specific therapeutic models. Our account is thus generic, but we write with a number of explicitly attachment-influenced therapies in mind. These include mentalization-based treatments (Allen, Fonagy, & Bateman, 2008), short-term psychodynamic therapies (Fosha & Slowiaczek, 1997; Frederickson, 2014), experiential treatments such as emotionally focused therapy for couples (see Johnson, Chapter 41, this volume), more cognitive approaches influenced by Bowlby's work (e.g., Guidano & Liotti, 1983), as well as various approaches of relational psychoanalysis influenced by attachment research (Eagle, 2013; Holmes, 2001).

Establishing a Secure Base

It is easy to be misled into thinking that "offering a secure base" (Bowlby, 1988) consists of little more than creating a warm, reliable, collaborative relationship in which patients will be duly receptive to therapeutic interventions. Given Bowlby's profound gift for theory, he undoubtedly had more in mind than these basic conditions. Trust is a two-way process. In his model, secure children turn to their "wiser and stronger" attachment figures when distressed, but they also expect that caregivers will trust them: be attuned to their feelings, validate their perceptions, and be appropriately responsive. Under ideal conditions, these two forms of trust feed each other, creating a virtuous cycle. In AIP the same principles apply.

This emphasis on *mutual* trust has considerable technical implications. While there is an implicit asymmetry or "natural pedagogy" (Csibra & Gergely, 2009) in the therapeutic relationship, the attachment-informed psychotherapist eschews the role of the expert or that of the teacher. AIP therapists' preferred role is that of a trusted companion for patients' autonomous attempts to make meaning of and affectively regulate their experiences, both negative and positive. The sensitivity, nonjudgmental understanding, and acceptance AIP embodies represent an attempted "corrective experience" for patients who have been consistently rejected or misunderstood.

Establishing a secure base is thus the first step in AIP, and it is arguably a curative ingredient in its own right. But as any therapist knows, this is no easy task. First, due to their adverse developmental experiences, patients may struggle to learn from others or be receptive to their communications (Fonagy & Allison, 2014). Second, due to their patients' insecure interpersonal strategies, therapists may find themselves pushed into mistrusting or unconsciously rejecting patients. As in Collodi's Pinocchio, patients' problems in inspiring trust in others go hand in hand with difficulties in trusting others. Often therapeutic ruptures may result in diagnostic terms misused to legitimize therapeutic failures—"narcissism," "borderline," and so on. In what follows, we outline a number of ways in which AIP tries to overcome these difficulties.

Repairing Ruptures

No matter how carefully a therapist treads, there will invariably be occasions where patient–therapist trust seems broken and communication stymied. However, if patient and therapist are able to *meta-communicate* (i.e., to communicate about communication), these disjunctures may also create therapeutic opportunities. Indeed, research suggests that successive cycles of rupture and repair lead to *stronger* therapeutic alliances than relationships that appear smooth throughout (Eubanks-Carter, Muran, & Safran, 2018). This is consistent with research showing that infant–caregiver dyads later judged "secure" in the Strange Situation Procedure (SSP) are characterized not by consistently synchronous interactions, but by repeated cycles of mild misattunement and *repair* (Beebe & Lachmann, 2013).

In AIP, relational ruptures are defined as events that signal decreased trust in therapy or the therapeutic relationship, in either the patient or the therapist. They can occur in one of two situations: *withdrawal* or *confrontation* (Safran & Muran, 2000). In our opinion, these loosely correspond with the paradigmatic insecure *attachment styles* described in the branch of attachment-informed psychotherapy research stemming from personality and social psychology (Daly & Mallinckrodt, 2009; Mikulincer & Shaver, 2007). In the *avoidant* style, the patient has low expectations of being understood or believed by the therapist. This manifests itself through *withdrawal* and diminished emotional closeness, through efforts to limit their communications, and by shifting attention away from immediate experience or problematic affect. In the *anxious* style, patients mistrust the authenticity and relevance of therapists' communication. This can lead to *confrontation* as the patient appears to discount or violently rebut their therapist's perspectives—perhaps in the service of counteracting imagined distractedness. In both scenarios, the AIP therapist tries to focus on the patient's and their own subjective experience of the rupture in open and nonblaming ways. Such ruptures perpetuate but also highlight self-defeating aspects of patients' relational styles; resolving them becomes a significant goal of AIP.

Adapting Communication Patterns

Another set of clinically relevant individual differences, termed *attachment patterns,* have been demarcated by attachment research based on detailed infant observation and discourse analysis. Attachment patterns are acquired in early development and continue to shape how people communicate their experience and make meaning of it with others. The SSP reveals how, adapting to their parents' way of communicating, infants communicate their attachment needs in very different ways (Ainsworth, Blehar, Waters, & Wall, 1978). Following brief separations, secure infants seek proximity to the caregiver and are easily pacified, avoidant infants tend to ignore him/her, ambivalent infants insistently seek and resist attempts at soothing, while disorganized infants display various conflicted, disoriented, or fearful behaviors. The Adult Attachment Interview (AAI) identifies parallel categories in adult autobiographical narrative styles—secure-autonomous, dismissing, preoccupied, and unresolved (Main, Kaplan, & Cassidy, 1985).

Recent research has studied these same patterns in the psychotherapy context. The Patient Attachment Coding System (PACS; Talia, Miller-Bottome, & Daniel, 2017) is an assessment validated with the AAI that yields an attachment classification based on the patient's discourse in any given psychotherapy session, and in any therapeutic modality. The PACS reveals striking differences in communication patterns between the organized attachment classifications. Secure patients are able to be open and share their attitudes with candor, and to support these by clear examples and cogent reports of internal experiences; in so doing, they make their communication easy to understand and to accept as true. Dismissing patients' attempt to maximize the chances of being understood by being concise, but undermine their communication by offering barren, etiolated narratives devoid of affective color. Preoccupied patients strive to elicit therapists' support but express themselves in rambling ways that make it hard for their listener to "get their point."

The PACS interprets these stable communicative patterns as reflecting basic—and not inherently pathological—attachment-related attempts to *enhance trust,* regardless of the topic discussed or of the therapist's activity. Consistent with this, AIP therapists aim to validate and work with, rather than summarily change, these patterns. Dismissing patients' minimalistic responses can be thought of not as avoidance, but as an invitation to add more. Preoccupied patients' prolix or confusing replaying of past episodes might be seen not in terms of attempts to devalue or ignore the therapist's comments, but instead as attempts to provide maximum information, and to open a window into their inner world. Holmes (2010) has advocated a two-stage therapeutic approach in which the therapist initially goes with, and to an extent mirrors the patient's communication style, and then gradually, through a combination of validation and challenge, moves to a freer and more coherent conversational mutuality.

Implicit is the AIP view that, at least initially, the therapist will adapt to the patient's style in order to minimize the possibility of ruptures (Daly

& Mallinckrodt, 2009); yet typically this is not sufficient in the long run. Insecure attachment patterns constrain patients' capacity for open affective communication, and thus impede therapeutic work. Such difficulties are especially problematic during ruptures, whose resolution rests on both therapist and patient being able to express their experiences of the problem. This perspective is confirmed by recent research suggesting that secure attachment is characterized by the capacity to communicate openly with the therapist even or especially when problems arise (Miller-Bottome, Talia, Eubanks, Safran, & Muran, 2019). At these junctures, therapists need to work hard to help insecure patients express themselves with the clarity and vividness typical of secure attachment.

Note that this dialogic way of conceptualizing different attachment *patterns* does not cohere with the tradition of research on attachment *styles* referred to in the previous section (Roisman et al., 2007). Although psychotherapy research has often tended to conflate results emerging from the two research traditions, they are likely to tap into different constructs (see, e.g., Daniel, 2006, for a similar point of view). Attachment *styles* can be thought of as reflecting tendencies toward experiencing relationships. Attachment *patterns* (as seen in the AAI and the PACS) reflect differing ways in which we attempt to communicate such experiences; they may influence one's relational experience, but they are distinct from it. For example, secure patients may openly disclose feeling anxious, angry, or distant from their therapist, reflecting on possible sources of these negative emotions and stating their needs in present terms. Such disclosures can be misrecognized as a sign of attachment insecurity when in fact they facilitate deeper connection (Miller-Bottome et al., 2019). Clarifying the relationship between attachment *patterns* and attachment *styles* requires further research, but we advocate assessing and conceptualizing separately these two aspects of attachment-related differences in case formulations (see Talia, Taubner, & Miller-Bottome, 2019).

From Interpersonal to Intrapersonal

The aim of AIP could be summarized as the attempt to help people to know themselves in order that they may relate to and communicate with others. At the same time, *being known* is a precondition for knowing oneself; AIP deploys a continuing dialectic between the interpersonal and the intrapsychic.

Bowlby developed the idea of "defensive exclusion" to capture the distortions in attention, cognitions, and perception that have an interpersonal origin but now serve to rupture communication *within* oneself. AIP translates these processes into *in vivo* relational configurations in the actual patient–therapist relationship and in the matrix of patients' and therapists' past experiences brought into the present by it. These, in turn, act as a nidus for patients' gradually emerging self-knowledge.

A Difference That Makes a Difference

AIP tends to recommend interventions that reproduce aspects of security-promoting parenting. A crucial component here is the idea of "sensitivity," first identified by Mary Ainsworth (see Holmes & Slade, 2017). Transposed into a therapy context, therapist sensitivity refers to their ability to interpret accurately and help regulate patients' affective states.

Therapists, too, vary in their attachment security. In fact, the recent introduction of the Therapist Attunement Scales (TASc; Talia, Muzi, Lingiardi, & Taubner, 2020) has shown that it is possible to predict a therapist's attachment pattern (as assessed with the AAI) based on how his or her interventions foster attunement with the patient in any given session. In the TASc, coders rate the frequency and intensity of different intervention markers, which leads them to assign a global classification to the therapist's attachment. Initial evidence suggests that such classification may not be significantly influenced by what the patient does in session, but it reflects a therapist's trait-like disposition toward connecting to others (Talia et al., 2020).

Dismissing therapists are distinguished by their attempts to make explicit the patient's current beliefs without relating these to their own views. Preoccupied therapists tend to focus more consistently on real details of the patient's life and evaluate the patient's experience independently from the patient. Secure therapists, finally, are characterized by a seeming ability to retain balance and affective even-handedness, without being coldly neutral or diminishing their expertise. They communicate that they understand what the patient says and partly agree with it, but posit their own perspective without detachment, overidentification, or omniscient coerciveness.

This is also the essence of the "mentalizing stance": the ability to see the other as an autonomous, goal-seeking, feeling being, described by Holmes (2010) as "to see oneself from the outside and the other from the inside." Not limiting themselves to open questions and banal repetition nor all-knowingly informing the patient about "how things really are," secure therapists espouse empathic not-knowing and gentle encouragement to ever-further emotional exploration. Their "triple listening stance" entails therapists' (1) creating within themselves a receptive listening space in which to represent and contain the patient's discourse, (2) being able to listen to themselves listening (i.e., "countertransference"), and (3) listening to their comments as they are listened to by the patient. AIP sees these "third-ear" listening skills as a key to selection and training of therapists.

Conclusion

The TASc has shown that, no less than their patients, therapists are shaped by their attachment histories and conversational styles. These individual differences will influence all the core components of AIP discussed so far: establishing a secure base, repairing ruptures, reciprocally adapting one's own and the patient's ways of communicating, and transposing patients' inner worlds in an interpersonal context. This then raises the question about the optimal therapist–patient match, and its impact on therapy outcome; more research is needed on these topics. Secure attachment may be ideal, but a sizable minority of therapists will have insecure attachment tendencies. If through personal therapy, reading, and supervision therapists can better learn to know themselves, we can be encouraged that a degree of acknowledged insecurity may even enhance rather than diminish therapeutic efficacy. The implications for our patients are similarly hopeful.

REFERENCES

Ainsworth, M. S., Blehar, M. C., Waters, E., & Wall, S. (1978). *Patterns of attachment: A psychological study of the Strange Situation*. Hillsdale, NJ: Erlbaum.

Allen, J. G., Fonagy, P., & Bateman, A. W. (2008). *Mentalizing in clinical practice*. Washington, DC: American Psychiatric Publishing.

Beebe, B., & Lachmann, F. M. (2013). *Infant research and adult treatment: Co-constructing interactions*. London: Routledge.

Bowlby, J. (1988). *A secure base: Clinical applications of attachment theory*. London: Routledge.

Csibra, G., & Gergely, G. (2009). Natural pedagogy. *Trends in Cognitive Sciences, 13*(4), 148–153.

Daly, K. D., & Mallinckrodt, B. (2009). Experienced therapists' approach to psychotherapy for adults with attachment avoidance or attachment anxiety. *Journal of Counseling Psychology, 56*(4), 549.

Daniel, S. I. (2006). Adult attachment patterns and individual psychotherapy: A review. *Clinical Psychology Review, 26*(8), 968–984.

Eagle, M. N. (2013). *Attachment and psychoanalysis: Theory, research, and clinical implications*. New York: Guilford Press.

Eubanks, C. F., Muran, J. C., & Safran, J. D. (2018). Alliance rupture repair: A meta-analysis. *Psychotherapy, 55*(4), 508.

Fonagy, P., & Allison, E. (2014). The role of mentalizing and epistemic trust in the therapeutic relationship. *Psychotherapy, 51*(3), 372.

Fosha, D., & Slowiaczek, M. L. (1997). Techniques to accelerate dynamic psychotherapy. *American Journal of Psychotherapy, 51*(2), 229–251.

Frederickson, J. (2014). *Co-creating change: Effective dynamic therapy techniques*. Kansas City: Seven Leaves Press.

Guidano, V. F., & Liotti, G. (1983). *Cognitive processes and emotional disorders: A structural approach to psychotherapy*. New York: Guilford Press.

Holmes, J. (2001). *The search for the secure base: Attachment theory and psychotherapy*. London: Routledge.

Holmes, J. (2010). Integration in psychoanalytic psychotherapy—an attachment meta-perspective. *Psychoanalytic Psychotherapy, 24*(3), 183–201.

Holmes, J., & Slade, A. (2017). *Attachment in therapeutic practice*. London: SAGE.

Main, M., Kaplan, N., & Cassidy, J. (1985). Security in infancy, childhood, and adulthood: A move to the level of representation. In I. Bretherton & E. Waters (Eds.), Growing points of attachment theory and research. *Monographs of the Society for Research in Child Development, 50*(1–2, Serial No. 209), 66–104.

Mikulincer, M., & Shaver, P. R. (2007). *Attachment in adulthood: Structure, dynamics, and change*. New York: Guilford Press.

Miller-Bottome, M., Talia, A., Eubanks, C. F., Safran, J. D., & Muran, J. C. (2019). Secure in-session attachment predicts rupture resolution: Negotiating a secure base. *Psychoanalytic Psychology, 36*(2), 132–138.

Roisman, G. I., Holland, A., Fortuna, K., Fraley, R. C., Clausell, E., & Clarke, A. (2007). The Adult Attachment Interview and self-reports of attachment style: An empirical rapprochement. *Journal of Personality and Social Psychology, 92*(4), 678.

Safran, J. D., & Muran, J. C. (2000). Resolving therapeutic alliance ruptures: Diversity and integration. *Journal of Clinical Psychology, 56*(2), 233–243.

Talia, A., Miller-Bottome, M., & Daniel, S. I. (2017). Assessing attachment in psychotherapy: Validation of the Patient Attachment Coding System (PACS). *Clinical Psychology and Psychotherapy, 24*(1), 149–161.

Talia, A., Muzi, L., Lingiardi, V., & Taubner, S. (2020). How to be a secure base: Therapists' attachment representations and their link to attunement in psychotherapy. *Attachment and Human Development, 22*(2), 189–206.

Talia, A., Taubner, S., & Miller-Bottome, M. (2019). Advances in research on attachment-related psychotherapy processes: Seven teaching points for trainees and supervisors. *Research in Psychotherapy: Psychopathology, Process and Outcome, 22*(3).

CHAPTER 41

Attachment Principles as a Guide to Therapeutic Change
The Example of Emotionally Focused Therapy

Susan M. Johnson

Not long before he died, John Bowlby noted (1988, pp. ix–x) that he was "disappointed that clinicians have been slow to test the theory's uses." Indeed, the use of attachment theory to guide clinical intervention, especially with adults, has been slow in coming, even though the links between insecure attachment and mental health problems have become increasingly clear (Mikulincer & Shaver, 2016). Changes resulting from therapeutic outcomes have been found in a few therapies explicitly guided by attachment science, notably in individual psychodynamic therapy (Rost, Luyten, Fearon, & Fonagy, 2019) and in emotionally focused therapy (EFT) (Burgess-Moser et al., 2015)—which is best known as a couples intervention but is also used as an intervention for individual and family distress. Both of these models have been shown to positively impact key mental health factors such as depression, and can be linked to changes in adults' attachment security (Johnson, 2019). When we consider this kind of change, however, the picture is somewhat complicated by the fact that even though models may use a common frame of reference on attachment, they often focus on different factors and pathways to change. For example, Wallin (2007) suggests that attachment theory leads naturally to a focus on teaching mindfulness, whereas Fonagy (Fonagy & Bateman, 2006) emphasizes shaping reflective functioning (i.e., the capacity to think about mental states in oneself and others) and the generation of "representational coherence" as key change factors. EFT focuses more on the corrective emotional experience as the royal route to change and emotional balance as a key transformational factor (Johnson, 2019). This chapter will discuss lessons learned about shaping clinical change from the extensive research studies on EFT (see also *www.iceeft.com* for a comprehensive list of studies of this model).

Attachment theory does not exactly spell out how to move clients from distress and dysregulation into a state of health. It does, however, provide a clear sense of dysfunction (what needs fixing) and a clear picture of healthy functioning (what to aim for). Health is a felt sense of connection with others, maintained through actual interactions or mental representations, which in turn fosters emotional balance and regulation, the construction of a coherent inner world, positive models of self and other, and full flexible engagement with the world (Johnson, 2019). The most essential feature of ongoing distress and dysfunction is emotional isolation resulting in helplessness—vulnerability without solution. The great strength of attachment theory is that it links self and relational system into a whole. Bowlby was a systems theorist, always noting the circular feedback loops between the "inner ring" of cognitive and emotional processing and the "outer ring" of interactional patterns. As a therapy that integrates humanistic, experiential, and systemic relational interventions, EFT seems, to this author, to capture the essence of attachment science (Johnson, 2019).

EFT's Grounding: Six Core Attachment Principles

For the EFT therapist, there are six core principles of attachment that translate directly into protocols for intervention. First, there is continual focus on the processing and regulation of emotions, especially, as Bowlby termed them, "frightening, alien or unacceptable" emotions. The goal here is emotional balance, best achieved by coregulation with others that allows full engagement with emotion and the ability to render it into a coherent whole, rather than leaving it denied, fragmented, or blocked. Emotion organizes people's inner worlds and key interactions with others.

Second, EFT emphasizes the creation and maintenance of in-session safety in a collaborative nonpathologizing alliance. Bowlby's stories of interventions, for example with a potentially abusive young mother or with an angry widow, always show this nonpathologizing tendency and offer a model of an alliance where, in a way that parallels the work of Rogers (1951), the father of experiential therapy, the therapist is genuinely present. Like a safe attachment figure, the therapist is accessible, responsive, and engaged. Change evolves with the client; it is not something done to the client.

Third, in all modalities of treatment, there is a constant back and forth of within and between perspectives. The self is a process constantly created in the space between inner experience, the signals sent to others, and the interpretation of responses from others. The therapist shapes new inner experience with the client and turns this into new dramas that redefine existential pain and loss, fears and needs, as described below.

Fourth, the view of health and thus the direction of EFT is clear. It is always to help clients deal constructively with vulnerability and remove blocks to openly engaging with experience and with others. The EFT therapist does not have to teach coping or relational skills per se. These skills will naturally emerge in an organic fashion in a safe environment where a secure base is offered for exploration. Thus, empathy for others naturally emerges once affect regulation improves and the fear of others becomes less overwhelming.

Fifth, the therapist focuses on present process, on the here and now. Core elements of past experience emerge in the present as emotions are evoked. Modern attachment theory acknowledges that working models are "hot," emotionally loaded, and much more fluid than previously thought (Mikulincer & Shaver, 2016). During every session, the therapist creates interpersonal dramas that disconfirm or expand constricted working models and affect regulation patterns.

Sixth, Bowlby based attachment on ethology, the science of observed animal behavior, and EFT is profoundly empirical in its operation. Like attachment theory, EFT focuses on the process of observation and the delineation of patterns of behavior. EFT also includes a comprehensive research program detailing the outcome of within-session processes.

The EFT Intervention Tango

These six core attachment principles are operationalized in the three main stages of EFT—stabilization, the restructuring of attachment and the sense of self, and consolidation—and in the key, constantly reoccurring macro-intervention sequence in EFT called the EFT tango (Figure 41.1). This tango, so named because the tango is a dance of constant attunement with another, has five moves. These moves may vary in pacing and intensity across stages.

In Move 1 the therapist reflects present process, both within and between—that is, inner emotional processes and interactional realities and responses. The therapist might say, "*I notice, Amy, that you try to explain to Mark about your 'upset' and when this doesn't seem to move him, you speak faster and faster and more loudly and tell him about what he calls his 'mistakes,' until you finally explode and point your finger at him. My sense is that you get frantic to be heard here. And Mark, you give Amy reasons why she should not be upset and when this does not work you turn your body away from her and shut down.*" Mark nods. "*And the more silent you become, the more agitated and insistent Amy becomes. This plays out until both of you withdraw. It seems like this dance defeats both of you and leaves you both alone here.*"

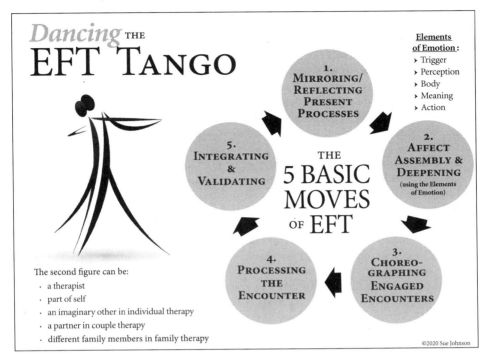

FIGURE 41.1. The EFT tango.

Move 2 involves the therapist assembling and deepening emotion beyond reactive surface emotions to more core responses. This involves engaging with the key elements of emotion—trigger, body sensations, meaning dimensions, and action tendencies—in a visceral way rather than talking about emotions. The word emotion comes from the Latin *emovere,* "to move," and the accessing of new emotions evokes new meanings and new action tendencies. Changing the emotional music changes how adults "dance" with others in an organic, naturally occurring fashion. The therapist evokes emotion and orders and regulates it at the same time. The therapist might say, *"Mark, what happens to you when Amy begins to detail your 'mistakes'?"* Mark states that he feels nothing. *"As she says, 'You are an emotional cripple like your dad,' your face goes flat and still and you turn away. That must be hard to hear."* (The therapist notes a specific trigger and body response.) *"How does it feel when she says that?"* Mark replies that he feels sick. The therapist asks, *"And what do you say to yourself in your head?"* Mark replies that he will never please Amy and so he just gives up and shuts down. (He gives the meaning and his action tendency.) The therapist then puts all these elements together and validates how hard it is to hear that Mark's wife is disappointed with him, that for most of us this is scary. (Mark nods emphatically and adds that he is overwhelmed by Amy's emotion remarks.)

In Move 3 these core responses are used to transform key interactions with others, in session with others (in couples or family therapy) or by bringing alive images of attachment figures and ways of connecting with parts of the self (in individual therapy). Here the therapist will distill Mark's emotional responses and ask, *"Can you turn to Amy now and tell her, 'It is hard to hear your disappointment with me, scary even. So I do shut down. I just get so overwhelmed'?"* This new drama is then reflected on and made coherent in Move 4. The therapist checks what it is like for Mark to say this and he states that he feels good because this captures his reality. Then the therapist asks how Amy responds. Amy weeps and replies that she never knew he was overwhelmed; she thought he was indifferent. The therapist repeats the whole process of Moves 1–3 and frames the dance and the distance it creates as the couples' mutual enemy.

The therapist then, in Move 5, summarizes this whole process in ways that validate the person and highlight the elements that Bowlby suggests protect against dysfunction, a sense of competence and worth. The therapist might comment on Mark's courage in opening up to his partner and Amy's honesty in how she responded, the obvious feeling they have for each other and how they are already delineating the pattern—the dance—that keeps them stuck in distress. The therapist normalizes Amy's anger as desperation at loss of connection with Mark and Mark's attempts to protect himself from feeling rejected by Amy.

The therapist uses micro interventions, empathic reflection, evocative questions focused on the *how* of experience, validation, and deepening emotion with techniques such as repetition and imagery. The therapist also uses small interpretations, such as framing aggressive responses as desperate calls for attention, to reframe the pattern of emotional regulation and interactional cycle of responses people are caught in as the problem, rather than their personal failings, thus choreographing new kinds of interactions. In all of these interventions, the therapist emulates parenting behaviors associated with attachment security. The ideal mother responds to a child's fear or blocked exploration by titrating risks, naming and validating the fear, and encouraging small steps forward. We have learned, for example, that the secret to having clients engage with what Bowlby (1988, p. 138) called "frightening, alien and unacceptable emotions" is to stay soft, slow, and specific. Recent research on emotion shows that making emotions specific and concrete aids in emotion regulation (Barrett, 2004). Of course, attuning to and outlining emotion with specificity is made infinitely simpler by the map to human misery and motivation supplied by attachment science. Sensitivity to abandonment and rejection, thwarted longings for connection and care, and the desperate avoidance of pain that begins as a search for protection and then becomes a prison are common across all clients.

Therapeutic Change in EFT

At present, there are nine studies of change processes within EFT couples interventions (Greenman & Johnson, 2013) and one in progress as part of a study of EFT for individuals with emotional disorders (EFIT). The findings are consistent and are hypothesized to remain the same for the EFIT study. Consistent with the theory of EFT, success at the end of therapy and at follow-up—whether this means increased marital satisfaction or intimacy, less depression, or more attachment security—is routinely predicted by two factors: the depth of the client's emotional processing, and authentic encounters with others or key parts of self associated with attachment figures (such as the disapproving self-dialogue learned from a rejecting father). These are coded on formal measures such as the 7-level Experiencing Scale (Klein, Mathieu, Gendlin, & Kiesler, 1969) in key sessions identified by the therapist as significant in terms of change in Stage 2 of EFT. These change events have been titled "softenings" in that vulnerability is accessed and dealt with in a different, more open way, or, in couples therapy, "Hold me tight" conversations where attachment fears and needs are specified and expressed in ways that pull the partner close and evoke responsiveness (Johnson, 2008). These events are viewed as corrective existential dramas. Fears and needs are accessed and engaged, and basic questions as to the worth of self and the competence to define inner experience are answered affirmatively. New ways to relate to self and other can then be explored.

Summary

Attachment theory tells us that expanding emotion regulation and patterns of engagement with others in moments of constructive dependency enables clients to move into belonging and becoming. A felt sense of safe haven and secure base connection with the therapist and with the other partner allows for a new kind of engagement with ongoing experience and a revision of negative working models of self and other. The clinical vignettes offered by Bowlby (1988, p. 155) reflect the same focus on accepting and staying with a client's emotional experience and leading the client through this experience into deeper connection with self and other as is advocated by Rogers (1951) and epitomized in EFT (Johnson, 2019). A task for the future is to examine if and how that this change process, outlined in our couples therapy research, also predicts successful outcome in EFIT and in EFFT (EFT with distressed families).

The field of psychotherapy is in dire need of a coherent unifying vision of the essential elements of what it means to be human, a vision that takes us beyond simply coping but rather toward growth and what Rogers (1961) called full "existential living," where individuals have "this underlying confidence in themselves as trustworthy instruments for encountering life" (p. 195). Over 30 years of clinical practice and research studies in EFT send a clear message, that attachment science has an enormous contribution to make in terms of integrating the field of psychotherapy. In particular, more than insight or coping skills, change is essentially about new emotional experience and new ways to truly connect with others.

REFERENCES

Barrett, L. F. (2004). Feelings or words: Understanding the content in self-reported ratings of experienced emotion. *Journal of Personality and Social Psychology, 61,* 226–244.

Bowlby, J. (1988). *A secure base: Parent–child attachment and healthy human development.* New York: Basic Books.

Burgess Moser, M., Johnson, S. M., Dalgleish, T., Lafontaine, M. F., Wiebe, S. A., & Tasca, G. (2015). Changes in relationship specific romantic attachment in emotionally focused couple therapy. *Journal of Marital and Family Therapy, 42,* 231–245.

Fonagy, P., & Bateman, A. W. (2006). Mechanisms of change in mentalization based treatment of BPD. *Journal of Clinical Psychology, 62,* 411–430.

Greenman, P., & Johnson, S. M. (2013). Process research on emotionally focused therapy for couples: Linking theory to practice. *Family Process, 52,* 46–51.

Johnson, S. M. (2008). *Hold me tight: Seven conversations for a lifetime of love.* New York: Little Brown.

Johnson, S. M. (2019). *Attachment theory in practice: EFT with individuals, couples and families.* New York: Guilford Press.

Klein, M. H., Mathieu, P. L., Gendlin, E. T., & Kiesler D. J. (1969). *The Experiencing Scale: A research and training manual* (Vol. 1). Madison, WI: Psychiatric Institute.

Mikulincer, M., & Shaver, P. (2016). *Attachment in adulthood: Structure, dynamics and change* (2nd ed.). New York: Guilford Press.

Rogers, C. (1951). *Client-centered therapy.* Boston: Houghton Mifflin.

Rogers, C. (1961). *On becoming a person.* New York: Houghton Mifflin.

Rost, F., Luyten, D., Fearon, R., & Fonagy, P. (2019). Personality and outcome in individual therapy with treatment resistant depression: Exploring differential treatment effects in the Tavistock Adult Depression study. *jJournal of Consulting and Clinical Psychology, 87,* 433–445.

Wallin, D. J. (2007). *Attachment in psychotherapy.* New York: Guilford Press.

TOPIC 9

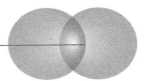

ATTACHMENT, SYSTEMS, AND SERVICES

- How are attachment theory and research relevant to systems and services for children and families?

- What lessons can we learn from these programs?

CHAPTER 42

Attachment and Child Care

Margaret Tresch Owen
Cynthia A. Frosch

Classic theories on parent–child relationships stress the hazards of early separations, and a basic tenet of attachment theory is that a child's early separation from an attachment figure can cause despair, anxiety, and withdrawal. From a theoretical perspective, as well as from cultural beliefs about the importance of maternal care, concerns have been widely expressed among researchers and parents alike about the effects of daily separations from the mother on the development of child–mother attachment. Early research findings on maternal employment and attachment fueled these concerns (e.g., Belsky, 1988), although evidence for attachment insecurity when mothers were employed may have reflected other variables, such as the quality of nonmaternal care, mothers' accessibility and sensitivity with their infants, or maternal desires related to independence (Clarke-Stewart, 1988). Parents have expressed similar concerns regarding separations along with fears that they might have less influence on their child if their young child experienced child care outside the home. Few have voiced similar concerns about fathers' employment-related absences in the child's early years.

In this chapter, we review foundational evidence from longitudinal research on early child care and attachment within a relational context. Next, we examine the multiple attachment relationships children may share with parental and nonparental caregivers. We highlight the possibility of the parent–caregiver partnership as an important but often overlooked contributor to children's attachment security. Finally, we offer recommendations for research, policy, and practice.

Foundational Evidence: The NICHD Study of Early Child Care and Youth Development

A major impetus behind the launching of the National Institute of Child Health and Human Development (NICHD) Study of Early Child Care and Youth Development (SECCYD) was debate about the risks of extensive and early entry into nonmaternal care for the development of a secure infant–mother attachment, and recognition of the inadequacies of the existing literature. The NICHD SECCYD, with its extensive and careful measurement of multiple, longitudinal features of child care experiences, parent, parenting, and home characteristics, and child outcomes, including state-of-the-art measures of attachment, became the largest, most extensive, and best documented study of early child care experience in the United States. Major studies have also been conducted in other developed countries, including Canada and Israel (e.g., Baker, Gruber, & Milligan, 2008; Sagi, Koren-Karie, Gini, Ziv, & Joels, 2002).

Notably, in the first major study examining multiple features of child care, the NICHD SECCYD found no main effects of the quantity, quality, or stability of nonmaternal care in 10 sites across the United States on the security of infant–mother attachment measured at 15 months (NICHD Early Child Care Research Network [ECCRN], 1997). Findings also indicated the Strange Situation was equally valid for children who experienced child care and those who did not. Main effects of the quantity and quality of nonmaternal care were also unrelated to attachment security measured subsequently at 24 and 36 months. The strongest predictor of attachment security at all ages was observed maternal sensitivity toward the child (NICHD ECCRN, 1997, 2001). Notably, maternal sensitivity moderated links between child care experience and attachment security. When maternal sensitivity was low (i.e., bottom third of the sample) more hours, low quality, and less stable child care increased the risk of insecure infant–mother attachment. When maternal sensitivity was higher, child care hours and the quality of child care caregiving were unrelated to attachment security. Effect sizes were small at all ages, but the same pattern of findings was found for attachment security measured at 24 and 36 months.

The longitudinal findings from the NICHD SECCYD strongly suggested that daily separation from mother associated with child care experience, in and of itself, did not undermine child–mother attachment security. Even the experience of lower quality child care, observed as prevalent in the SECCYD (NICHD ECCRN, 2000), was unrelated to attachment security except when coupled with low maternal sensitivity. Thus, scholars' and parents' concerns about the effects of child care on children's attachment security with their mothers should have been at least partially assuaged by results from this major U.S. longitudinal study, in which early entry into child care for extensive hours was common. Moreover, the added risk of low-quality child care, which is prevalent in the United States, was and is cause for continued concern. Indeed, in another large study of child care effects in Israel, center-based child care was associated with attachment insecurity (Sagi et al., 2002). The authors ascribed this effect to the poor quality of center-based care in Israel (e.g., high child–adult ratios, lack of professional training). Thus, the issue of child care quality remains an important consideration, especially given cross- and within-country variability in care quality.

The concern that maternal sensitivity might be negatively affected when children experience more nonmaternal care was also addressed in the SECCYD (NICHD ECCRN, 1999, 2003a). Results were mixed. More hours and lower quality care were each associated with somewhat less maternal sensitivity across infancy and early childhood, controlling for multiple selection factors, particularly among White families. By age 3 years, among non-White (predominantly African American) families, more hours of care was positively associated with maternal sensitivity. In contrast, for White children, maternal sensitivity was negatively associated with hours of care, both in infancy and across early childhood. In addition, higher quality care across infancy and early childhood related uniquely to more sensitive mother–child interactions, regardless of race or ethnicity (NICHD ECCRN, 1999, 2003a).

In secondary analyses of these data, using a fixed-effects panel model that relies on within-child and parent variation over time (essentially using each child and parent as its own control), Nomaguchi and DeMaris (2013) found no evidence that the amount of child care was associated with maternal sensitivity, even within the SECCYD's large White subsample. Similarly, a recent study of age of entry into child care in Norway found no evidence of effects on either maternal or paternal sensitivity (Zachrisson, Owen, Nordahl, Ribeiro, & Dearing, 2020). Thus, these studies fail to support clearly the hypothesis that early and extensive child care has detrimental effects on parental sensitivity. However, prevalent conditions of lower quality child care provide an element of risk, and higher quality care may provide benefits.

Parents Matter Regardless of Child Care Experience

Another concern expressed by parents, and investigated by researchers, is whether early full-time child care will diminish parents' influence. This is based on the issue of diminished time with parents (i.e., time with mother is the expressed concern) when care is shared with child care providers, especially during infancy. Results of several early studies were mixed. In the SECCYD, however, essentially no differences were found in associations between maternal sensitivity and child outcomes in comparisons between two extreme groups—those experiencing more than 30 hours per week of nonmaternal care and those who received no nonmaternal care (NICHD ECCRN, 2003b). Moreover, comparisons of effect sizes of parenting and child care quality indicated that parenting was the stronger predictor by far of child outcomes across early childhood, including measures of expressive language, behavior problems, social competence, and preacademic skills (NICHD ECCRN, 2006). Together, the evidence suggests that parenting behavior matters, regardless of children's child care experience.

Children's Multiple Attachment Relationships with Parental and Nonparental Caregivers

The importance of high-quality caregiving for child–mother and child–father attachment security extends to the security of attachment with child care providers. It is well established that children form attachments to nonmaternal caregivers (see also chapter by Ahnert, Chapter 4, this volume), although the quality of these attachment relationships may be unrelated. For example, in a study of low-income children of Mexican heritage and their mothers and nonmaternal child care providers, Howes and Guerra (2009) found relative independence between attachment relationships with mothers and child care providers, although higher quality caregiving was associated with more secure attachment, whether with mother or the care provider.

Consistent with attachment theory, these findings indicate the critical importance of high-quality caregiving across children's different relationships. For practitioners providing care for children with insecure attachments with their parents, one key question may be whether a secure attachment with a child care provider can help buffer effects of insecure attachments with parents. Moreover, what remains unknown are the links between caregiving quality and attachment security in child–caregiver dyads that comprise members of different socioeconomic and racial/ethnic backgrounds. Differing attitudes about childrearing may affect children's attachments with nonparental caregivers, as these differences may generate stress and strain upon the parent–caregiver partnership and undermine the child's attachment security.

Parent–Caregiver Partnerships and the Attachment-Related Experiences of Children in Child Care

Pawl (1992) noted astutely that "relationships between people are not necessarily conceptualized as the centrally important factor in day care, and the various continuities which are based on the adult relationship are often insufficiently appreciated" (p. 9). While maternal sensitivity consistently predicts infant–mother attachment security for children experiencing early child care, the quality of the parent–caregiver partnership may be important for attachment-supportive caregiving behavior toward children in child care settings. Owen, Ware, and Barfoot (2000) argued that the partnership between parent and caregiver, operationalized in this study as the "sharing and seeking of information about the child" (p. 415), helps provide links between the child's experiences both at home and in child care and promotes more responsive, supportive caregiving behavior in both mothers and child care providers. In a study of 53 3-year-old children in center-based and less formal child care settings, they found more frequent parent–caregiver information-seeking and -sharing, as reported by the mothers and the care providers, was associated with observational ratings of higher quality caregiving by child care providers and mothers alike. Mothers and caregivers were each more supportive, respectful of the child's autonomy, and stimulating of cognitive development when they reported asking about and sharing information about the child's behavior on a more frequent basis. Within a Korean sample of 1- to 3-year-old children, positive mother–caregiver relationships were associated with less parenting stress (Kim, Moon, Kim, & Ahn, 2013), possibly by means of a recognition of the child care provider as an important relational partner in the child's life.

Surprisingly, little attention has focused on the broader system of relationships among mothers, fathers, and children's nonparental caregivers. Moreover, father–caregiver partnerships and the impact of relationship-focused interventions on the parent–caregiver partnership and the child's network of attachment relationships remain understudied. For example, how might both parents' and caregivers' representations of their own attachment histories relate to the quality of the parent–caregiver partnership? And how might interventions for high-risk families, such as Attachment and Biobehavioral Catch-up (ABC), support positive parent–caregiver partnerships? Despite these gaps, evidence suggests that attachment-influenced practices in child care environments—such as use of family groupings and the continued presence of the same primary caregiver—are associated with more supportive caregiving behaviors (e.g., Owen, Klausli, Mata-Otera, & Caughy, 2008).

Child Care through the Lens of Attachment Theory

Attachment theory has been applied to intervention work in child care settings. For example, Biringen and colleagues (2012) found that participation in a brief emotion education training for caregivers improved emotional availability in child–caregiver dyads and increased child–caregiver attachment security. Control group providers, in comparison, showed greater detachment and less structuring behavior with children over time. The authors concluded that positive changes in the child–caregiver relationship may have benefits for providers (e.g., greater job satisfaction) as well as for children.

Beyond indices of high-quality caregiving, caregiver turnover and instability of care warrant additional consideration when studying child care and children's attachments. For example, using the Fragile Families and Child Well-Being data set, Pilarz and Hill (2014) found that multiple changing child care arrangements across the first three years of life were associated with more child externalizing behavior problems, regardless of family income or child care type. Potential proximal processes related to changing arrangements and their influence on relationship systems across caregivers, parents, and children remain to be explored in greater depth.

Summary and Conclusions

In summary, evidence reviewed in this chapter highlights the interplay of attachment and early child care. While foundational evidence indicated few main effects of child care experience on attachment security, the importance of high quality and stable child care remains central to children's development. In addition, caregiving sensitivity, a consistent predictor of child–parent attachment security, is relevant for the study of children's multiple attachment relationships, including those with child care providers. Although evidence is emerging slowly, the parent–caregiver partnership may hold promise for supporting the security of children's multiple attachment relationships.

Despite several decades now of careful study, questions about child care and children's attachment relationships, as well as the processes involved in the formation and maintenance of these relationships across contexts, still merit further study. Moreover, applications of attachment theory to the disparate child care system and to the broad range of caregiving arrangements that parents use remain critical areas of inquiry, particularly in the context of family stress, instability, and/or low socioeconomic status. In the United States, policies have been enacted at the state level to support improvements in the availability and quality of child care, but far greater supports for parents and the child care system alike are needed. For example, how can early child care providers, teachers, and parents better support children as they transition into and out of early child care and education environments? And how can child care systems best support children through the experiences of loss that they inevitably will encounter, given the relatively high rates of caregiver turnover within most child care settings? A center (and teacher) that pays attention to these experiences of loss and transition may be in a better position to support security within children's systems of attachment relationships. For children experiencing early child care, much of learning is relationally embedded. Therefore, promoting secure attachment relationships must be a primary focus of early childhood research, practice, and policy.

REFERENCES

Baker, M., Gruber, J., & Milligan, J. (2008). Universal child care, maternal labor supply, and family well-being. *Journal of Political Economy, 116,* 709–745.

Belsky, J. (1988). The "effects" of infant day care reconsidered. *Early Childhood Research Quarterly, 3,* 235–272.

Biringen, Z., Altenhofen, S., Aberle, J., Baker, M., Brosal, A., Bennet, S., . . . Swaim, R. (2012). Emotional availability, attachment, and intervention in center-based child care for infants and toddlers. *Development and Psychopathology, 24,* 23–34.

Clarke-Stewart, K. A. (1988). "The 'effects' of infant day care reconsidered" reconsidered: Risks for parents, children, and researchers. *Early Childhood Research Quarterly, 3,* 293–318.

Howes, C., & Guerra, A. G. W. (2009). Networks of attachment relationships in low-income children of Mexican heritage: Infancy through preschool. *Social Development, 18,* 896–914.

Kim, J. M., Moon, S. M., Kim, Y. K., & Ahn, S. H. (2013). The effects of maternal parenting knowledge and mother–caregiver relationship on parenting stress. *Korean Journal of Child Studies, 34,* 79–98.

NICHD Early Child Care Research Network. (1997). The effects of infant child care on infant–mother attachment security: Results of the NICHD Study of Early Child Care. *Child Development, 68,* 860–879.

NICHD Early Child Care Research Network. (1999). Child care and mother–child interaction in the first three years of life. *Developmental Psychology, 35,* 1399–1413.

NICHD Early Child Care Research Network. (2000). Characteristics and quality of child care for toddlers and preschoolers. *Applied Developmental Science, 4,* 116–135.

NICHD Early Child Care Research Network. (2001). Child care and family predictors of preschool attachment and stability from infancy. *Developmental Psychology, 37,* 847–862.

NICHD Early Child Care Research Network. (2003a). Early child care and mother–child interaction from 36 months through first grade. *Infant Behavior and Development, 26,* 345–370.

NICHD Early Child Care Research Network. (2003b). Families matter—even for kids in child care. *Journal of Developmental and Behavioral Pediatrics, 24,* 58–64.

NICHD Early Child Care Research Network. (2006). Child care effect sizes for the NICHD Study of Early Child Care and Youth Development. *American Psychologist, 61,* 99–116.

Nomaguchi, K. M., & DeMaris, A. (2013). Nonmaternal care's association with mother's parenting sensitivity: A case of self-selection bias? *Journal of Marriage and Family, 75,* 760–777.

Owen, M. T., Klausli, J. F., Mata-Otera, A. M., & Caughy, M. O. (2008). Relationship-focused child care practices: Quality of care and child outcomes for children in poverty. *Early Education and Development, 19,* 302–329.

Owen, M. T., Ware, A. M., & Barfoot, B. (2000). Caregiver–mother partnership behavior and the quality of caregiver–child and mother–child interactions. *Early Childhood Research Quarterly, 15,* 413–428.

Pawl, J. H. (1992). Infants in day care: Reflections on experiences, expectations and relationships. In S. Provence, J. Pawl, & E. Fenichel (Eds.), *The ZERO TO THREE child care anthology 1984–1992* (pp. 7–13). Arlington, VA: ZERO TO THREE/National Center for Clinical Infant Programs.

Pilarz, A. R., & Hill, H. D. (2014). Unstable and multiple child care arrangements and young children's behavior. *Early Childhood Research Quarterly, 29,* 471–483.

Sagi, A., Koren-Karie, N., Gini, M., Ziv, Y., & Joels, T. (2002). Shedding further light on the effects of various types and quality of early child care on infant–mother attachment relationship: The Haifa Study of Early Child Care. *Child Development, 73,* 1166–1186.

Zachrisson, H. D., Owen, M. T., Nordahl, K. B., Ribeiro, L., & Dearing, E. (2020). Too early for early education?: Effects on parenting for mothers and fathers. *Journal of Marriage and Family.* [Epub ahead of print]

CHAPTER 43

Attachment and Early Childhood Education Systems in the United States

Bridget K. Hamre
Amanda P. Williford

Most young children in the United States spend significant time in early childhood education (ECE) settings before the age of 5. Children's experiences in these settings influence the development of early social-emotional, self-regulatory, and cognitive skills that are foundational to long-term success. Although young children's experiences within their families have larger impacts on development and learning (Parcel & Bixby, 2016), ECE settings are of particular interest because they represent a system that can be influenced more readily by policy. Attachment theory and research have powerfully influenced ECE systems' policies and practices. In this chapter, we briefly review the research at the intersection of attachment and ECE systems and discuss several key opportunities and challenges in designing systems to best support children's relational development in out-of-home settings prior to kindergarten.

ECE Systems in the United States

In the United States, ECE is not a single system, but a patchwork of systems regulating out-of-home settings. Four major sectors provide ECE to young children: family child care homes, private child care centers, federally funded Early Head Start and Head Start programs, and state and community prekindergarten (PreK) programs. Although services in all four sectors aim to provide safe, reliable care for children, they often serve children from different sociodemographic backgrounds and have varying regulatory structures, revenue sources and funding levels, expectations concerning the most important "outcomes" for children and families, and approaches to defining and measuring quality. The potential for these systems to impact children's development is tremendous given the numbers of children spending substantial time in them from birth through kindergarten. In 2016, 73% of 3- to 5-year-olds and 54% of 1- to 2-year-olds spent at least 1 day a week in nonparental care, averaging between 21 and 27 hours a week (U.S. Department of Education, 2016).

Teacher–Child Relationships in ECE Settings

There is strong and consistent evidence that children's experiences in ECE settings influence development in ways that have long-term impacts. Children with closer and less conflictual relationships with their teachers have stronger social-emotional outcomes (Hamre, 2014) and demonstrate lower levels of stress measured by cortisol across the day (Hatfield & Williford, 2017). Young children's positive relationships with teachers enhance their classroom engagement and support their language and academic development, particular among children at risk due to challenges with behavioral regulation (Williford, Whittaker, Vitiello, & Downer, 2013).

Attachment theory has informed the conceptualization of high-quality teacher–child relationships (Williford, Carter, & Pianta, 2016). High-quality teacher–child relationships are defined in terms of the warmth, sensitivity, and support for autonomy that a teacher provides to children in his or her classroom—this parallels the attachment concept of a secure base. The level of security achieved through the child–parent bond is theorized to directly influence the child's ability to successfully interact in and navigate new ECE environments (Williford et al., 2016).

Most young children in the United States experience warm supportive relationships with teachers and caregivers. In a study of 3,062 preschool children, Howes and Ritchie (1999) found that 65% of children were in secure or "near-secure" relationships with their teachers as measured via independent observations using the Attachment Q-set. Warm and supportive teacher–child relationships provide students with the emotional security necessary to engage in learning activities and develop the full range of skills needed to be successful in school—academic, behavioral, emotional, and social (Pianta, 1999). A strong teacher–child relationship is particularly salient for students who experience the classroom setting as challenging (Baker, Grant, & Morlock, 2008). Unfortunately, the very children most likely to benefit from strong and positive relationships with teachers are often least likely to have those types of relationships. For example, children who display externalizing behaviors in the classroom are at risk for experiencing negative interactions with teachers and are described by teachers as having more conflict and less closeness with them (Hamre, 2014).

ECE Systems Policy and Practices That Support Positive Teacher–Child Relationships

How might we design ECE settings that are most likely to support the development of positive relationships among teachers and children? Teacher–child relationships are established and maintained through daily reciprocal interactions that provide information to both the teacher and the child (Hamre, 2014). Consistent with attachment theory, the daily relational interactions between a teacher and child contribute to the creation of the child's internal working model, or schema, of the relationship that informs expectations and guides subsequent perceptions by both the teacher and the child (Pianta, 1999). Among these daily exchanges, *how* the teacher and child interact with each other is viewed as the main source of information used to build their relationship. A teacher's sensitivity and responsiveness to a child's needs, consistency of availability, tone of voice, timing of responsiveness, and level of acceptance and emotional warmth conveyed are critical to the formation of positive teacher–child relationships. When children consistently experience these types of relationships in classrooms, they learn to "see" teachers as a secure base for engaging in other classrooms tasks such as peer play and learning activities. Children's feelings of trust in their teachers promote their exploration in the classroom. In moments of stress (e.g., frustration with a task, difficult interactions with peers) children rely on the secure base of their teacher to navigate the demands of the classroom. Two recent studies provide empirical support for using an attachment framework to conceptualize the ECE classroom: 3- and 4-year-old children's representation of their relationship with their teachers, assessed through children's narratives, moderated the link between observed teacher–child interactions and their classroom task engagement such that children with more emotionally negative and less emotionally positive representations were more dependent on positive interactions with their teachers to remain oriented to tasks (Wolcott, Williford, & Hartz-Mandell, 2019). Furthermore, the quality of teacher–child dyadic interactions was directly linked with teacher-reported task engagement, and indirectly linked, through child security, with observed task engagement (Alamos & Williford, 2020).

The challenge, then, is to create policies and practices that improve children's daily interactions with teachers in ECE settings to improve the nature and quality of teacher–child relationships. We suggest two potential pathways: Quality Rating and Improvement Systems (QRISs) and the use of evidence-based curricula and professional development models. We briefly review the evidence for each approach and discuss some of the challenges inherent in scaling the impacts of these policies and practices.

Quality Rating and Improvement Systems

QRISs assess, report, and improve the level of quality in an ECE system across ages and sectors, usually at the state level, and are one of the primary regulatory mechanisms for ECE quality in the United States. Most states have a QRIS that can be voluntary, although an increasing number are being mandated for programs that accept public funding or that are licensed, expanding their influence on many of the settings where young children spend time out of the home. Although each state's QRIS is unique, most rate programs on some type of scale (e.g., a five-star system) and commonly assess programs in areas such as staff qualifications and training, curriculum, family engagement, environment, teacher–child interactions, and use of assessments. Most include observational measures of classroom quality, providing an opportunity to directly measure and improve the nature of children's daily interactions with teachers.

One observational measure used in over half of the QRISs across states was developed in large part based on attachment theory—providing a direct example of the way developmental research can influence policy and practice at large scale. The Classroom Assessment Scoring System (CLASS; Pianta, La Paro, & Hamre, 2008), measures the quality of teacher–child interactions across three broad domains—emotional support, classroom organization, and instructional support. There is substantial conceptual and empirical overlap among the domain scores, indicating an underlying emphasis on a teacher's ability to effectively respond to students through warm, sensitive, and contingent interactions across domains. The emotional support domain is most relevant to the current discussion. Classrooms scoring high on emotional support have teacher–child interactions characterized by high levels of warmth and responsiveness—the same elements demonstrated to support positive student–teacher relationships. Numerous studies directly link children's experiences of emotional support, as measured by CLASS, and the development of more positive and less conflictual relationships among teachers and children (Hamre, 2014).

By using a developmentally informed measure such as the CLASS in a state or federal policy system, policymakers can support changes in teaching practice in ways that are most likely to support positive child outcomes. Work using CLASS in Louisiana provides a compelling case for the potential impact of this type of ECE policy reform. In 2014, Louisiana began rolling out a universal QRIS that uses the CLASS as the primary measure of quality. Recent data suggest notable improvements in the quality of emotional support children experience in ECE settings across the state, as well as evidence that children in center-based child care, who typically experience lower quality than children in Head Start or state PreK programs, are seeing the most dramatic increases (Bassok, Magouirk, & Markowitz, 2020). These findings are notable given the scale of the work, with over 15,000 CLASS observations occurring in infant, toddler, and preschool classrooms across the state each year. Early results demonstrate significant associations between quality, as rated by the CLASS in the Louisiana system, and children's self-regulatory and early learning outcomes (Vitiello, Bassok, Hamre, Player, & Williford, 2018) and the value of aligning accountability policies such as QRISs to developmental theory and research.

Evidence-Based Curricula and Professional Development

Another pathway for ECE systems to enhance the quality of teacher–child relationships is through scaling evidence-based curricula and interventions targeted to improve teacher–child interactions. A recent meta-analysis of interventions that included educators in center and home-based child care as well as state-funded preschool showed positive effects at the classroom, educator, and child levels (Werner, Linting, Vermeer, & van IJzendoorn, 2016). The largest effects were improvements in teacher–child interaction skills, followed by classroom quality and more modest improvements in children's social-emotional behavior. A number of interventions demonstrated improvement in the quality of teacher–child relationships, including those focused on the teacher–child dyad, such as Banking Time (Williford et al., 2017) and Playing-2-gether (Vancraeyveldt, Verschueren, Van Craeyevelt, Wouters, & Colpin, 2015), teacher coaching models such as MyTeaching Partner (Pianta, Mashburn, Downer, Hamre, & Justice, 2008), parent engagement models such as Getting Ready (Sheridan et al., 2019), and universal social-emotional curricula such as PATHS (Greenberg, Domitrovich, Karabay, Tuncdemir, & Gest, 2017). The extent to which these interventions and curricula explicitly use attachment theory in their theory of change varies. However, consistent with attachment theory, these interventions build from an understanding that for young children, sensitive and responsive interactions support children's autonomy, help children feel secure in the classroom, allow them to take learning risks, and thus stimulate their social-emotional and academic learning.

Many of these intervention approaches could be scaled through existing policies that require ECE programs to use evidence-based curricula and teachers to complete systematic professional development activities for accreditation or licensing. Unfortunately, the majority of ECE classrooms do not use evidence-based curricula and few teachers have access to high-quality professional development (Hamre, Partee, & Mulcahy, 2017). To date, few of the professional development models that have been tested in smaller, university-run randomized controlled trials have been tested when delivered in scaled-up implementations.

Challenges in Supporting Positive Relationships in ECE Settings

There are significant challenges to policy efforts designed to change the nature of children's experiences in ECE settings. Most notably, the ECE workforce is characterized by low pay, highly variable educational requirements, and high workplace stress (National Research Council, 2015). Teachers feeling stressed and depressed report more conflictual relationships with children, which can, in turn, increase stress and burnout (Gagnon, Huelsman, Kidder-Ashley, & Lewis, 2019). Better supporting ECE teachers' own well-being and economic security will play a crucial role in policy solutions designed to support children's relational functioning in these settings.

Despite the reach of policy reforms such as those in Louisiana, the ECE system in the United States is quite fragmented, leaving many of most vulnerable children in settings not touched by current policies, such as kith and kin and family child care. Although research demonstrates that children in family child care settings do experience strong emotional bonds with their caregivers, the fragmentation of the system itself limits the ways policy can positively impact all children's experiences. There is a great need for research on how to support caregivers in these less formal settings (Garner, Parker, & Prigmore, 2019).

The Future of Attachment and ECE Settings

Federal, state, and local policymakers are focused as never before on ECE. Increased funding across sectors will result in greater ECE access, but most importantly, there is the potential to ensure that more young children experience high-quality programs. The research reviewed demonstrates the importance of aligning the definition of "quality" with developmental research on the components of children's daily experiences in classrooms that best support positive relationships with teachers. QRISs and other ECE policies are potential levers to guarantee that curricula and professional development are used to promote contingent and sensitive teacher–child interactions for all children. Given increased pressure to support early academic development for young children, and evidence of the "push down" of highly academic instruction into kindergarten, it will be important to keep a focus on the critical role of early teacher–child relationships as these policies evolve in coming years.

REFERENCES

Alamos, P., & Williford, A. P. (2020). Teacher–child emotion talk in preschool children displaying elevated externalizing behaviors. *Journal of Applied Developmental Psychology, 67,* 101–107.

Baker, J. A., Grant, S., & Morlock, L. (2008). The teacher–student relationship as a developmental context for children with internalizing or externalizing behavior problems. *School Psychology Quarterly, 23*(1), 3–15.

Bassok, D., Magouirk, P., & Markowitz, A. (2020). Systemwide changes in the quality of early childhood education: Trends in Louisiana from 2015–16 to 2018–19. Retrieved from *https://curry.virginia.edu/sites/default/files/uploads/ epw/Systemwide%20Changes%20in%20the%20Quality%20of%20Early%20 Childhood%20Education_Final.pdf.*

Gagnon, S. G., Huelsman, T. J., Kidder-Ashley, P., & Lewis, A. (2019). Preschool student–teacher relationships and teaching stress. *Early Childhood Education Journal, 47*(2), 217–225.

Garner, P. W., Parker, T. S., & Prigmore, S. B. (2019). Caregivers' emotional competence and behavioral responsiveness as correlates of early childcare workers' relationships with children in their care. *Infant Mental Health Journal, 40*(4), 496–512.

Greenberg, M., Domitrovich, C., Karabay, S. O., Tuncdemir, A., & Gest, S. (2017). Focusing on teacher–children relationship perception and children's social emotional behaviors—the PATHS preschool program. *International Journal of Educational Research Review, 3*(1), 8–20.

Hamre, B. K. (2014). Teachers' daily interactions with children: An essential ingredient of effective early childhood programs. *Child Development Perspectives, 8,* 223–230.

Hamre, B. K., Partee, A., & Mulcahy, C. (2017). Enhancing the impact of professional development in the context of preschool expansion. *AERA Open, 3*(4), 2332858417733686.

Hatfield, B. E., & Williford, A. P. (2017). Cortisol patterns for young children displaying disruptive behavior: Links to a teacher–child, relationship-focused intervention. *Prevention Science, 18,* 40–49.

Howes, C., & Ritchie, S. (1999). Attachment organizations in children with difficult life circumstances. *Development and Psychopathology, 11,* 251–268.

National Research Council. (2015). Transforming the workforce for children birth through age 8: A unifying foundation. Retrieved from *www.fcd-us.org/ transforming-workforce-children-birth-age-eight-unifying-foundation.*

Parcel, T. L., & Bixby, M. S. (2016). The ties that bind: Social capital, families, and children's well-being. *Child Development Perspectives, 10*(2), 87–92.

Pianta, R. C. (1999). *Enhancing relationships between children and teachers.* Washington, DC: American Psychological Association.

Pianta, R. C., La Paro, K., & Hamre, B. K. (2008). *Classroom Assessment Scoring System (CLASS)*. Baltimore: Brookes.

Pianta, R. C., Mashburn, A. J., Downer, J. T., Hamre, B. K., & Justice, L. (2008). Effects of web-mediated professional development resources on teacher–child interactions in pre-kindergarten classrooms. *Early Childhood Research Quarterly, 23*(4), 431–451.

Sheridan, S. M., Knoche, L. L., Boise, C. E., Moen, A. L., Lester, H., Edwards, C. P., . . . Cheng, K. (2019). Supporting preschool children with developmental concerns: Effects of the Getting Ready intervention on school-based social competencies and relationships. *Early Childhood Research Quarterly, 48,* 303–316.

U.S. Department of Education. (2016). National Center for Education Statistics, Early Childhood Program Participation Survey of the 2016 National Household Education Surveys program. Retrieved from *https://nces.ed.gov/pubs2017/2017101REV.pdf.*

Vancraeyveldt, C., Verschueren, K., Van Craeyevelt, S., Wouters, S., & Colpin, H. (2015). Teacher-reported effects of the Playing-2-gether intervention on child externalizing problem behavior. *Educational Psychology, 35,* 466–483.

Vitiello, V. E., Bassok, D., Hamre, B. K., Player, D., & Williford, A. P. (2018). Measuring the quality of teacher–child interactions at scale: Comparing research-based and state observation approaches. *Early Childhood Research Quarterly, 44,* 161–169.

Werner, C. D., Linting, M., Vermeer, H. J., & van IJzendoorn, M. H. (2016). Do intervention programs in child care promote the quality of caregiver–child interactions?: A meta-analysis of randomized controlled trials. *Prevention Science, 17*(2), 259–273.

Williford, A. P., Carter, L. M., & Pianta, R. C. (2016). Attachment and school readiness. In J. Cassidy & P. R. Shaver (Eds.), *Handbook of attachment: Theory, research, and clinical applications* (3rd ed., pp. 966–982). New York: Guilford Press.

Williford, A. P., LoCasale-Crouch, J., Whittaker, J. V., DeCoster, J., Hartz, K. A., Carter, L. M., . . . Hatfield, B. E. (2017). Changing teacher–child dyadic interactions to improve preschool children's externalizing behaviors. *Child Development, 88*(5), 1544–1553.

Williford, A. P., Whittaker, J. V., Vitiello, V. E., & Downer, J. T. (2013). Children's engagement within the preschool classroom and their development of self-regulation. *Early Education and Development, 24,* 162–187.

Wolcott, C. S., Williford, A. P., & Hartz-Mandell, K. (2019). The validity of narratives for understanding children's perceptions of the teacher–child relationship for preschoolers who display elevated disruptive behaviors. *Early Education and Development, 30*(7), 887–912.

CHAPTER 44

An Attachment Theory Approach to Parental Separation, Divorce, and Child Custody

Michael E. Lamb

Since its derivation and articulation by John Bowlby and his colleagues, such as Mary Ainsworth and the Robinsons, in the three decades after the end of World War II, attachment theory has come to dominate scholarly understanding of close relationships, especially those between parents and children. The relevant literature is now voluminous and the goal of this chapter is to highlight, mostly by reference to review articles and other secondary sources, the many ways in which an appreciation of attachment theory can usefully highlight and elucidate the key issues that arise when parents separate and decisions must be made about the care of their children.

Attachment to Mothers and Fathers

According to attachment theory, infants progressively learn to discriminate among adult caregivers, develop preferences, and gradually develop emotional attachments to those who care for them (Bowlby, 1969). From the very beginning, fathers are as competent to care for their infants as mothers are; when they emerge, gender differences in parental sensitivity appear attributable to differences in the amount of practical experience (Branger, Emmen, Woudstra, Alink, & Mesman, 2019; Lamb, 2002; Parke, 2013). At around 7 or 8 months of age, attachments become increasingly apparent as infants begin to protest when separated and preferentially seek specific caregivers by whom they are most easily soothed. Most infants in two-parent families form attachments to both parents at this age, even though fathers typically spend less time with their infants than mothers do (for reviews, see Lamb, 2002; Lamb & Lewis, 2015). However, most infants come to prefer the parents who take primary responsibility for their care (typically mothers) and those preferred relationships tend to have a greater impact on subsequent behavior and development, albeit not clearly in direct proportion to the relative levels of involvement. Furthermore, relationships with both parents remain psychologically important even when there are disparities in the two parents' levels of participation in child care.

Individual differences in responsiveness (but not differences in levels of involvement) affect the quality or security of the attachment relationships that form, and the quality of both mother–child and father–child interaction remain the most reliable predictors of individual differences in later psychosocial adjustment (Lamb & Lewis, 2015). Preferences for primary caregivers diminish with age and often disappear by 18 months of age (Lamb, 2002). Although toddlers may resist transitions between parents in the second year, they generally comfort quite quickly once the transition is accomplished. This is particularly likely when both parents continue to have the opportunity to engage in normal parenting activities (feeding, playing, soothing, putting to bed, etc.).

Infants and toddlers need regular interaction with their "attachment figures" in order to foster, maintain, and strengthen their relationships with them. This means that young children need to interact with both parents in a variety of contexts (feeding, playing, diapering, soothing, reading, putting to bed, etc.) to ensure that the relationships are consolidated and strengthened. In the absence of such opportunities for regular interaction across a broad range of contexts, infant–parent relationships may weaken. Extended separations from parents with whom children have formed meaningful attachments are thus undesirable because they unduly stress developing attachment relationships, which can gradually erode. The increased cognitive and language abilities of 2- to 3-year-olds enable them to tolerate somewhat longer separations but their very primitive sense of time limits their ability to understand and cope with lengthy separations (Kelly & Lamb, 2000).

Relationships with parents continue to play a crucial role in shaping children's development beyond toddlerhood. Not surprisingly, therefore, children appear better adjusted when they enjoy warm positive relationships with two actively involved parents (Lamb, 2012). Children are better off with insecure attachments than without attachment relationships, however, because these enduring ties play essential formative roles in later social and emotional functioning (Bowlby, 1973). There is also a substantial literature documenting the adverse effects of disrupted parent–child relationships on children's adjustment (e.g., Amato & Dorius, 2010; Clarke-Stewart & Brentano, 2006). There is a clear relation between age of separation and later attachment quality in adolescents such that the "weakest" attachments to nonresident parents are reported by those whose parents separated in the first 5 years of their lives (e.g., Woodward, Ferguson, & Belsky, 2000).

When Parents Separate

On average, children benefit from being raised in two-parent families rather than separated, divorced, or never-married single-parent households (e.g., Amato & Dorius, 2010; Clarke-Stewart & Brentano, 2006; Lamb, 2016). However, there is considerable variability within groups, and the differences between groups—with respect to psychosocial adjustment; behavior and achievement at school; educational attainment; employment trajectories; income generation; involvement in antisocial, delinquent, or criminal behavior; and the ability to establish and maintain intimate relationships—are relatively small (Lamb, 2016). In fact, the majority of children with separated parents enjoy average or better-than-average social and emotional adjustment as young adults.

Approximately 20–25% of children have adjustment problems post-separation, however, compared to 12% in two-parent families. Such individual differences in outcomes force us to identify more precisely the ways in which parental separation may affect children's lives. Five interrelated factors appear to be especially significant (Lamb, 2016):

1. Typically, single parenthood is associated with a variety of social and financial stresses with which custodial parents must cope, and economic stresses or poverty appear to account (statistically speaking) for many effects of single parenthood.

2. Because single parents need to work more extensively outside the home than partnered parents do, parents spend less time with children in single-parent families and the levels of supervision and guidance are lower and less reliable.

3. Conflict between the parents commonly precedes, emerges, or increases during separation and divorce processes, and often continues for some time beyond them. Interparental conflict is an important correlate of children's psychosocial maladjustment, just as partner harmony, its conceptual inverse, appears to be a reliable correlate of positive adjustment. Indeed, some of the effects of separation can be viewed as the effects of preseparation conflict and violence (Booth & Amato, 2001; Kelly, 2000).

4. As noted earlier, the quality and type of parenting are important influences on the postseparation adjustment of children and adolescents. Many parents are preoccupied, stressed, emotionally labile, angry, and depressed around and after separation, and their "diminished parenting" includes less positive involvement and affection as well as more coercive and harsh discipline.

5. Parental separation also commonly disrupts one of the child's most important and enduring relationships, that with the father, although the bivariate associations between father absence and children's adjustment are much weaker than one might expect (Amato & Gilbreth, 1999).

However, children's well-being is significantly enhanced when their relationships with nonresident fathers are positive, when nonresident fathers engage in active parenting, and when contact with nonresident fathers is frequent. By contrast, reduced levels of paternal involvement are associated with declines in the salience and closeness of child–father relationships and commensurate increases in the probability of psychological distress and maladjustment. Numerous studies have shown that shared parenting arrangements are associated with better child adjustment than single-parent arrangements postseparation (Nielsen, 2018). As in two-parent families, in other words, the quality of continued relationships with both parents is crucial. The better (richer, deeper, and more secure) the parent–child relationships, the better the children's adjustment, whether or not the parents live together.

Overall, then, a number of factors help account for individual differences in the effects of parental separation. However, the ability to maintain meaningful relationships with both parents appears to be of central importance, both in its own right and as a correlate of some of the other factors.

How to Minimize the Adverse Effects of Parental Separation?

Writing on behalf of 18 experts on the effects of divorce and contrasting parenting plans, Lamb, Sternberg, and Thompson (1997) observed two and a half decades ago that

> to maintain high-quality relationships with their children, parents need to have sufficiently extensive and regular interactions with them, but the amount of time involved is usually less important than the quality of the interaction that it fosters. Time distribution arrangements that ensure the involvement of both parents in important aspects of their children's everyday lives and routines . . . are likely to keep nonresidential parents playing

psychologically important and central roles in the lives of their children. (p. 400)

Consistent with this view, studies of children's and young adults' perceptions of their postdivorce living arrangements indicate that the majority express strong wishes and longing for more time with their fathers, a desire for more closeness, and favorable views of shared physical custody as their preferred schedule (Braver, Ellman, Votruba, & Fabricius, 2011; Fabricius, 2003; Fabricius, Sokol, Diaz, & Braver, 2012).

Embracing a view of relationships rooted in attachment theory, my colleagues and I (Lamb, 2016; Lamb et al., 1997) have argued that it is important for parents to be integral parts of their children's lives in order to ensure the maintenance of relationships over time. This remains especially important as children get older and greater portions of their time are occupied outside the family by virtue of friendships, extracurricular activities, and education/training. At all ages, it is important for parents to know teachers and friends, what is happening at school or preschool, how relationships with peers are going, what other activities are important or meaningful to children, and about daily ups and downs in their children's emotional lives. It is hard to do this without regular and extensive firsthand involvement with their children in a variety of contexts.

The evening and overnight periods (as with extended days that include naptimes) with nonresidential parents are especially important psychologically for infants, toddlers, and young children. They provide opportunities for crucial social interactions and nurturing activities, including bathing, soothing hurts and anxieties, bedtime rituals, comforting in the middle of the night, and the reassurance and security of snuggling in the morning that brief visits cannot provide. According to attachment theory, these everyday activities promote and maintain trust and confidence in the parents, while deepening and strengthening child–parent attachments, and thus they need to be encouraged when decisions about nonresidential parental access and contact are made (Lamb, 2016; Lamb et al., 1997).

Such recommendations were initially controversial. Neo-psychoanalysts and clinicians who clung to an outdated view of attachment that held that infants formed a single primary relationship, rather than relationships with both parents, argued that infants and young children should not be separated for long, and certainly not overnight, from their primary attachment figures. In fact, the evidence shows that most infants are attached to both of their parents, and that when this is the case, they benefit from opportunities to spend time, including overnights, with both parents, for the reasons explained above (Lamb, 2016; Warshak, 2014). As Warshak (2014) pointed out, the prohibition of overnight visitation has been justified by prejudices and beliefs rather than by empirical evidence. When both parents have established significant attachments and both have been actively involved in the child's care, overnight visits consolidate attachments and promote child adjustment. Not surprisingly, therefore, the studies often cited in opposition to overnights for young children do not actually show what has been claimed, as explained in a recent review of all the studies of the impacts of overnight "visits" on infant– and toddler–parent attachments (Lamb, 2018).

To minimize the deleterious impact of extended separations from either parent in early childhood, attachment theory tells us there should be more frequent transitions than would perhaps be desirable with older children to ensure the continuity of both relationships and to promote the children's security and comfort (Lamb, 2016; Lamb et al., 1997). Interestingly, psychologists have long recognized the need to minimize the length of separations from attachment figures when devising parenting plans for young children, but they have typically focused only on separations from mothers, thereby revealing their presumption that young children are not meaningfully attached to their fathers, or that paternal involvement is a peripheral influence. It is little wonder that such arrangements as weekly visits for a few hours or every other shortened weekend lead to attenuation of the relationships between nonresident parents and their children (Lamb, 2016; Lamb et al., 1997).

Of course, the quality of the relationships between nonresidential parents and their children is also crucial when determining whether to sever or promote relationships between separated parents and their children. Sadly, there are many families in which nonresident fathers and children have sufficiently poor relationships—perhaps because of the fathers' psychopathology, substance or alcohol abuse, or violent abusive behavior—that "maintenance" of interaction or involvement may not be of net benefit to the children. The number of relationships like this is difficult to estimate; research suggests that they may comprise around 20% of separating families (Cashmore et al., 2010; Johnston & Roseby, 1997; Maccoby & Mnookin, 1992). This suggests that more than three-quarters of the children experiencing their parents' separation could benefit from having and maintaining relationships with both of their parents.

Conclusion

Research on early social development and on the correlates of parental separation have together yielded a clearer understanding of the ways in which parental separation and subsequent parenting patterns can affect children's well-being. Crucially, most children benefit from supportive relationships with both of their parents, whether or not those parents live together. However, a minority of children do not have supportive relationships with one or both parents, so restrictions on the amount of contact are advisable. For perhaps 75% of separating families, post-separation parenting plans that encourage regular participation by two psychologically healthy parents in as broad as possible an array of social contexts can foster committed and meaningful child–parent attachment relationships.

REFERENCES

Amato, P. R., & Dorius, C. (2010). Fathers, children, and divorce. In M. E. Lamb (Ed.), *The role of the father in child development* (5th ed., pp. 177–200). Hoboken, NJ: Wiley.

Amato, P. R., & Gilbreth, J. G. (1999). Non-resident fathers and children's well-being: A meta-analysis. *Journal of Marriage and the Family, 61,* 557–573.

Booth, A., & Amato, P. R. (2001). Parental predivorce relations and offspring postdivorce well-being. *Journal of Marriage and the Family, 63,* 197–212.

Bowlby, J. (1969). *Attachment and loss: Vol. 1. Attachment.* New York: Basic Books.

Bowlby, J. (1973). *Attachment and loss: Vol. 2. Separation.* New York: Basic Books.

Branger, M. C. E., Emmen, R. A. G., Woudstra, M. J., Alink, L. R. A., & Mesman, J. (2019). Context matters: Maternal and paternal sensitivity to infants in four settings. *Journal of Family Psychology, 33*(7), 851–856.

Braver, S. L., Ellman, I., Votruba, A., & Fabricius, W. V. (2011). Lay judgments about child custody after divorce. *Psychology, Public Policy and Law, 17,* 212–240.

Cashmore, J., Parkinson, P., Weston, R., Patulny, R., Redmond, G., Qu, L., & Katz, I. (2010). *Shared care parenting arrangements since the 2006 Family Law Reforms: Report to the Australian Government Attorney-General's Department.* Sydney, Australia: University of New South Wales Social Policy Research Centre.

Clarke-Stewart, K. A., & Brentano, C. (2006). *Divorce: Causes and consequences.* New Haven, CT: Yale University Press.

Fabricius, W. V. (2003). Listening to children of divorce: New findings on living arrangements, college support and relocation that rebut Wallerstein, Lewis and Blakeslee (2000). *Family Relations, 52,* 385–396.

Fabricius, W. V., Sokol, K. R., Diaz, P., & Braver, S. L. (2012). Parenting time, parent conflict, parent–child relationships, and children's physical health. In K. Kuehnle & L. Drozd (Eds.), *Parenting plan evaluations: Applied research for the family court* (pp. 188–213). New York: Oxford University Press.

Johnston, J. R., & Roseby, V. (1997). *In the name of the child: A developmental approach to understanding and helping children of conflict and violent divorce.* New York: Free Press.

Kelly, J. B. (2000). Children's adjustment in conflicted marriage and divorce: A decade review of research. *Journal of the American Academy of Child Psychiatry, 39,* 963–973.

Kelly, J. B., & Lamb, M. E. (2000). Using child development research to make appropriate custody and access decisions for young children. *Family and Conciliation Courts Review, 38,* 297–311.

Lamb, M. E. (2002). Infant–father attachments and their impact on child development. In C. S. Tamis-LeMonda & N. Cabrera (Eds.), *Handbook of father involvement: Multidisciplinary perspectives* (pp. 93–117). Mahwah, NJ: Erlbaum.

Lamb, M. E. (2012). Mothers, fathers, families, and circumstances: Factors affecting children's adjustment. *Applied Developmental Science, 16,* 98–111.

Lamb, M. E. (2016). Critical analysis of research on parenting plans and children's well-being. In L. Drozd, M. Saini, & N. Olesen (Eds.), *Parenting plan evaluations: Applied research for family court* (2nd ed., pp. 170–202). New York: Oxford University Press.

Lamb, M. E. (2018). Does shared parenting by separated parents affect the adjustment of young children? *Journal of Child Custody, 15,* 16–25.

Lamb, M. E., & Lewis, C. (2015). The role of parent–child relationships in child development. In M. H. Bornstein & M. E. Lamb (Eds.), *Developmental science: An advanced textbook* (7th ed., pp. 535–586). New York: Psychology Press.

Lamb, M. E., Sternberg, K. J., & Thompson, R. A. (1997). The effects of divorce and custody arrangements on children's behavior, development, and adjustment. *Family and Conciliation Courts Review, 35,* 393–404.

Maccoby, E. E., & Mnookin, R. H. (1992). *Dividing the child: Social and legal dilemmas of custody.* Cambridge, MA: Harvard University Press.

Nielsen, L. (2018). Joint versus sole physical custody: Children's outcomes independent of parent–child relationships, income, and conflict in 60 studies. *Journal of Divorce and Remarriage, 59,* 247–281.

Parke, R. (2013). *Future families.* Hoboken, NJ: Wiley.

Warshak, R. A. (2014). Social science and parenting plans for young children: A consensus report. *Psychology, Public Policy, and Law, 20,* 46–67.

Woodward, L., Ferguson, D. M., & Belsky, J. (2000). Timing of parental separation and attachment to parents in adolescence: Results of a prospective study from birth to age 16. *Journal of Marriage and the Family, 62,* 162–174.

CHAPTER 45

Child Protective Systems

Jody Todd Manly
Anna Smith
Sheree L. Toth
Dante Cicchetti

Attachment and Child Maltreatment

Research findings indicate that maltreated children are more likely to have insecure attachments than nonmaltreated children and are at particular risk for developing disorganized attachments, which may result from inconsistent and frightening interactions with their parents (Cyr, Euser, Bakermans-Kranenburg, & van IJzendoorn, 2010). Maltreated children with disorganized attachments may lack a coherent attachment strategy because their parents are a source of both fear and protection (Cicchetti & Toth, 2016). In some samples, 80–90% of maltreated children were classified with a disorganized attachment pattern, compared with 15% of children in normative samples (Cicchetti & Toth, 2016; van IJzendoorn, Schuengel, & Bakermans-Kranenburg, 1999). Although genetic variations have been linked to insecure attachment, Cicchetti, Rogosch, and Toth (2011) found that child abuse and neglect may overpower genetic risk, as genetic variation did not predict disorganized attachment in a maltreated sample, suggesting that maltreatment may be a particularly salient risk factor for developing disorganized attachments. Translational research on attachment in maltreated children is especially relevant for Child Protective Services (CPS), family court, and child welfare systems. This chapter briefly reviews implications of attachment research for these systems to inform placement and intervention decisions, ideally to support families in preventing child abuse and neglect, or, alternately, to improve relationships with biological parents and alternative caregivers. Policy implications and future directions are discussed.

Placement in out-of-home care is likely to further disrupt attachment relationships. Efforts are often made to maintain parent–child relationships through visitation when possible, but visitation can increase the likelihood of loyalty conflicts in children's relationships with biological and new caregivers, and repeated separations from both caregivers may further strain the child's attachment representations (Mennen & O'Keefe, 2005; see also Zeanah & Dozier, Chapter 46, this volume). Maltreated children lacking a coherent attachment strategy may have difficulty forming close relationships with new caregivers because strategies that were somewhat functional within the context of their relationship with their maltreating parent may no longer be adaptive with an alternative caregiver (Mennen & O'Keefe, 2005). Although children can form secure attachments with new caregivers regardless of their attachment status with their biological parent, the new caregiver's own attachment representations and expectations may lead them to miss cues from the child or incorrectly interpret the child's actions as rejection, increasing the likelihood of an insecure attachment with the new caregiver (Lawler, Shaver, & Goodman, 2011).

Relevance of Attachment to CPS and Family Court

Because maltreated children are at higher risk for insecure, especially disorganized, attachments with their biological parents (Cicchetti & Toth, 2016), they need particular attention to their interpersonal development in service and placement decisions. Although ensuring safety in their home environments is critical, removal from biological parents and placement with alternative caregivers can further disrupt vulnerable relationships and pose challenges for children who are then expected to form relationships with unfamiliar caregivers while adjusting to new routines, rules, and expectations. Those with decision-making authority must be fully informed regarding the implications of both the impact of trauma and the need for relationship support for these children's functioning when making risk-benefit analyses that affect children's and families' futures, as these decisions can have lifelong consequences for children's development (Mennen & O'Keefe, 2005).

Some training and information on attachment is available to professionals in the CPS and family court systems. For example, the National Council of Juvenile and Family Court Judges has hosted attachment training for judges. CPS workers can access workshops and resources through organizations such as the U.S. Children's Bureau. However, scattered workshops and tip sheets do not create widespread understanding or uptake of attachment theory and research.

More specifically, even for those who understand attachment, evaluating attachment relationships for individual children requires in-depth training in observation with sophisticated understanding of subtle cues in children's interpersonal development and time for comprehensive assessment of attachment that is not readily available in court and CPS settings. Attachment classifications are not easily ascertained, may vary for specific relationships, and may change over time. Caution should be exercised with regard to use of attachment information as well because presence of a disorganized attachment with a biological parent is not a diagnostic indicator of the presence of maltreatment, and assessment procedures developed for group differences in research contexts should not be extrapolated to make clinical decisions (Granqvist et al., 2017). Principles of equifinality in developmental psychopathology underscore that there may be multiple pathways through which a child develops a disorganized attachment classification, including socioeconomic risk factors, parental psychopathology, substance abuse, and combined genetic and environmental variables (Cyr et al., 2010; Granqvist et al., 2017). Partnerships between CPS and court teams with therapists knowledgeable in attachment, however, can enhance decision-making processes and service delivery.

Intervention Approaches with Families Connected to the Child Welfare System

A number of evidence-based attachment theory-informed interventions are available that can prevent maltreatment occurrence and/or support healing from trauma after abuse and neglect have occurred (Facompré, Bernard, & Waters, 2018; Zeanah & Dozier, Chapter 46, this volume). To facilitate positive outcomes, interventions should wrap services around children and families and nurture parent–child relationships within a supportive ecological context that promotes healthy interactions and builds trust and healing. Within birth families, services that support healthy parent–child relationships and reduce risks associated with attachment disruption may promote secure attachment relationships and prevent maltreatment and trauma. Such risks include multiple and cumulative socioeconomic and demographic characteristics such as poverty, single parenthood, racism and discrimination, exposure to violence, parental stress or psychopathology leading to withdrawal from parent–child interactions, chaotic home environments, and parental trauma and loss (Cyr et al., 2010). Families who are involved with CPS whose children remain home can benefit from support of parent–child relationships and remediation of factors that led to maltreatment. Beyond teaching parenting skills, services should address intergenerational patterns of trauma and conflictual relationships and resulting psychopathology to support secure attachment development (Mennen & O'Keefe, 2005). If children are placed with alternative caregivers, such as foster parents, kinship caregivers, or other nonrelative caregivers, then therapeutic services can be implemented to improve parent–child relationships and promote healing, not only from maltreatment, but also from disruptions in the relationships caused by separation.

When placement with alternative caregivers occurs, these adults can play important roles in promoting healing from trauma and can serve as alternative attachment figures to provide corrective emotional experiences and nurturing care. Foster parents with histories of secure states of mind with respect to attachment and adequate resources and supports are best positioned to promote secure attachment relationships with the children in their care (Dozier, Stovall, Albus, & Bates, 2001). Alternative caregivers need training in attachment and trauma as well as support for managing challenging behaviors and interpersonal difficulties in caring for traumatized children who have experienced relationship disruption (Lawler et al., 2011). Without an understanding of attachment and the impact that trauma and disrupted relationships can have on behavioral and emotional dysregulation, alternative caregivers are likely to misunderstand children's behavior and misattribute signs of insecure attachment as rejection or inability to form positive relationships (Dozier et al., 2001). With services designed to support alternative caregivers, placements are more likely to be stabilized and children's outcomes are more likely to improve.

Evidence-Based Interventions Supporting Attachment Security for Children in Child Welfare

Although a number of intervention models have been developed and evaluated for promoting secure attachment, improving parent–child relationships, and supporting healing from trauma (see Dozier & Bernard, 2019; Lawler et al., 2011; Toth, Alto, & Warmingham, Chapter 39, this volume), not all have been evaluated with children who are involved with CPS and/or placed out of the home. A few that have been evaluated in this context warrant particular mention here. For example, Child–Parent Psychotherapy (CPP) has demonstrated efficacy at improving security of attachment in a maltreated sample (Toth, Michl-Petzing, Guild, & Lieberman, 2017). By incorporating CPP within a family court setting and providing integrated care for young maltreated children, Safe Babies Court

Teams have utilized attachment knowledge and evidence-based treatment through partnerships among CPS, early intervention, mental health, judicial, and legal systems that have improved outcomes for children in the child welfare system (Osofsky & Lieberman, 2011). The Safe Babies Court Teams integrate training on trauma and attachment, joint multidisciplinary treatment planning, coordinated case management and referrals for services, frequent hearings and case reviews, communication, and information sharing that have been shown to reduce recidivism, expedite permanency, and improve outcomes for parents and children (Osofsky & Lieberman, 2011).

A meta-analysis of parenting interventions for foster and adoptive parents found that a number of treatment models demonstrate evidence for improving parenting sensitivity, knowledge, discipline practices, and parental stress for alternative caregivers (Schoemaker et al., 2020). Although the results showed reductions in children's behavior problems, they did not demonstrate improvements in attachment security. This may reflect intervention foci (as not all are focused specifically on attachment), treatment duration, and/or outcomes assessed.

Attachment and Biobehavioral Catch-up (ABC) is noteworthy because it has been evaluated with both foster parents and children in their care and with biological parents and their children who were involved with CPS and at risk of foster placement. With the former, improvements in foster parent sensitivity have been documented, and with the latter, improvements in attachment security with biological parents have been demonstrated (Dozier & Bernard, 2019). Thus, ABC potentially can be implemented preventively to avoid out-of-home placements or after placement to improve caregiver–child relationships and child outcomes.

Policy Implications

Implementing policies that support CPS-involved children and families to improve attachment security may involve a substantial reworking of child welfare and family court systems to provide a more supportive rather than adversarial and punitive approach. Ideally, preventive strategies such as universal home visitation, access to financial and health care services, affordable child care, and other policies that support families in culturally respectful ways may reduce the number of children who experience maltreatment and other adverse events and avoid their placement in out-of-home care.

Some have argued that policies such as mandatory reporting laws that are intended to protect children may serve as disincentives for families to seek help and may therefore reduce rather than increase access to services (Raz, 2017). Other countries without mandated reporter laws focus on connecting families with services that promote prevention and treatment with a less criminalizing approach. Positive relationships between foster and biological families should be encouraged when possible, with ongoing contact occurring after placement changes to maintain positive connections among children and the important people in their lives (see Zeanah & Dozier, Chapter 46, this volume). Placement changes and disruptions should be avoided as much as possible. For any child, disruptions in placements are likely to be extremely stressful, but for young children during formative years for developing attachment relationships, they are likely to be devastating. Evidence from adoption studies documenting better outcomes with early placements suggest that decisions should be made as quickly as possible, especially for young children, to avoid missing important developmental opportunities when attachments are being formed (Mennen & O'Keefe, 2005).

While CPS and family court are planning for permanency that may include terminations of parental rights, they are simultaneously preparing for returning children to their biological parents. To support reunification, frequent visits with parents should be encouraged, with services to address healing and trauma treatment for the disruptions to the relationships that separations are likely to have caused for both children and caregivers (Mennen & O'Keefe, 2005).

When changes of placement are necessary, it is essential to explain what is happening to children in developmentally appropriate ways, with adequate time and preparation for the transition (Mennen & O'Keefe, 2005). CPS staff trained in attachment, trauma, and appropriate developmental expectations with reflective supervision and adequate secondary traumatic stress prevention resources in place will be better positioned to support children and families through child welfare processes. Alternative caregivers who are prepared for the likelihood of children's mistrust, attachment difficulties, behavior problems, and posttraumatic stress reactions will be more able to provide sensitive and nurturing care. Although CPS involvement often closes shortly after permanency goals are achieved, both biological and resource families and the children in their care are likely to need ongoing supports postreunification or adoption.

Future Directions and Recommendations

Recommendations for the future include the following:

1. Provide consistent, comprehensive training and education on attachment and trauma for all professionals who touch the lives of children in the child protective system, including judges, attorneys, CPS staff, court-appointed special advocates/guardian ad litem (CASA/GAL)

volunteers, law enforcement, domestic violence shelter staff, child care providers, educators, medical professionals, mental health providers, and the like. This training could occur as part of educational programs (e.g., law school courses) as well as ongoing professional development to help providers stay abreast of new learning in the fields of attachment, trauma, cultural sensitivity, and evidence-based intervention (Osofsky & Lieberman, 2011).

2. Continue research addressing the impact of CPS intervention and foster care on attachment development as well as the most effective preventive and treatment approaches, and disseminate this research to facilitate rapid uptake in real-world implementation.

3. Improve access to evidence-based trauma treatment for children who have experienced maltreatment, including more frequent screening for symptoms of posttraumatic stress and attachment or interpersonal difficulties.

4. Improve training and access to services for alternative caregivers that support understanding of children's attachment needs, management of emotional and behavioral dysregulation, cultural considerations, and improved sensitivity and nurturance to respond to the challenges of the children in their care, especially for children with special needs.

REFERENCES

Cicchetti, D., Rogosch, F. A., & Toth, S. L. (2011). The effects of child maltreatment and polymorphisms of the serotonin transporter and dopamine D4 receptor genes on infant attachment and intervention efficacy. *Development and Psychopathology, 23*(2), 357–372.

Cicchetti, D., & Toth, S. L. (2016). Child maltreatment and developmental psychopathology: A multilevel perspective. In D. Cicchetti (Ed.), *Developmental psychopathology: Vol. 3. Maladaptation and psychopathology* (pp. 1–55). Hoboken, NJ: Wiley.

Cyr, C., Euser, E. M., Bakermans-Kranenburg, M. J., & van IJzendoorn, M. H. (2010). Attachment security and disorganization in maltreating and high-risk families: A series of meta-analyses. *Development and Psychopathology, 22*(1), 87–108.

Dozier, M., & Bernard, K. (2019). *Coaching parents of vulnerable infants: The Attachment and Biobehavioral Catch-Up approach.* New York: Guilford Press.

Dozier, M., Stovall, K. C., Albus, K. E., & Bates, B. (2001). Attachment for infants in foster care: The role of caregiver state of mind. *Child Development, 72*(5), 1467–1477.

Facompré, C. R., Bernard, K., & Waters, T. E. A. (2018). Effectives of interventions in preventing disorganized attachment: A meta-analysis. *Development and Psychopathology, 30*(1), 1–11.

Granqvist, P., Sroufe, L. A., Dozier, M., Hesse, E., Steele, M., van IJzendoorn, M., . . . Duschinsky, R. (2017). Disorganized attachment in infancy: A review of the phenomenon and its implications for clinicians and policy-makers. *Attachment and Human Development, 19*(6), 534–558.

Lawler, M. J., Shaver, P. R., & Goodman, G. S. (2011). Toward relationship-based child welfare services. *Children and Youth Services Review, 33*(3), 473–480.

Mennen, F. E., & O'Keefe, M. (2005). Informed decisions in child welfare: The use of attachment theory. *Children and Youth Services Review, 27*(6), 577–593.

Osofsky, J. D., & Lieberman, A. F. (2011). A call for integrating a mental health perspective into systems of care for abused and neglected infants and young children. *American Psychologist, 66*(2), 120–128.

Raz, M. (2017). Unintended consequences of expanded mandatory reporting laws. *Pediatrics, 139*(2), e21063511.

Schoemaker, N. K., Wentholt, W. G. M., Goemans, A., Vermeer, H. J., Juffer, F., & Alink, L. R. A. (2020). A meta-analytic review of parenting interventions in foster care and adoption. *Development and Psychopathology, 32*(3), 1149–1172.

Toth, S. L., Michl-Petzing, L. C., Guild, D., & Lieberman, A. (2017). Child–parent psychotherapy: Theoretical bases, clinical applications, and empirical support. In H. Steele & M. Steele (Eds.), *Handbook of attachment-based interventions* (pp. 296–317). New York: Guilford Press.

van IJzendoorn, M. H., Schuengel, C., & Bakermans-Kranenburg, M. J. (1999). Disorganized attachment in early childhood: Meta-analysis of precursors, concomitants, and sequelae. *Development and Psychopathology, 11*(2), 225–250.

CHAPTER 46

Attachment and Foster Care

Charles H. Zeanah
Mary Dozier

Attachment and Maltreatment

Attachment relationships between parents and children are especially salient in the context of maltreatment. Maltreatment impacts the young child's sense of safety and security, which are at the core of the child–caregiver attachment. One major pathway to disorganized attachment is through frightening and frightened caregiver behavior that places children in the untenable situation in which the source of comfort is also the source of fear (Main & Hesse, 1990). Disorganized attachment is posited to reflect the child's inability to resolve simultaneous conflicting urges to approach and to withdraw. Maltreatment is associated with at least a threefold increase in the risk for disorganized attachment (van IJzendoorn, Schuengel, & Bakermans-Kranenburg, 1999).

Severe deprivation also seems to be an especially potent predictor of disorganized attachment, as documented in studies of children being raised in large, impersonal, and depriving institutions (Bakermans-Kranenberg et al., 2011). Severe deprivation/neglect may even lead to nonattachment, or what is clinically defined as reactive attachment disorder, and to disinhibited social engagement disorder (Oosterman & Schuengel, 2007; Zeanah, Smyke, Koga, Carlson, & BEIP Core Group, 2005).

Foster care is the preferred societal intervention for children who cannot be raised by their parents. Children younger than age 5 represent the largest proportion of children in foster care. Thus, the role of the attachment relationship between foster parents and young maltreated children is especially important but remains important even when children are older. Despite its importance, focusing on the centrality of attachment relationships as a mechanism to support recovery in children who have previously experienced serious disturbances and disorders of attachment is often overlooked. Though attachment for school-age children and adolescents in foster care also matters, in this chapter we focus primarily on younger children, for whom foster parents must be primary attachment figures.

Attachment and Foster Care

When children are not safe with their birth parents, they are often removed and placed with foster parents. For infants and young children, such placement changes are accompanied by disruptions in attachments to primary attachment figures at an age when they are unable to sustain attachments in the absence of substantial amounts of physical contact (i.e., older children are better able to sustain attachments even through long separations). Young children in foster care are faced simultaneously with experiencing a disruption to their original attachment figures and then forming attachments to caregivers with whom they do not have a prior relationship. These are clearly significant challenges; at a point when a primary developmental task is to keep and maintain access to attachment figures, children must negotiate new caregiving relationships.

Infants younger than about a year of age appear to establish attachments quickly. Within a week or less of being placed with new foster parents, infants appear to consolidate attachment behaviors, approaching foster parents when distressed in ways that are consistent with and predicted by foster parents' responsiveness (Stovall-McClough & Dozier, 2004). When infants are older than 12 months of age, such consolidation takes longer. Children often show avoidant and/or resistant behaviors over several months before showing a stable pattern of attachment. Nonetheless, both younger and older infants eventually develop attachments that match their new attachment figures' responsiveness (as assessed by the foster parents' state of mind with regard to attachment) with proportions of secure and insecure attachment similar to children from intact dyads (52% in each case) (Dozier, Stovall, Albus, & Bates, 2001; van den Dries, Juffer, van IJzendoorn, & Bakermans-Kranenburg, 2009; van IJzendoorn, 1995).

An important and as yet unanswered question is what the child carries forward from relationships that are subsequently disrupted. Vulnerability from previous experiences is evident in that rates of disorganized attachment are elevated as children form attachments to new caregivers (about 30–35%, as contrasted with about 15% in low-risk samples) (Dozier et al., 2001; van den Dries et al., 2009). Moreover, children who have experienced multiple disruptions show increased risk for problem behaviors (Almas et al., 2020; Oosterman & Schuengel, 2007).

Foster Care as an Attachment-Based Intervention

Foster care is intended to be a relatively short-term intervention, with preference for permanency clearly evident in law and in practice. Nevertheless, in the earliest years of life, when young children are initially forming and consolidating attachments, it is imperative to recognize and support the role of foster parents as the young child's primary attachment figures.

Foster parents differ in the extent to which they feel committed to their foster children, that is, the extent to which they think of a child as "their own." Foster parents have a variety of reasons for keeping some emotional distance, such as concern that the child will be removed from their care, having fostered many children previously, or experiencing the child's behavior as pushing them away. Children, though, are best served by caregivers who feel committed to them because children need to feel that parents will protect them at all costs—stand between them and danger—and that they are therefore safe in their parents' care.

Our view is that foster care must be embraced seriously as an intervention following maltreatment. Placement of children in foster families is the most common intervention provided to maltreated children in the United States and in many other countries. Though an imperfect and often underdeveloped intervention, foster care is demonstrably superior to alternative approaches such as family preservation efforts (Al et al., 2012) or group care (Zeanah, Smyke, & Settles, 2006).

Without question, foster parents can make a dramatic difference in the lives of young children, and yet, augmentations to "usual foster care" almost always show better outcomes than "usual foster care" alone. This raises the question of why societies have not more fully invested in those elements of foster care that are linked to better outcomes.

Important data on this question come from the Bucharest Early Intervention Project (BEIP). Infants who had been abandoned by their families in the first few months of life were placed in large impersonal institutions with inadequate levels of staffing and care. With one caregiver typically assigned to care for 12–15 children, and caregivers working rotating 8-hour shifts, the care provided was nonindividualized and often insensitive. For all these reasons, the young children raised in these conditions of psychosocial deprivation had limited opportunities to form robust attachments and rarely did (Zeanah et al., 2005). The BEIP study randomized 136 infants and toddlers to care as usual or to placement in the BEIP-supported foster care program and followed them through 54 months of age. The BEIP foster care model emphasized full psychological investment by foster parents to children in their care, as well as sensitive responsiveness and emotional availability (Smyke, Zeanah, Fox, & Nelson, 2009)..

Results at the conclusion of the trial showed that, across developmental domains, young children randomized to foster care had significantly more favorable outcomes than children who were randomized to usual care, despite the fact that the children in foster care had experienced an average of 22 months of exposure to deprived institutional rearing (Zeanah et al., 2017). Attachment security (49% foster care and 17% care as usual, $p < .001$) and organization (77% foster care and 54% care as usual, $p < .01$) were more prevalent, and signs of disorders of attachment were reduced for children placed in foster care ($p < .001$). Security of attachment mediated the effects of caregiving quality on total psychiatric symptoms across both groups (McGoron et al., 2012). In other words, attachment mattered for all children, but those in foster care were almost four times more likely to have secure attachment relationships with their caregivers than those who had more prolonged institutional rearing (thus more severe deprivation).

Dozier and colleagues have demonstrated that foster care may be augmented with a brief, in-home parenting intervention called Attachment and Biobehavioral Catch-Up (ABC; Dozier & Bernard, 2019; see also chapters by Dozier & Bernard, Chapter 38, and by Berlin, West, & Jones Harden, Chapter 47, this volume). A randomized controlled trial compared the ABC augmentation administered to foster parents and the children ages 1–24 months in their care to a comparably intensive in-home psychoeducational intervention targeting cognitive and language skills. Investigators demonstrated increased sensitive behaviors in the foster parents who received ABC. The foster parents who received ABC also reported more secure and less avoidant attachment behaviors in their foster children (Bick & Dozier, 2013), and children demonstrated stronger language development (Raby, Freedman, Yarger, Lind, & Dozier, 2019) and stronger inhibitory control (Lind, Bernard, Yarger, & Dozier, 2020) than children in the control condition.

Zeanah and Smyke (2005) reported on a community-based intervention for maltreated children in foster care that emphasized the foster parent's role as the primary attachment figure for young children (birth to 5 years) in care. Because young children in foster care spend only a few hours a week with their biological parents, and because young children need actual physical comfort when their attachment needs are activated, it is essential that the child form an attachment to foster parents who are their primary caregivers. This program worked simultaneously to build secure attachments in the foster children to their foster parents while also reconstructing (to increase security) the attachments of the young children to their biological parents, often implementing multiple evidence-based interventions including ABC, Child–Parent Psychotherapy (Lieberman, van Horn, & Ghosh Ippen, 2005), and Circle of Security (Hoffman, Marvin, Cooper, & Powell, 2006) to enhance attachment security. These treatments were applied based on individualized assessments. Results from this intervention showed reductions in maltreatment recidivism for the target child and for subsequent siblings (Zeanah & Smyke, 2005).

Enhancing Systems Collaboration

Given the importance of attachment as an essential therapeutic ingredient of foster care for young children, attachment ought to be a central focus of the systems affecting children in care. Unfortunately, our experience is that attachment is poorly understood, and its principles are often ignored by both Child Protective Services (CPS) and the legal system. For example, transitions from one caregiver to another—including transitions from one foster parent to another and returns to biological parents—are often abrupt and not well planned. Foster placements are often disrupted after months of stability because a relative willing to take the child has been identified, without prioritizing the child's best interest. Young children are transported to visits by drivers who have no meaningful relationships with them, and then children may have stressful visits with biological parents without having an attachment figure present with them. These are all unnecessary additional burdens placed on young children who are already at the extreme of the risk continuum.

In our view, decision makers in these systems are uninformed rather than callous or malicious. This suggests that an important task for researchers, clinicians, and policymakers is to make attachment principles more accessible to child protection professionals, lawyers, and judges, so that their decisions may be better informed by developmental science. The challenge is how best to accomplish this.

One approach is to develop training efforts in graduate schools, postgraduate training, and continuing education programs for CPS staff and legal students and professionals. Scattered efforts to date seem mostly aimed at professional continuing education audiences. Introducing more information about attachment into graduate programs in social work, followed by more advanced intensive training and sustained consultation about application as a part of child protection training, would be helpful.

In addition to training, another approach is to provide ongoing expert consultation to child protection professionals and to legal professionals. For example, mental health professionals from Southwest Human

Development in Phoenix who are well versed in attachment spend time weekly in CPS offices to offer case-specific consultation. Similarly, professionals versed in attachment from the Jewish Board of Families and Children in New York meet regularly for "lunch and learn" sessions with judges in which they can discuss hypothetical dilemmas based on actual cases.

A more comprehensive approach is provided by the Quality Parenting Initiative (Shauffer, 2012). This approach, implemented in a dozen states, involves encouraging foster parents to commit fully to their foster children, while *simultaneously* supporting birth parents and collaborating with efforts to reunify parents and children. In exchange, foster parents are treated as full-fledged professionals and members of the collaborative team of child protection workers and community providers. One manifestation of foster parents' role is to have them not only attend visits between children and their biological parents but also receive coaching in following the child's lead (i.e., to follow the child's interests versus the parent's "agenda") during visits.

Fostering Relationships (see Dozier & Bernard, 2019), a visitation support program used in conjunction with the Quality Parenting Initiative, seeks to encourage collaboration between the two sets of caregivers. Foster parents commit to participation in visits with birth parents, thus providing support to children. Birth parents are coached before each visit, helping them to anticipate that their children may not show feelings of closeness to them, and helping them to practice interacting in responsive ways to children's cues (thus making them interesting play partners). Also, foster parents (after brief training) are coached to make positive comments to birth parents about their ability to follow children's lead during interactions. Preliminary data suggest that this approach enhances the quality of birth parent interactions with their children and increases the likelihood that birth parents will persist in visits.

Conclusions

Foster care, though often not well regarded, is the most effective intervention for orphaned, maltreated, and abandoned young children that has been developed (Al et al., 2012; Zeanah et al., 2017). Indeed, foster care serves as a regulating environment for children, since young children are significantly more likely to develop secure attachments with foster parents than with maltreating birth parents. Foster care could be improved if attachment principles were better appreciated and integrated into training so that foster parents have skills, resources, and roles to support them in providing the care vulnerable young children need. Determining how best to facilitate these improvements represents an important next step.

REFERENCES

Al, C. M. W., Stams, G. J. J. M., Bek, M. S., Damen, E. M., Asscher, J. J., & van der Laan, P. H. (2012). A meta-analysis of intensive family preservation programs: Placement prevention and improvement of family functioning. *Children and Youth Services Review, 34,* 1472–1479.

Almas, A. N., Woodbury, M. R., Papp, L. J., Nelson, C. A., Zeanah, C. H., & Fox, N. A. (2020). The impact of caregiving disruptions experienced by previously institutionalized children on multiple outcomes in late childhood. *Child Development, 91,* 96–109.

Bakermans-Kranenburg, M. J., Steele, H., Zeanah, C. H., Muhamedrahimov, R. J., Vorria, P., Dobrova-Krol, N. A., . . . Gunnar, M. R. (2011). Attachment and emotional development in institutional care: Characteristics and catch-up. In R. B. McCall, M. H. van IJzendoorn, F. Juffer, C. J. Groark, & V. K. Groza (Eds.), Children without permanent parents: Research, practice, and policy. *Monographs of the Society for Research in Child Development, 76*(4), 62–91.

Bick, J., & Dozier, M. (2013). The effectiveness of an attachment-based intervention in promoting foster mothers' sensitivity toward foster infants. *Infant Mental Health Journal, 34,* 95–103.

Dozier, M., & Bernard, K. (2019). *Coaching parents of vulnerable infants: The Attachment and Biobehavioral Catch-up approach.* New York: Guilford Press.

Dozier, M., Stovall, K. C., Albus, K. E., & Bates, B. (2001). Attachment for infants in foster care: The role of caregiver state of mind. *Child Development, 72,* 1467–1477.

Hoffman, K., Marvin, R., Cooper, G., & Powell, B. (2006). Changing toddlers' and preschoolers' attachment classifications: The Circle of Security intervention. *Journal of Consulting and Clinical Psychology, 74,* 1017–1026.

Lieberman, A., van Horn, P., & Ghosh Ippen, C. (2005). Toward evidence-based treatment: Child–parent psychotherapy with preschoolers exposed to marital violence. *Journal of the American Academy of Child and Adolescent Psychiatry, 44,* 1241–1248.

Lind, T., Bernard, K., Yarger, H. A., & Dozier, M. (2020). Promoting compliance in children referred to Child Protective Services: A randomized clinical trial. *Child Development, 91,* 563–576.

Main, M., & Hesse, E. (1990). Parents' unresolved traumatic experiences are related to infant disorganized attachment status: Is frightened and/or frightening parental behavior the linking mechanism? In M. T. Greenberg, D. Cicchetti, & E. Cummings (Eds.), *Attachment in the preschool years: Theory, research, and intervention* (pp. 161–182). Chicago: University of Chicago Press.

McGoron, L., Gleason, M. M., Smyke, A. T., Drury, S. S., Nelson, C. A., Gregas, M. C., . . . Zeanah, C. H. (2012). Recovering from early deprivation: Attachment mediates effects of caregiving on psychopathology. *Journal of the American Academy of Child and Adolescent Psychiatry, 51,* 683–693.

Oosterman, M., & Schuengel, C. (2007). Autonomic reactivity of children to separation and reunion with foster parents. *Journal of the American Academy of Child and Adolescent Psychiatry, 46,* 1196–1203.

Raby, K. L., Freedman, E., Yarger, H. A., Lind, T., & Dozier, M. (2019). Enhancing the language development of toddlers in foster care by promoting foster parents' sensitivity: Results from a randomized control trial. *Developmental Science, 22,* e12753.

Shauffer, C. (2012, May/June). The Quality Parenting Initiative: Fostering in the 21st century. *Fostering Families Today,* pp. 24–25.

Smyke, A. T., Zeanah, C. H., Fox, N. A., & Nelson, C. A. (2009). A new model of foster care for young children: The Bucharest Early Intervention Project. *Child and Adolescent Psychiatric Clinics of North America, 18*(3), 721–734.

Stovall-McClough, K. C., & Dozier, M. (2004). Forming attachments in foster care: Infant attachment behaviors in the first two months of placement. *Development and Psychopathology, 16,* 253–271.

van den Dries, L., Juffer, F., van IJzendoorn, M. H., & Bakermans-Kranenburg, M. J. (2009). Fostering security?: A meta-analysis of attachment in adopted children. *Children and Youth Services Review, 31,* 410–421.

van IJzendoorn, M. H. (1995). Adult attachment representations, parental responsiveness, and infant attachment: A meta-analysis on the predictive validity of the adult attachment interview. *Psychological Bulletin, 117,* 387–403.

van IJzendoorn, M. H., Schuengel, C., & Bakermans-Kranenburg, M. J. (1999). Disorganized attachment in early childhood: Meta-analysis of precursors, concomitants, and sequelae. *Development and Psychopathology, 11*(2), 225–249.

Zeanah, C. H., Humphreys, K. L., Fox, N. A., & Nelson, C. A. (2017). Alternatives for abandoned children: Lessons from the Bucharest Early Intervention Project. *Current Opinion in Psychology, 15,* 182–188.

Zeanah, C. H., & Smyke, A. T. (2005). Building attachment relationships following maltreatment and severe deprivation. In L. J. Berlin, Y. Ziv, L. Amaya-Jackson, & M. T. Greenberg (Eds.), *Enhancing early attachments: Theory, research, intervention and policy* (pp. 195–216). New York: Guilford Press.

Zeanah, C. H., Smyke, A. T., Koga, S. F. M., Carlson, E., & BEIP Core Group. (2005). Attachment in institutionalized and community children in Romania. *Child Development, 76,* 1015–1028.

Zeanah, C. H., Smyke, A. T., & Settles, L. (2006). Orphanages as a developmental context for early childhood. In K. McCartney & D. Phillips (Eds.), *Blackwell handbook of early childhood development* (pp. 424–454). Malden, MA: Blackwell.

CHAPTER 47

Attachment and Early Home Visiting
Toward a More Perfect Union

Lisa J. Berlin
Allison West
Brenda Jones Harden

The landmark Affordable Care Act of 2010 established the Maternal, Infant, and Early Childhood Home Visiting (MIECHV) Program that in turn galvanized an unprecedented expansion of early home visiting in the United States. In 2018, over 286,000 families received a total of more than 3 million home visits (National Home Visiting Resource Center, 2019). Typically targeted toward low-income or at-risk families, home visiting services consist of professional or paraprofessional visitors providing regular home-based sessions to pregnant women and new parents. Home visitors' activities include instructing mothers in basic infant care, connecting families to community services, and promoting supportive parenting. Home visiting provides a unique opportunity to observe and guide infant–parent interaction in the environment in which it most often occurs. Home visiting is thus an ideal context in which to strengthen infant–parent relationships and promote the development of infant attachment security.

The MIECHV Program supports both home visiting services and research–practice partnerships to improve the effectiveness and efficiency of home visiting. For example, the "precision home visiting" approach centers on data-driven alignment of participants' needs, intervention foci, and intervention content (Supplee & Duggan, 2019). Like the precision home visiting approach, attachment theory and research emphasize precise concepts and assessments. Of particular relevance to home visiting, attachment theory and research highlight *sensitive* parenting as a key driver of infant attachment security. Originally defined by Ainsworth and her colleagues (Ainsworth, Blehar, Waters, & Wall, 1978), sensitivity refers to parents' accurate interpretations of their infants' cues (e.g., crying) and prompt and contingent responsiveness to these signals. Attachment research has identified caregiver sensitivity as the major precursor of infant attachment security (Zeegers, Colonnesi, Stams, & Meins, 2017). Parental sensitivity has in turn become a target of virtually all attachment-based interventions (Steele & Steele, 2018).

In this chapter, we consider the roles of attachment theory, attachment-focused intervention models, and attachment-related assessments in early home visiting in the United States. We offer three recommendations designed to improve early home visiting: expand the use of attachment-focused intervention models; tailor home visiting services according to attachment-relevant information; and increase the assessment of parental sensitivity.

Expand the Use of Attachment-Focused Intervention Models in Early Home Visiting

MIECHV funds are competitively awarded to states and territories to provide home visits to pregnant women and parents with young children. MIECHV grantees must spend at least 75% of their funds to implement one of 18 pre-approved "evidence-based" home visiting models, all of which aim to encourage "positive" parenting (Health Resources and Services Administration [HRSA], 2019). MIECHV grantees must also document annual improvements in at least four of six "benchmark" domains (HRSA, 2019).

The MIECHV Program's largest research initiative, the Mother and Infant Home Visiting Program Evaluation (MIHOPE), is a randomized trial of 4,229 families and 88 programs in 12 states implementing one of the four most widely used MIECHV-approved home visiting models: the Early Head Start home-based option, the Nurse–Family Partnership, Healthy Families America, or Parents as Teachers (Michaelopoulos et al., 2019). Notably, three of these four programs trace their roots at least partially to attachment theory (Donelan-McCall & Olds, 2018; Harding, Galano, Martin, Huntington, & Schellenbach, 2007; U.S. Department of Health and Human Services, 1994). All four programs explicitly target parenting as a critical lever for supporting early child development (Michaelopoulos et al., 2019). The Healthy Families America program, moreover, defines one of its aims as to "promote . . . healthy attachment" (Healthy Families America, 2019).

The MIHOPE trial included a video-recorded semistructured play assessment from which maternal sensitivity toward their 15-month-old infants was reliably rated. Home-visited mothers demonstrated more sensitivity than control mothers (p = .05). The intervention effect was small (d = 0.07) and comparable to effects from prior single-model evaluations (Avellar & Supplee, 2013), thus suggesting an opportunity to better align program goals and results. Notably, no model's impacts on sensitivity approached a medium effect size (d = 0.50), an effect size identified in a seminal meta-analysis of attachment-focused interventions as necessary to improve attachment security (Bakermans-Kranenburg, van IJzendoorn, & Juffer, 2003). Moreover, the one study of which we are aware that tested the impacts of one of these four home visiting models (Healthy Families) on infant attachment security indicated a null effect (Berlin et al., 2017). Given the stated goals of these (indeed, most) home visiting models, it is critical to increase home visiting's effects on parental sensitivity. In this regard, findings from several attachment-focused home visiting models are instructive.

Among its 18 approved home visiting models, the MIECHV Program includes two that are based predominantly on attachment theory and target infant attachment security. The first, Attachment and Biobehavioral Catch-up (ABC), focuses on parental sensitivity and consists of 10 weekly parent coaching sessions delivered to the mother and child together (see Dozier & Bernard, Chapter 38, and Zeanah & Dozier, Chapter 46, this volume). Both experimental and quasi-experimental studies have found ABC to be associated with pre- to postintervention changes in observed maternal sensitivity. ABC has also demonstrated positive effects on infant attachment security and organization (see Dozier & Bernard, 2019, for a full review).

Minding the Baby (MTB) provides comprehensive nurse and social worker home visits for over 2 years, from pregnancy through the child's second birthday (Sadler et al., 2013; Slade et al., 2020). MTB is based in part on adult attachment research emphasizing parents' own representations of attachment and their abilities to understand their children's internal states as important precursors of both sensitive parenting and child attachment security (Verhage et al., 2016; Zeegers et al., 2017). One of MTB's key intervention targets is, thus, mothers' reflectiveness or "mentalizing" capacity. Two randomized trials of MTB have revealed positive impacts on maternal "reflective functioning" and on infant attachment security and organization (effect sizes were not reported and maternal sensitivity was not assessed).

Both of these attachment-focused home visiting models target infant attachment security, and both models' intervention foci draw directly on the findings of attachment research pertaining to key antecedents of infant attachment, especially sensitive parenting. Both models, thus, exemplify a precise alignment between intervention targets and content. In addition to positive impacts on infant–mother attachment and, for ABC, positive impacts on sensitivity, ABC and MTB have shown positive impacts in other domains highlighted by MIECHV, such as child health (e.g., pediatric immunizations; Sadler et al., 2013) and school readiness (e.g., executive functioning; Dozier & Bernard, Chapter 38, this volume). Their results suggest that service providers concerned with parenting and infant–parent attachment seriously consider implementing one of these attachment-focused models, either alone or in combination with other home-based models.

One option is to braid one of the major MIECHV models with a brief, evidence-based, attachment-focused intervention. One such braided option recently tested by our research team consisted of home-based Early Head Start services as usual supplemented with ABC (Berlin, Martoccio, & Jones Harden, 2018). In a randomized trial, this "Early Head Start plus ABC" model had a medium-sized effect ($d = 0.47$) on a composite index of maternal sensitivity. Other brief (six- to eight-session) attachment-focused interventions delivered in the home to caregivers and their young children include the Video-Feedback Intervention to Promote Positive Parenting (VIPP; Bakermans-Kranenburg & Oosterman, Chapter 37, this volume) and the Attachment Video-Feedback Intervention (AVI; Moss et al., 2018). Both programs have shown positive effects on sensitivity and infant attachment (see Steele & Steele, 2018, for reviews of these and other attachment-focused interventions).

Tailor Home Visiting According to Attachment-Relevant Information

As noted, the precision home visiting approach emphasizes careful consideration of participants' needs and the potential tailoring of services according to these needs. Our recommendations for tailoring build on evidence of moderated impacts of home visiting services. For example, our team found stronger impacts of our Early Head Start plus ABC model for those mothers who demonstrated greater baseline intrusiveness (i.e., less sensitivity; Berlin et al., 2018). It may be useful for parents initiating home visiting services to participate in brief observational assessments of sensitivity, the results of which could then be used to triage the relatively less-sensitive parents into an attachment-focused model or option.

A second recommendation comes from several studies examining the roles of mothers' and home visitors' attachment security in the course and outcome of home visiting. Although somewhat fragmented in approach, these studies point to the relevance of adult attachment as a screening and/or tailoring factor. For example, in our Early Head Start plus ABC trial, in addition to finding positive effects overall, we found that mothers who classified themselves as secure or anxious according to Hazan and Shaver's (1987) Adult Attachment Style assessment showed stronger positive effects on maternal sensitivity than mothers who classified themselves as avoidant. Also relevant are results from a study of the Healthy Start program in which both mothers' and home visitors' self-reported attachment avoidance and anxiety were related to program engagement (McFarlane et al., 2010).

Given the highly intimate and relational nature of home visiting, it is consistent with what is known about adult attachment (i.e., its relevance to comfort with dependence on others, fears of abandonment, and relational openness; see Shaver & Mikulincer, Chapter 33, this volume) that parents' and/or home visitors' own attachment security could influence the success of a home visiting intervention. It may be valuable, thus, to screen incoming participants' self-reported attachment and to use this information to inform program approaches. For example, mothers with relatively high levels of attachment avoidance may be especially difficult to engage and may require special up-front efforts to build the therapeutic alliance with the home visitor. Mothers with relatively high levels of attachment anxiety may require especially gentle tapering of services at program termination. With respect to home visitors' attachment security, results from a recent ABC study illustrated the value of screening parent coaches on the basis of their self-reported attachment security or related constructs: ABC parent coaches' scores on a pretraining assessment of "valuing of attachment/openness" predicted their ability to provide ABC with high fidelity (Dozier & Bernard, 2019).

Increase the Assessment of Parental Sensitivity in the Development and Evaluation of Home Visiting Models

Given that many home visiting programs aim to promote supportive parenting, we recommend increasing the assessment of parental sensitivity in the context of program development and evaluation. First, with respect to program development, the MIECHV program's HomVEE initiative regularly reviews home visiting models and findings of their efficacy (Sama-Miler et al., 2018). Models are deemed eligible for MIECHV funding on the basis of positive effects in at least one of eight outcome domains, one of which is "positive parenting practices." Outcome assessments are carefully documented and ranked, with both observational and standardized self-report assessments ranked "primary." Few of these parenting measures consist of observational assessments of parental sensitivity, however. To increase precision as well as a focus on attachment, we recommend that HomVEE highlight home visiting models with documented effects on observed parenting sensitivity. For example, it would be valuable for such models to receive an asterisk in the parenting domain.

Second, with respect to program evaluation, each of the statutorily defined "benchmark" domains in which MIECHV grantees must demonstrate annual improvement includes at least one specific performance measure. "Parent–child interaction" is one of the performance measures in the school readiness domain. To demonstrate improvement, a grantee must have increased the "percent of primary caregivers enrolled in home visiting who receive an observation of caregiver–child interaction by the home visitor using a validated tool" (Labiner-Wolfe, Vladutiu, Peplinski, Cano, & Willis, 2018). We recommend increasing technical assistance for MIECHV grantees to generate actual ratings of caregiver sensitivity using brief observational measures (e.g., the 25-item Maternal Behavior Q-Set; Tarabulsy et al., 2009).

Conclusions

A consideration of the roles of attachment theory, attachment-focused intervention models, and attachment-related assessments in early home visiting in the United States informed three recommendations: expand the use of attachment-focused intervention models; tailor home visiting services according to attachment-relevant information; and increase the assessment of parental sensitivity. We emphasize that we offer our recommendation to expand the use of attachment-focused intervention models, either alone or in combination with other models, as (1) one way to prioritize support for the crucial child–parent attachment relationship and (2) a strategy to leverage the combined strengths of broad-based home visiting services with attachment-focused interventions known to promote sensitive caregiving and/or infant attachment security. In cases where it is not feasible to implement or add an attachment-focused intervention model, the use of attachment-relevant assessments for screening, tailoring, and program development and evaluation stand to add value. Ideally, the use of such assessments will occur in the context of research–practice partnerships. For example, researchers could collaborate with program staff to identify assessments that are both well validated and feasible. Similarly, program staff could partner with researchers to analyze and interpret such assessment data. Accumulating evidence about what works for whom can in turn be fed back to guide the effectiveness and precision of early home visiting.

REFERENCES

Ainsworth, M. D. S., Blehar, M. C., Waters, E., & Wall, S. (1978). *Patterns of attachment: A psychological study of the Strange Situation*. Hillsdale, NJ: Erlbaum.

Avellar, S. A., & Supplee, L. H. (2013). Effectiveness of home visiting in improving child health and reducing child maltreatment. *Pediatrics, 132*(2), 90–99.

Bakermans-Kranenburg, M. J., van IJzendoorn, M. H., & Juffer, F. (2003). Less is more: Meta-analyses of sensitivity and attachment interventions in early childhood. *Psychological Bulletin, 129*(2), 195–215.

Berlin, L. J., Martoccio, T. L., Appleyard Carmody, K., Goodman, W. B., O'Donnell, K., William, J., . . . Dodge, K. A. (2017). Can typical U.S. home visits affect infant attachment?: Preliminary findings from a randomized trial of Healthy Families Durham. *Attachment and Human Development, 19*(6), 559–579.

Berlin, L. J., Martoccio, T. L., & Jones Harden, B. (2018). Improving Early Head Start's impacts on parenting through attachment-based intervention: A randomized controlled trial. *Developmental Psychology, 54*, 2316–2327.

Donelan-McCall, N., & Olds, D. (2018). The Nurse–Family Partnership: Theoretical and empirical foundations. In H. Steele & M. Steele (Eds.), *Handbook of attachment-based interventions* (pp. 79–103). New York: Guilford Press.

Dozier, M., & Bernard, K. (2019). *Coaching parents of vulnerable infants: The Attachment and Biobehavioral Catch-Up approach*. New York: Guilford Press.

Harding, K., Galano, J., Martin, J., Huntington, L., & Schellenbach, C. J. (2007). Healthy Families America effectiveness: A comprehensive review of outcomes. *Journal of Prevention and Intervention in the Community, 34*(1–2), 149–179.

Hazan, C., & Shaver, P. (1987). Romantic love conceptualized as an attachment process. *Journal of Personality and Social Psychology, 52*(3), 511–524.

Health Resources and Services Administration. (2019). Home visiting. Retrieved from *mchb.hrsa.gov/programs/homevisiting*.

Healthy Families America. (2019). The Healthy Families America strategy. Retrieved from *www.healthyfamiliesamerica.org*.

Labiner-Wolfe, J., Vladutiu, C., Peplinski, K., Cano, C., & Willis, D. (2018). Redesigning the Maternal, Infant, and Early Childhood Home Visiting Program performance measurement system. *Maternal and Child Health Journal, 22*, 467–473.

McFarlane, E., Burrell, L., Fuddy, L., Tandon, D., Derauf, C., Leaf, P., & Duggan, A. (2010). Association of home visitors' and mothers' attachment style with family engagement. *Journal of Community Psychology, 38*, 541–556.

Michaelopoulos, C., Faucetta, K., Hill, C. J., Portilla, X. A., Burrell, L., Lee, H., . . . Knox, V. (2019). *Impacts on family outcomes of evidence-based early childhood home visiting: Results from the Mother and Infant Home Visiting Program Evaluation* (OPRE Report 2019-07). Washington, DC: Office of Planning, Research, and Evaluation, Administration for Children and Families, U.S. Department of Health and Human Services.

Moss, E., Tarabusly, G. M., Dubois-Comtois, K., Cyr, C., Bernier, A., & St-Laurent, D. (2018). The Attachment Video-Feedback Intervention program. In H.

Steele & M. Steele (Eds.), *Handbook of attachment-based interventions* (pp. 318–338). New York: Guilford Press.

National Home Visiting Resource Center. (2019). *2019 home visiting yearbook.* Arlington, VA: James Bell Associates and the Urban Institute.

Sadler, L. S., Slade, A., Close, N., Webb, D. L., Simpson, T., Fennie, K., & Mayes, L. C. (2013). Minding the Baby: Enhancing reflectiveness to improve early health and relationship outcomes in an interdisciplinary home-visiting program. *Infant Mental Health Journal, 34*(5), 391–405.

Sama-Miler, E., Akers, L., Mraz-Esposito, A., Zukiewicz, M., Avellar, S., Paulsell, D., & Del Grosso, P. (2018). *Home visiting evidence of effectiveness review.* Washington, DC: Office of Planning, Research, and Evaluation, Administration for Children and Families, U.S. Department of Health and Human Services.

Slade, A., Holland, M. L., Ordway, M. R., Carlson, E. A., Jeon, S. Close, N., . . . Sadler, L. S. (2020). Minding the Baby: Enhancing parental reflective functioning and infant attachment in an attachment-based, interdisciplinary home visiting program. *Development and Psychopathology, 32*(1), 123–137.

Steele, H., & Steele, M. (Eds.). (2018). *Handbook of attachment-based interventions.* New York: Guilford Press.

Supplee, L. H., & Duggan, A. (2019). Innovative research methods to advance precision in home visiting for more efficient and effective programs. *Child Development Perspectives, 13*(3), 173–179.

Tarabulsy, G. M., Provost, M. A., Bordeleau, S., Trudel-Fitzgerald, C., Moran, G., Pederson, D. R., . . . Pierce, T. (2009). Validation of a short version of the maternal behavior Q-set applied to a brief video record of mother–infant interaction. *Infant Behavior and Development, 32*(1), 132–136.

U.S. Department of Health and Human Services. (1994). *Statement of the Advisory Committee on Services for Families with Infants and Toddlers* (DHHS Publication No. 1994-615-032/03062). Washington, DC: U.S. Government Printing Office. Retrieved from *www.bmcc.edu/Headstart/Advse_Commtte/index.html.*

Verhage, M. L., Schuengel, C., Madigan, S., Fearon, R. M., Oosterman, M., Cassibba, R., . . . van IJzendoorn, M. H. (2016). Narrowing the transmission gap: A synthesis of three decades of research on intergenerational transmission of attachment. *Psychological Bulletin, 142*(4), 337–366.

Zeegers, M. A. J., Colonnesi, C., Stams, G.-J. J. M., & Meins, E. (2017). Mind matters: A meta-analysis on parental mentalization and sensitivity as predictors of infant–parent attachment. *Psychological Bulletin, 143,* 1245–1272.

CONCLUDING COMMENTARY

CHAPTER 48

Assembling the Puzzle
Interlocking Pieces, Missing Pieces, and the Emerging Picture

Ross A. Thompson
Lisa J. Berlin
Jeffry A. Simpson

A recent comprehensive exam given by a prominent attachment scholar posed this question: *Attachment theory has been influential for a longer period than most other psychological theories, now more than 50 years, and it shows no signs of diminishing importance. What can account for its enduring influence?* Although we might sympathize with the student taking this exam, the chapters of this volume answer the professor's query well. The continuing generativity of attachment theory derives from the breadth of its relevance to issues in developmental, social, and personality psychology, its broad applications to clinical and social policy concerns, and its capacity to address classic questions in psychology. Moreover, the theory has lifespan applications, connects behavioral with representational processes, and has introduced new measurement approaches. Finally, no small reason for the theory's endurance has been the capacity of attachment researchers to pose new, interesting questions that expand the reach of both theoretical and empirical inquiry. Each of these aspects of attachment theory is reflected in the pages of this volume. These chapters also illustrate some of the contradictions, inconsistencies, limitations, and unanswered questions that will be important for the next generation of attachment scholars to address.

In this concluding commentary, we reflect on the chapters that addressed each of the nine fundamental questions that organize this volume. Our primary purpose is to note points of convergence and divergence, describe what we can (and cannot) conclude about each question, and identify future directions for theory and research. Like assembling a jigsaw puzzle, our goal is to identify the emerging picture created collectively by these contributors and also to consider what is still missing. In the final section, we offer our own proposals for what will significantly advance the field by discussing the need for a truly lifespan theory of attachment with a focus on the development of internal working models (IWMs).

Defining Attachment and Attachment Security

Few questions are more central to attachment theory than the two that introduce the opening section of this book: *What kinds of relationships "qualify" as attachment relationships?* and *What are the origins and nature of security?* The authors who addressed these questions represent different areas of psychology and examine different types of attachment relationships at different stages of life.

In the first chapter, Sroufe initiates a through-line of this collection of essays as a whole. He describes the unique features that define attachment relationships in both children and adults, reminding us that Bowlby viewed infant–caregiver attachments as prototypical, a view that strongly influenced the developmental study of attachment. Sroufe also emphasizes that attachments involve specific relationships and that we need to discover how early attachment experiences are combined with later ones to shape secure or insecure attachment orientations in adulthood. Fearon and Schuengel discuss intersections between Hinde's (1997) conceptualization of relationships and Ainsworth's (1991) view of attachment as a specific kind of affectional bond. They also note that the presence of attachment behavior does not necessarily imply the presence of a deep affectional bond. Likewise, Sroufe and Shaver and Mikulincer note that there can be strong emotional ties between individuals that are not attachments. Ahnert focuses on patterns of attachment between children and child care providers (caregivers), how these attachments may develop differently than child–parent attachments, and how the quality of child–caregiver attachment (or child–teacher closeness) is associated with children's cognitive performance, behavioral adjustment, and stress management in educational settings. Shaver and Mikulincer discuss the criteria for attachment figures and attachment relationships in adulthood and summarize the signature cognitive and emotional features of security in adults. Focusing primarily on adult patterns of attachment based on the Adult Attachment Interview (AAI), Jacobvitz and Hazan review the developmental origins of attachment security in adults, the kinds of relationships that represent bona fide attachments, and how early attachment patterns may change as individuals move toward adulthood. Aviles and Zeifman encourage future attachment scholars to investigate a wider range of close relationships, particularly platonic friendships, which might fulfill attachment functions in adulthood similar to those fulfilled by romantic pair-bonded relationships.

Several core themes reverberate across the chapters in this section. To begin with, regardless of relationship type (e.g., child–parent, child–caregiver, adult romantic partners, close friends), all of the authors tend to define attachment relationships as well as their basic functions similarly. Early in life, attachments between children and their primary caregivers are viewed as a relationship-specific construct (Sroufe) that becomes a more trait-like orientation by adulthood. Attachments are also conceptualized as a special type of relationship that serves the primary attachment functions of safe haven and secure base provision. Additionally, most adult attachment scholars emphasize proximity maintenance as a key attachment function (Simpson, Rholes, Eller, & Paetzold, 2021). Attachment relationships are also defined by the preference for specific attachment figure(s) in certain situations, particularly when an individual is distressed, is separated from, or loses an attachment figure. Finally, attachments patterns (in children) and orientations (in adults) differ in their quality (i.e., whether they are secure or insecure, including whether they are higher/lower on attachment avoidance and/or anxiety), but not necessarily in their strength. Thus, for both children and adults, there is reasonably good consensus regarding what constitutes an attachment relationship and what promotes a sense of security.

There is some divergence, however, in how the authors conceptualize and measure attachment. Developmental and clinical scholars, for example, most frequently use "indirect" measures (e.g., the AAI) to examine how adults reflect on their childhood relationships with their parents, whereas most social/personality scholars investigate how adults directly perceive and report on the nature of their prior or current adult romantic relationships. These differences may partly explain why these different measures (e.g., the AAI and the adult romantic attachment measures) correlate rather weakly (Topic 2), an issue we discuss at greater length in the next section. There is also variability in how the authors portray development and change in attachment over the life course, ranging from models that emphasize the formative influences of infant–caregiver attachment (Sroufe) to those emphasizing that life stress, therapy, and other experiences can modify adult attachment representations (Jacobvitz & Hazan) to the view that people acquire multiple representations of relationships that shape their overall attachment orientation (Shaver & Mikulincer; see Collins, Guichard, Ford, & Feeney, 2004). These are significant differences important to attachment theory.

A final theme touches on the evolutionary origins of attachment theory (Bowlby, 1969/1982; Simpson & Belsky, 2016). Most attachment theorists acknowledge that the attachment system evolved because it helped infants and young children survive the many perils of childhood (Ainsworth, 1991; Bowlby, 1969/1982). Simply surviving childhood, however, means nothing in terms of reproductive fitness unless individuals also reproduce and successfully raise their own children to reproductive age. Given the numerous challenges and demands of our ancestral environments, sustained biparental care (Fletcher, Simpson, Campbell, & Overall, 2015; Zeifman, 2019) along with alloparental care (Hrdy, 2009) was almost certainly needed to raise children to reproductive age. Thus, the cognitive, affective, and behavioral features of the attachment system, which initially evolved to increase survival during childhood, may have been exapted (i.e., "borrowed" for another purpose) to facilitate other attachment bonds later in life, particularly those between mates who needed to remain together long enough to rear their children successfully. Although neither Bowlby nor Ainsworth discussed this possible additional evolutionary force, it most likely undergirds adult romantic attachment bonds. This supposition is supported by recent evidence indicating that adult romantic relationships and childhood attachments involving parents have similar neurochemical processes (e.g., Feldman, 2017).

Collectively, the authors of this section pose a variety of insightful questions that deserve closer theoretical and empirical attention. Chief among these is the question of how early attachment experiences "combine" with later attachment experiences to form attachment orientations in adulthood. How, for instance, are attachment experiences beyond elementary school incorporated into working models, which then shape adult attachment security, avoidance, and anxiety? How, and in what contexts, do these adult orientations guide a person's behavior? Additional questions raised by the chapters in this section are also worthy of further scrutiny. For example, if attachment behaviors do not always reflect or result in the development of strong affectional bonds, why do some relationships become deep affectional bonds whereas others do not? What are the critical conditions needed for attachment bonds to form in children, adolescents, and adults, especially given the varied conditions in which these relationships develop, including orphanage care, foster care, child care, and parental care? How do different motivational systems, such as attachment, mating, and caregiving, independently and/ or jointly influence how people relate to their romantic partners, their children, and other significant people in their lives? How do attachment bonds form between close, platonic friends? Are the neurochemical processes underlying these relationships the same as those for romantic pair-bonded relationships? Addressing these questions will advance multiple aspects of attachment theory and research.

Measuring the Security of Attachment

From its inception, methodological advances have propelled the attachment field. Bowlby's theory was influential before Ainsworth's Strange Situation, but the significance of attachment theory was certainly magnified by the development of this procedure and the organizational view of attachment it instantiated. So important is the Strange Situation to attachment research that, for many, it is the gold standard for developmental research, with subsequent measures of attachment being convergently validated by their concordance with attachment classifications derived from it. Both Hazan and Shaver's (1987) development of an adult romantic attachment questionnaire and the creation of the AAI (Main, Kaplan, & Cassidy, 1985) inaugurated profound advances in attachment research in adulthood. Indeed, the history of attachment research is written by advances in the measurement of attachment, in part because advances in assessment have benchmarked developing conceptions of attachment and its behavioral manifestations.

The chapters in this section do not profile all of the available attachment measures, but rather they survey the range of measurement approaches sufficiently to frame some of the important issues of this field. The authors were asked to discuss *How should attachment security be assessed?* and *What are the advantages and challenges of alternative measurement approaches?* We were also interested in whether there is a central element of attachment relationships captured by each of these diverse approaches. Contributors to this section profiled narrative assessments and self-report questionnaires (Crowell), representational measures (Waters), and priming methods (Gillath & Ai), with broader reflections on the strengths and limitations of categorical (Steele & Steele) and dimensional (Raby, Fraley, & Roisman) assessments of attachment.

One clear conclusion that frames the discussion of attachment methodology is that different assessments are not highly correlated, either concurrently or across time. Crowell states the matter directly with respect to the AAI and the Experiences in Close Relationships (ECR) scale: "Although both measures predict important aspects of close relationship functioning in adulthood, they do not predict the same outcomes in the same ways." Waters offers a similar conclusion with respect to the AAI and secure base script methods, even though they are significantly but modestly correlated (see also Mikulincer & Shaver, 2016, for a broader review). Viewed longitudinally, there is a weak and often nonsignificant association between different attachment assessments across developmental periods (Booth-Laforce & Roisman; Fraley & Dugan), even though this confounds measurement consistency with the stability of attachment over time. Thus, attachment quality indexed by one well-validated measure is not necessarily highly convergent with attachment quality indexed by another.

This conclusion is unsurprising in some respects. After all, the measures profiled in this section differ significantly in measurement approach (e.g., behavioral vs. self-report vs. narrative interview vs. semiprojective probes) and thus in the criteria that distinguish different attachment patterns or orientations. Attachment is behavioral, representational, and intrapsychic, and current measures differentially index these different features of attachment functioning. It is also true that existing measures were created for different purposes, such as studying attachment in infants, children, or adults, in typical versus at-risk samples, or to broaden inquiry by activating security through priming. Finally, different measures sometimes assess different attachment relationships using different conceptualizations of the IWMs associated with these relationships.

The conclusion that different attachment measures do not necessarily share considerable common variance is consequential, however, for at least two reasons. First, conclusions concerning some issues that are central to attachment theory, such as stability and change in the security of attachment (Topic 4) and the continuing influence of early attachment (Topic 5), both discussed in more depth below, must be qualified by the particular measure(s) of attachment on which research conclusions are based. As we note in our discussion of stability and change, for example, the strongest conclusions concerning the consistency of attachment across relationships and time are those that are based on the same attachment measure assessing the same relationships (or the same type of relationship) on each measurement occasion. Second, different measures of attachment are also likely to have somewhat different correlates because they capture different (as well as common) sources of variance. Taken together, generalizations across different measures about the nature of attachment security must be made cautiously.

In light of this, how should attachment researchers decide on their measurement approach? One answer is that it depends on which aspects of attachment functioning are of greatest interest. Priming is an obvious example of a methodology uniquely suited to eliciting secure or insecure representations, but priming may not be as useful to those who are interested in a person's characteristic attachment orientation, and it is not suitable for studying infants and young children. Representational measures differ in the depth of their assessment, ranging from self-reports to script methodology to interview protocols designed to "surprise the unconscious" (Main & Goldwyn, 1984). Moreover, measures of attachment differ in whether they are designed to assess partner-specific attachment functioning or a person's generalized attachment orientation. Crowell's conclusion concerning the AAI and the ECR—that these are different measures and do not predict the same outcomes in the same ways— generalizes to the full range of attachment assessments.

A broader answer is that the psychometric characteristics of attachment measures should guide researchers' choices. As Raby and colleagues note, dimensional approaches have advantages over the traditional categorical orientation of developmental attachment research because they maximize variance and enable enhanced statistical power. On this basis, citing the field's "reliance on evidence drawn from underpowered studies," Roisman and Groh urge a revisiting of fundamental methodological commitments such as the categorical classification system. At the same time, while acknowledging the psychometric benefits of dimensional measures, Steele and Steele argue, consistent with the organizational view (Sroufe & Waters, 1977), that differences in attachment are fundamentally differences in quality rather than quantity along some dimension. To illustrate, they point to infant disorganization and adult unresolved loss and trauma, which are not easily captured by current dimensional approaches. According to them, a categorical approach will always be part of thinking about variation in attachment. An important subtext to this colloquy is the question of whether attachment studies are primarily modeling typical variations or clinically relevant variations in attachment functioning because, for the latter, variability in the origins and consequences of attachment organization is especially multidimensional and complex. Thus here, again, the choice of measurement strategy may depend on the goals of study.

An additional appeal to the use of dimensional measures of attachment is that they permit comparability of measurement across different stages of life by establishing a two-factor structure to variability in attachment—one dimension tapping attachment anxiety and a second dimension tapping attachment avoidance—from infancy through adulthood. However, Waters's script methodology can also be used across a wide developmental range. He proposes that secure base scripts develop through dual processes of elaboration and generalization, with the result that early individual differences in secure base script knowledge are categorical in nature (secure vs. insecure), but then develop into more continuous dimensions (reflecting different degrees of security). Testing this view in future research will help inform the largest issue raised collectively by the chapters of this book: the need for a model outlining how IWMs develop and change across the life course. In addition, we urge attachment researchers to make more explicit the theoretical assumptions underlying the design and use of attachment measures. These assumptions are central to how measures are designed and interpreted and should be of fundamental importance to attachment researchers.

The Nature and Function of IWMs

We asked the authors of chapters for this section to consider these key questions: *What are internal working models?* and *How do they operate?* Our goal was to determine whether there are common elements to diverse conceptualizations that might lead us toward a more theoretically consistent portrayal of working models. Doing so could help us identify the most interesting and important issues that could inform a lifespan understanding of IWMs.

The five chapters on this topic—as well as other chapters in the volume—attest to the diverse portrayals of IWMs in attachment theory. According to some views (e.g., Waters, Waters, & Waters), IWMs are representations that are generalized across a person's experience of relationships, whereas to others (e.g., Girme & Overall), IWMs are relationship-specific and hierarchically organized. Shaver and Mikulincer refer to "a person's network of attachment-related memories and working models," and Gillath and Ai describe how this characterization is enlisted into priming methods in adult attachment research. To Cassidy, IWMs develop primarily to ensure safety in the context of threat, whereas Thompson emphasizes much broader functions of IWMs for self-understanding and relational interactions. Some descriptions of IWMs connect their development to other cognitive and social-cognitive processes, particularly cognitive scripts (Waters et al.; Cassidy) and autobiographical memory and emotion understanding (Oppenheim & Koren-Karie; Thompson), but others do not. There is also variability in whether IWMs are viewed as functioning primarily in a nonconscious or preconscious manner (Cassidy; Dykas & Cassidy, 2011; Oppenheim & Koren-Karie) or as operating primarily consciously to influence social information processing (Thompson).

Are all these attachment researchers referencing the same construct? As noted in several chapters, Bowlby's concept of the IWM was not well developed, leaving considerable uncertainty concerning his views of its defining characteristics, development, and proneness to stability over time. With researchers drawing on different aspects of Bowlby's theory to flesh out a portrayal of IWMs suitable to their work, it is easy to see how one's conception of mental working models can be much different from another's (Duschinsky et al., in press).

We might ask, therefore, what features each of these different formulations hold in common. Three come to mind. First, attachment researchers agree that IWMs arise from relationships with attachment figures and guide interactions with them. Furthermore, mental representations concerning an attachment figure's (1) availability as a secure base for exploration and (2) safe haven when threatened are prominent in working models based on attachment relationships, with some adding to these (3) mental representations of the attachment figure's proximity. Throughout life, these seem to be core elements of how individuals represent what they can expect from their attachment figures. Although attachment relationships extend representationally beyond these core features and IWMs are likely to become more complex, these features of IWMs are fundamental.

Second, attachment researchers agree that IWMs change developmentally and with relational experience. This is not an inconsequential consensus. Bowlby's concept of mental working models draws on object relations theory and the Freudian dynamic unconscious. Thus, one aspect of his IWM construct is a very early developing, prelinguistic perceptual-affective representation of caregiving experience that remains influential throughout life (Grossmann, 1999). But Bowlby also recognized the changes that occur in working models with the development of language, conceptual growth, and experience. This recognition has predominated in attachment theory. In his chapter for Topic 2, Waters elaborates this view to argue that Bowlby's concept is that IWMs "contain multiple constructs that unfold in a particular developmental sequence, change in latent structure, and undergo extensive generalization and elaboration across development." A number of chapters describing developmental changes in IWMs (Allen; Ahnert; Thompson) and the evolution of IWMs based on relational experience (Fraley & Dugan; Arriaga & Kumashiro; Girme & Overall) attest to this dynamic quality.

Thus, in our view, one of the most interesting and important issues for further study concerns the multifaceted ways that relational experiences influence growth and change in IWMs. Some researchers emphasize the content and quality of parent–child discourse on developing IWMs (Bretherton & Munholland, 2016; Oppenheim & Koren-Karie; Thompson), while others underscore how new relational experiences lead to the creation, consolidation, or revision of working models (Paetzold, Rholes, & George; Arriaga & Kumashiro; Girme & Overall), and there are other views (e.g., Kerns & Brumariu, 2016). These perspectives would benefit from greater cross-fertilization, especially as they contribute to conceptually unpacking the influence of relational experiences on attachment-related mental representations. One of several themes cutting across the literature as well as many of the chapters in the book is that different communication patterns and/or attachment "strategies" (e.g., Main, 1990) characterize secure and insecure attachments, particularly in terms of their development (Cassidy; Thompson), in the way people respond to loss (Shaver & Mikulincer), and in adult-based psychotherapeutic processes (Talia & Holmes). Also meriting further reflection are the interrelated questions of (1) how other aspects of the relationships that individuals share with their attachment figures (Fearon & Schuengel), especially those not associated with secure base and safe haven functions, affect attachment-related IWMs and (2) the potential impact of additional relational but nonattachment working models (e.g., Knee & Petty, 2013).

Third, attachment researchers agree that IWMs underlie a range of social, personality, and relational characteristics. They disagree, however, regarding the breadth of these associations—or, more specifically, on the breadth of characteristics associated with attachment that can be attributed to the influence of IWMs. This has led to some of the more serious criticisms of the IWM construct, including Hinde's (1988) concern that IWMs can "too easily explain anything" and Belsky and Cassidy's (1994) charge that IWMs constitute a "catch-all, post-hoc explanation" for any research finding linking attachment to other behavior. As research evidence documents a wider variety of external correlates of attachment, the IWM construct has consequently also expanded to "explain" these associations.

It is important to recognize, therefore, that there are many ways that attachment may be associated with other behaviors, independently of the functioning of IWMs. Chapters in this volume draw attention, for example, to the influences of attachment on physical health (Ehrlich & Cassidy), developing neurobiology (van IJzendoorn, Tharner, & Bakermans-Kranenburg), and the effects of environmental challenge and stress (Szepsenwol & Simpson). Harsh or supportive parental relationships that shape attachment may also contribute to other characteristics of individuals (e.g., self-esteem), and attachment security may moderate the effects of these relational influences (e.g., Kochanska & Kim, 2012). Attachment relationships may also foster a range of capabilities—social skills, sense of efficacy, cognitive competencies, self-regulation—that influence behavior independently of working models. In this light, a recommendation for the future is that, whenever IWMs are enlisted to explain empirical findings, researchers should specify precisely the aspect or understanding of IWMs that forms the basis of their explanation.

Consideration of the multiple avenues through which attachment can be influential suggests that understanding the association of IWMs with other social and personality characteristics requires not only a clear theoretical conceptualization of IWMs, but also the consideration of alternative explanations. For example, a direct association between the security of attachment and reading achievement in children could be construed as reflecting a secure IWM of the self, but researchers must also measure alternative mediators—such as parent involvement with schoolwork and positive child–teacher relationships—that are consistent with attachment theory and may be influential independently of IWMs (Sroufe, Egeland, Carlson, & Collins, 2005). It is easy to enlist IWMs as explanations of attachment-related behavior because they are usually unmeasured and thus flexible in application. We applaud the fact that studies of attachment outcomes are increasingly examining not only the direct associations of attachment with other behaviors, but also carefully conceptualized and measured mediators and moderators of their association (Thompson, 2016).

Including direct measures of IWMs in the research design would, of course, permit examination of their mediating influence most effectively.

One reason why some contemporary attachment researchers are drawn so strongly to script theory is that it presents a straightforward way of measuring cognitive processes related to IWMs. However, the usefulness of these and other emergent measures depends on their association with a well-developed model of IWMs that specifies the inclusive and exclusive features of the construct being measured (see Waters, Waters, & Waters). Thus, the development of theory and measurement of IWMs must proceed in concert.

Finally, we draw attention to another cross-cutting theme concerning developmental change in attachment and the IWMs with which it is associated. Many social/personality attachment scholars believe that, compared to young children, adults possess a more extensive network of working models that reflect the unique types of attachment relationships they have experienced across life (Fraley, 2019; Girme & Overall). This raises the possibility that specific working models within adults' more elaborate cognitive networks might become activated and guide their behavior in response to different attachment-relevant cues, events, or situations in adulthood. One major gap in the attachment literature involves understanding when (i.e., in response to what kinds of cues, events, or situations) certain types of working models uniquely predict certain attachment-relevant outcomes. For example, despite the fact that the AAI measures representations of how a person was treated by their parents during childhood—rather than how they have been treated by their romantic partners—greater security on the AAI uniquely predicts the quality of support that adults give to their romantic partners in stressful situations (e.g., Simpson, Rholes, Oriña, & Grich, 2002). In less stressful contexts, however, adult romantic attachment measures are stronger predictors than the AAI of different attachment-relevant outcomes, such as overall marital satisfaction and the quality of daily relationship functioning (Feeney, 2016; Mikulincer & Shaver, 2016). These findings suggest that adults possess a richer and more differentiated network of working models that reflect different types of attachment relationships forged at different developmental periods. Understanding the developmental processes leading to this, given that multiple attachments are typical for children, and their implications for the functioning of IWMs, is a major task for the future. We return to this theme at the end of the chapter.

Stability and Change in the Security of Attachment

Bowlby (1979, 1980) viewed both stability and change in attachment patterns (in children) and orientations (in adults) as basic processes that depended on continuity or changes in a person's environment, particularly their interactions with attachment figures. According to Bowlby, assimilation processes sustain attachment patterns/orientations, whereas accommodation processes allow them to change, primarily when new, significant interpersonal experiences or events contradict existing working models.

The five authors in this section of the book addressed two questions: *Should we expect attachment security to remain consistent over time?* and *Is there evidence for stability in attachment security?* Fraley and Dugan discuss how Bowlby and other attachment theorists conceptualize stability and change in attachment, the reasons why it is often difficult to draw clear inferences about attachment stability across social development and time, and what the best current evidence reveals. Booth-LaForce and Roisman focus on the key factors and variables that prospectively predict stability as well as change in attachment patterns/orientations from childhood into adulthood. Allen points out the numerous ways in which adolescents differ from young children, which challenges the search for patterns of continuity anticipated by attachment theory. Paetzold, Rholes, and George review recent research on the stability and change of adult romantic attachment orientations (i.e., anxiety and avoidance) during chronically stressful life events and discuss how stochastic models, which forecast the probability of various outcomes under different conditions using random variables, might shed light on when people's attachment orientations change or remain stable. Arriaga and Kumashiro review a new model—the attachment security enhancement model (Arriaga, Kumashiro, Simpson, & Overall, 2018)—which outlines ways in which romantic partners can help their insecure partners become less anxious or less avoidant, including the specific types of experiences that ought to induce change toward greater security.

Several basic themes run through these chapters. One involves the many challenges of attempting to document stability (or "continuity," as Allen prefers) versus change in attachment across development and over time. As several authors emphasize, secure and insecure working models as well as emotional and behavioral tendencies are manifest in different ways at different points of development, especially between birth and late adolescence (Allen). In addition, different attachment measures have been used to assess attachment security at different ages leading into adulthood, even when the quality of attachment to the same attachment figure (e.g., one's mother or father) is assessed. Moreover, determining the degree of stability in different types of attachment relationships (e.g., with one's parents, close friends, romantic partners) involves not only modeling different measures that often use different methods (e.g., behavioral observations, interviews, self-report, parent-report, or partner-report questionnaires), but also different attachment targets, which attenuates stability/continuity estimates (see Fraley & Dugan). Thus, it is fairly impressive that *any* systematic links—even rather weak ones—have been found between measures of early security with, or quality of caregiving from, parents and attachment patterns/orientations later in adulthood (see Booth-LaForce & Roisman). Not surprisingly, as we noted earlier, the best estimates of stability come from studies in which the same attachment assessment is used on more than one occasion with the same attachment figure.

Another major theme surrounds the relative emphasis on prototype versus revisionist views of attachment (Fraley & Dugan), which relates to the need for a lifespan model of how IWMs develop and change. Inspired by Bowlby, who was influenced by both psychoanalytic and ethological views of the enduring importance of early relationships, many developmental and clinical attachment scholars are influenced by the prototype hypothesis—the notion that early relationships with primary caregivers formatively shape how people think, feel, and behave in their later attachment relationships, including those that serve different functions than parent–child relationships, such as relationships with close friends and romantic partners. While there clearly are reliable empirical associations between early and later attachment patterns and behaviors, these effects tend to be small. Moreover, based both on Bowlby's (1973) discussions of developmental canalization and on contemporary life history theory (Del Giudice, Gangestad, & Kaplan, 2016; Simpson & Belsky, 2016), it makes sense for individuals to be influenced by adult experiences when determining whether they can or cannot form a secure relationship with new attachment figures. Recent empirical evidence indicates that adult attachment orientations change in systematic, predictable ways (Arriaga & Kumashiro; Fraley & Dugan; Paetzold et al.), such as when adults are chronically stressed or enter new life roles and either their own actions or their partner's actions strongly conflict with (i.e., counteract) their current working models.

The chapters in this section also draw attention to different patterns of stability and change. For example, children, adolescents, and adults can (1) remain stable in their attachment patterns/orientations across time, (2) change from being insecure to secure, or (3) change from being secure to insecure. Different factors/variables might be associated with each of these patterns of stability or change, and we are just beginning to learn from large, prospective studies which influences seem to promote stability or change in attachment. Reviewing findings from prospective studies involving children, Booth-LaForce and Roisman note that early maternal sensitivity and father presence are two salient variables that predict child security as well as its maintenance across time. Reviewing findings from studies of adults exposed to chronic stress, Paetzold and colleagues note that people who seek or give greater support to their romantic partners become less avoidant over time, whereas those who receive less support or more anger from their partners become more anxious. One core principle that underlies these findings is that people tend to maintain their current attachment orientations unless they have significant attachment-relevant experiences that strongly contradict their working models, which in turn launch accommodation processes (Arriaga & Kumashiro; Girme & Overall; Paetzold et al.).

The authors of this section also propose several important questions for future research on stability and change in attachment. For example, what are the specific conditions under which attachment security and insecurity change? Do people have to experience chronic stressors or enter new life roles for long-term changes to occur? How strongly must earlier and later measures of attachment be associated in order to support theoretical expectations of developmental continuity? How is attachment stability related to consistency and variation in IWMs? Do children and adults move with equal probability from one attachment pattern or orientation to another? Put another way, is it less likely that security or insecurity will change over time? Are some children or adults simply unable to move from one orientation to another due to specific traumatic experiences (e.g., maltreatment, betrayal, or chronic neglect)? Are there some conditions or experiences that help formerly insecure people to remain secure for longer periods of time and/or across different contexts?

Finally, and especially relevant to the lifespan development of IWMs, are the origins of attachment security (vs. insecurity) the same for children (in the context of child–parent relationships) as they are for adults (in the context of romantic pair bonds)? Might the primary sources of attachment security in early childhood, such as the quality of care received, be different than the primary sources of security in adulthood? For instance, could certain pivotal events that take place *after* a person enters a new type of attachment relationship—such as exposure to high levels of life stress, betrayal, or romantic partners who are undependable or unresponsive—mold adult attachment orientations with respect to that type of relationship? Answers to these intriguing questions await the next generation of attachment scholars.

The Continuing Influence of Early Attachment

Among attachment theory's most compelling questions are those pertaining to the enduring influence of early attachment quality on subsequent human development. The chapters that addressed this topic responded to these specific prompts: *What domains of later behavior should early attachment relationships predict, and why? For what domains should we not expect an association with early security?* and *What are, in other words, the boundary conditions for the influence of early attachment?* Three chapters (Roisman & Groh; van IJzendoorn et al.; Ehrlich & Cassidy) focus on the associations between early attachment and specific developmental outcomes, whereas one chapter (Mikulincer & Shaver) focuses predominantly on adult attachment orientations (assessed dimensionally) and one chapter (Szepsenwol & Simpson) examines the influence of attachment in the context of life-history theory.

Roisman and Groh's historical perspective emphasizes that more recent, large-scale and/or meta-analytic studies may require reevaluating earlier conclusions about the influence of early attachment quality along with the approaches used to analyze such effects. In particular, they characterize meta-analytic evidence linking early attachment security with greater social competence and fewer behavior problem symptoms as "modest." Interestingly, the age at which outcomes were assessed did not significantly moderate these effects, suggesting that attachment security may exert equally strong effects on early and later (e.g., adolescent) development. Roisman and Groh also illustrate attachment disorganization as the insecure category most strongly predictive of externalizing symptoms. Citing among other concerns that indicators of attachment disorganization and insecure-ambivalence/resistance load onto a common latent factor, they argue for increased use of continuous (instead of categorical) measures of individual differences in attachment (see also Raby et al.).

Both van IJzendoorn and colleagues and Ehrlich and Cassidy discuss the influence of early attachment in two more recently explored areas: brain development and physical health. Van IJzendoorn and coauthors describe associations between attachment disorganization and precociously early developing hippocampal volume (Cortes Hidalgo et al., 2019). They also describe evidence of associations between early parental sensitivity and insensitivity and childhood outcomes, such as brain volume and cortical thickness of the precentral frontal gyri, a brain area thought to be related to the development of empathy (Kok et al., 2015). Given the importance of empathy to peer relationships, these findings raise the question of whether the effects of early caregiving on brain development may underlie the effects of attachment quality on social competence discussed by Roisman and Groh.

In a similar vein, Ehrlich and Cassidy provide striking descriptions of associations between early attachment and both childhood and adult physical health. Their discussion raises questions about the interplay among attachment-related health and socioemotional outcomes. For example, could attachment-sensitive aspects of children's physical wellness affect the extent to which they participate more fully in activities that, in turn, promote the development of social skills and friendships? Another possibility discussed by Ehrlich and Cassidy is that attachment security affects individuals' stress regulation and health-promotive behaviors, which in turn affect health outcomes. Finally, in considering boundary conditions pertaining to attachment influences, both van IJzendoorn and colleagues and Ehrlich and Cassidy acknowledge the role of genetic predispositions that may interact with attachment experiences in ways that might both attenuate and intensify their effects.

Mikulincer and Shaver discuss a large body of evidence showing that adults' attachment orientations are not only forged in early caregiving experiences, but also are predictive of their functioning in three life domains: (1) close relationships, (2) emotion regulation and mental health, and (3) other behavioral systems, such as learning. They note that experiences in each of these life domains can also affect—and change—attachment orientations in adults. Thus, bidirectional associations between attachment and other developmental phenomena are important to acknowledge and assess.

Szepsenwol and Simpson argue that evidence of the influence of early attachment on (1) mating strategies, (2) parenting attitudes and behavior, (3) pubertal timing, and (4) health reflect multiply mediated pathways in a causal chain linking early caregiving to reproductive fitness outcomes. They also carefully exclude attachment-related outcomes that are not relevant to reproductive fitness. Rather, they link early attachment security to a "slow" life-history strategy defined by delayed puberty, a longer-term mating strategy, higher parental investment, and a longer, healthier life. A conversely "fast" life-history strategy enacted in response to a harsh early environment may help to explain precocious developmental phenomena such as the association between attachment disorganization and hippocampal volume described by van IJzendoorn and colleagues.

Mikulincer and Shaver provide important theoretical context for considering the cross-cutting issues raised by this group of chapters. They emphasize that individuals' attachment representations evolve in response to early *and* later attachment experiences, reflecting both early prototypes and later relational inputs. In this regard, similar to the evidence of stability in attachment patterns, it is impressive that there are, in aggregate, even "modest" links between early attachment patterns and important socioemotional outcomes. At the same time, again paralleling our preceding discussion of stability, we recognize the need for the field to define precisely the strength of the evidence necessary to demonstrate a theoretically meaningful effect of early attachment on later behavior. Complicating this issue is that many studies of the influence of early attachment loosely interchange predictions from attachment quality with predictions from its major precursor, parental sensitivity. The question thus arises as to when the effects of attachment are due "just" to prior or concurrent parenting and when they reflect a unique contribution of attachment quality per se (Fearon & Roisman, 2017). Studies of the outcomes of early attachment should attend rigorously to both influences (e.g., Raikes & Thompson, 2008) but rarely do. Another complication is that in some domains (e.g., brain development), attachment organization/

disorganization is a stronger predictor than attachment security/insecurity. Recognizing that developmental outcomes derive from a complex combination of predictors among which early attachment is only one, it is incumbent on attachment researchers to seriously consider, from carefully designed studies, the strength of the influence derived from attachment quality in relation to theoretical expectations concerning its formative effects.

On a related note, as discussed above, individual differences in attachment can be conceptualized and measured categorically, dimensionally, or in terms of attachment strategies (i.e., hyperactivating or "maximizing," and deactivating or "minimizing" strategies; Szepsenwol & Simpson; Main, 1990). Reconciling which approach(es) might be best suited for which research question(s) could help clarify the influence of early attachment patterns. Finally, it is important to define precisely not only which developmental phenomena are expected to derive from early attachment, but also which are considered adaptive both in the short term and long term. An improved understanding of the influence of early attachment can then be applied to services and systems for children and families with a long-term goal of promoting not only reproductive fitness, but also physical and mental health, writ large.

Culture and Attachment

Attachment theory and culture have been connected from the time of Ainsworth's (1967) pioneering studies in Uganda, but their association is complex. Bowlby's (1969/1982) theory described attachment in terms of evolutionarily adaptive processes that he believed were universal for humans. Although Bowlby's adaptational model has been critiqued and updated (Simpson & Belsky, 2016), the view that inclusive fitness requires species-typical behavioral adaptations has remained. But when it comes to understanding specifically what those behavioral adaptations constitute, critics from outside and within the attachment community have questioned the importance of caregiver sensitivity, the centrality of emotional security, and the model of caregiver–child interaction in which these processes occur. Thus, as attachment researchers widen the scope of their studies to encompass more diverse cultural contexts, the gulf between them and culturally oriented developmental researchers seems to widen.

The four chapters in this section exemplify this gulf, but also suggest potential ways of bridging it. The authors were asked to consider *How are attachment processes manifested in different cultures?* and *How does culture manifest itself in attachment processes?* Keller's chapter illustrates many of the criticisms of cultural researchers in arguing that (1) attachment researchers assume a specific type of caregiver–child relationship that is inapplicable to a large variety of cultural settings involving group care, (2) the methods of attachment research are relevant primarily to the experience of Western middle-class families and are less applicable to families in low- and middle-income agrarian communities, and (3) evolutionarily adaptive processes are context-sensitive and thus are not necessarily behaviorally universal. Keller also argues that attachment ideas have sometimes led to harmful interventions when applied to the practices of families from non-Western cultures. Morelli and Lu provide substantive illustrations of Keller's points from their observations of the cooperative social networks of early care by the Efe. As they describe, young children (as well as adults) "nimbly manage" these relational networks based on children's expectations concerning the solicitude of those who care for them because the child's survival depends on the continued reliability of others' care. Thus the biobehavioral synchrony of affect and behavior underlying attachment within the Efe is, in this view, a group rather than dyadic phenomenon.

In response to views like these, Mesman calls for greater modesty by attachment researchers in their claims about cross-cultural validity, urging their greater willingness to entertain uncomfortable questions arising from research findings, as well as resistance to the confirmation bias that can beset theory-driven researchers. Mesman goes as far as encouraging attachment scholars to search for the "black swans" in findings—those that would pose a genuine challenge to the theory. As the primary author of the chapter on culture in the most recent edition of the *Handbook of Attachment* (Mesman, van IJzendoorn, & Sagi-Schwartz, 2016), Mesman qualifies the conclusion of that review—that attachment theory can claim cross-cultural validity—by indicating that more difficult questions need to be asked before cross-cultural validity can be asserted.

In considering how the field can move forward, we begin by observing that there is considerable agreement on many issues between attachment researchers and their cultural critics. All agree that early relationships are important to children's survival and development. Most agree with Morelli and Lu that children form attachment relationships in all but the harshest circumstances, although other relationships are also developmentally important. As the first section of this book illustrates, attachment researchers have moved considerably beyond their early focus on maternal care to recognize, and study, the close relationships that young children develop with multiple caregivers (e.g., Ahnert and contributors to Topic 9). With respect to the sensitivity construct, Mesman and her colleagues (2017) have shown that when sensitivity is measured in a manner that provides latitude for culturally specific manifestations, sensitive responsiveness is observed in a range of low- and middle-income agrarian communities, although this conclusion has been disputed (Keller et al., 2018). Finally, when Morelli and Lu describe how Efe infants learn to manage their changing relational networks to obtain what they need given variability in the reliability and responsiveness of their adult caregivers, developing attachments to those they have learned to trust—especially when caregivers help to regulate infant distress and hunger—the process sounds similar to the influence of IWMs in attachment theory. Thus, the claims of attachment researchers and those who study development in the context of culture have more in common than some have suggested.

The Morelli and Lu findings also illustrate, however, that new questions should guide future studies to achieve a deeper understanding and intermingling of attachment and culture research. The challenge of defining what constitute attachment relationships (Topic 1) arises again: How do we determine which people in a young child's relational network are—or become—attachment figures? Meehan and Hawks (2013) documented that children in the Aka in the Congo Basin Rain Forest were cared for by more than 20 different people each day, as Mesman notes. But when they examined the children's differential display of attachment behaviors (such as proximity- and contact-seeking) toward these adults, the number of attachment figures thus identified was a much smaller subset of their relational network. Identifying the range of care providers, in other words, does not necessarily identify the number of attachment figures from the child's perspective. This observation illustrates that the gap between the questions posed by attachment researchers and the inquiries of culturally oriented developmentalists can be quite different, resulting in research findings that are not as mutually informative as they could be. As Thompson (2017, p. 318; original emphasis) wryly observed, "While culturally oriented researchers ask for greater *culturally informed attachment research,* attachment researchers sometimes wonder where they can find greater *attachment-informed cultural studies.*" Advancing research that more deeply integrates the questions posed by researchers in each community of scholars will also require methodological innovation that can benefit each field, such as considering the sensitivity of care at a group rather than a dyadic level (Morelli; Ahnert).

It may also be true that reframing the issue of culture and attachment is necessary. Establishing or refuting universality claims can become sterile and uninformative disputes over evidence. By contrast, the kinds of questions that might inspire more productive future thinking may need to consider Chisholm's claim that "no manifestation of culture could long exist that failed to meet infants' innate mammalian attachment needs." As Bowlby (1969/1982) originally proposed, we should ask how each culture solves the problem that *all* cultures must universally address: how to ensure that young survive to reproductive maturity and that their offspring do also (Thompson, 2020). Cultures must ensure infant survival to be viable, but how they accomplish this can encompass different normative practices of early care, different numbers of caregivers, different resources, different developmental goals for offspring, and so forth. What cultures *cannot* do is chronically ignore infant needs, regularly expose them to danger, or render them incapable of developing competencies relevant to their adult functioning. Viewed in this light, attachment is one of the universal developmental tasks that cultures must address (Keller & Kärtner, 2013). How they do so in diverse cultural contexts—and what practices they share in common—is a fundamental question that needs to be answered. The view that *we cannot understand attachment apart from an appreciation of culture* might offer new, provocative ways of understanding diverse human solutions to this universal cultural problem.

Chisholm's chapter provides an alternative reframing of the issue of culture and attachment by drawing on the "deep history" movement to propose that attachment both permeates and constrains culture. In this view, attachment is the evolved foundation for human fealty (or "we-ness") of all kinds, ranging from caregiving relationships to pair bonds to political allegiances. Viewed in this light, *we cannot understand culture apart from an appreciation of attachment.* Moreover, a view of attachment in this manner might contribute to a broader view of the influence of attachment in contemporary culture, focusing more attention on the significance of early relationships and the quality of care, and less attention (as Keller urges) on whether the specific constellation of caregiving relationships is consistent with the norms of one society or another. In this respect, the best applications of attachment theory and research to intervention, as illustrated by the contributions to Topics 8 and 9, are those that embrace the aspects of early relationships shared by different cultural systems, and, in so doing, enlist members of these cultural systems to help define and support appropriate patterns of care.

Separation and Loss

Separation (Bowlby, 1973) and loss (Bowlby, 1980) are twin pillars of attachment theory. Moreover, as Shaver and Mikulincer note, the sheer intensity of reactions to the separation or loss of an attachment figure provides some of the clearest evidence for the unquestionable power of attachment processes. Bowlby (1969/1982) began to realize that he was studying an important, evolved behavioral system when he observed the same basic sequence of reactions to separation and loss of attachment figures—protest, despair, detachment, and eventual reorganization (Bowlby, 1979)—in multiple species. Indeed, from an evolutionary standpoint, each stage of this sequence is an adaptive response to a "lost" attachment figure (Simpson & Belsky, 2016).

The authors for this section of the book were asked to address two questions: *How do people respond to the loss of an attachment figure?* and *What are the key processes and mechanisms involved?* They focus on different forms of separation and loss, ranging from the child's traumatic loss of a primary caregiver (Chu & Lieberman), to the breakup of romantic (Sbarra & Manvelian) and marital (Feeney & Monin) relationships, to normal (Shaver & Mikulincer) as well as pathological bereavement (Maccallum) in adults. Each chapter, in other words, addresses fundamental attachment processes associated with separation and loss at different stages of life and within different types of relationships, typically considering the attachment patterns/orientations of the bereaved person.

Chu and Lieberman focus on traumatic bereavement in young children following the prolonged separation or loss of their primary caregivers. Shaver and Mikulincer discuss the role of attachment hyperactivation and deactivation processes in normal as well as pathological grief and mourning. Sbarra and Manvelian review the psychological and biological ties that bind romantic partners together, focusing on various coregulation processes. Feeney and Monin address how the process and outcomes of divorce can be understood from an attachment perspective, emphasizing the persistence of attachment bonds that often remain following divorce. Maccallum examines how attachment theory informs our understanding of normal and especially pathological mourning processes, primarily in long-term romantic relationships.

Some prominent themes run across most or all of the chapters in this section. One salient theme is that variation in how people respond to separation and loss in relation to attachment has been well documented in adults, but less so in young children (see Chu & Lieberman). This disparity could be attributable to the extremity of loss to young children: (1) the severity of physical and psychological threat that young children experience when they lose a parent compared to when adults lose a romantic partner, (2) the "suddenness" with which separation or loss occurs in the minds of young children compared to adults, (3) the cognitive inability of young children to understand and make sense of why separation and loss has occurred, and (4) the fact that young children do not have the same knowledge, skills, or ability to find suitable replacement attachment figures as many adults do. Nevertheless, some variation in responses to separation and loss in relation to attachment does exist in young children beyond infancy, which remains a domain ripe for future inquiry.

Another salient theme highlighted by these chapters concerns detachment and reorganization processes (Bowlby, 1979). Neither construct has received sufficient theoretical or empirical attention, particularly given the paramount roles they assume in affecting grief and mourning outcomes. Moreover, this is an area within attachment theory where a fundamental normative (species-typical) process intersects with attachment-based individual differences to shape how grief and mourning unfold following separation or loss, especially in adults.

As highlighted by several authors, most notably Shaver and Miku-lincer, separation and loss activate attachment hyperactivation processes (also called a "maximizing" attachment strategy; Main, 1990) in children and adults, which are manifested in protest behaviors designed to literally or figuratively "retrieve" the lost attachment figure. If/when protest fails to accomplish this, attachment deactivation processes (a "minimizing" attachment strategy; Main, 1990) typically become manifested in detach-ment, which according to Bowlby (1979) helps individuals lessen or relin-quish the emotional bonds with their former attachment figure in order to facilitate the formation of subsequent attachment relationships. In other words, these two strategies, which are associated with anxious and avoidant attachment patterns/orientations in children and adults, tend to facilitate successful movement through the normative stages of grief en route to attachment reorganization following the loss of an attachment figure. When individuals stall or fail to progress through each of the grief stages, however, disordered mourning in the form of complicated grief (associated with dominating hyperactivation processes) or delayed grief (associated with dominating deactivation processes) can occur, as Mac-callum discusses. Moreover, as Feeney and Monin note, divorce can com-plicate movement through the normal stages of grief because divorced partners—many of whom remain in contact with each other due to joint child custody—frequently find it difficult to detach fully from their ex-partners.

A third cross-cutting theme involves whether the absence of grieving in adults reflects the true absence of distress versus a defensive reaction driven by chronic attachment deactivation processes. Some adults experi-ence little if any grief following the loss of a primary attachment figure, perhaps because their lost relationship did not meet their attachment needs, they "detached" emotionally from their former partners before the actual loss, they had alternative attachment figures who stepped in quickly either before or immediately following the loss, or they have social networks capable of meeting most of their key attachment needs. Further-more, some people may be buffered from experiencing intense distress following partner loss because they have positive (secure) IWMs or weaker needs for proximity, safe haven, or secure base contact with attachment figures. More needs to be understood about individuals who experience minimal distress or recover very quickly following the loss of an attach-ment figure; not all of them are likely to exhibit "defensive repression," which might produce pathological mourning.

Most importantly, the authors who addressed separation and loss raise several thoughtful questions for future research, such as the fol-lowing: (1) Similar to adults, does the preexisting quality of the attach-ment between a young child and their primary caregiver(s) predict the child's response to and recovery from separation and loss? (2) How does attachment reorganization occur, how are attachment functions transferred from the deceased partner to new attachment figures, and what role do memories of the deceased partner serve in promoting attachment security versus insecurity? (3) How do attachment hyperactivation and deactivation contribute to the attachment reorganization process? Do hyperactivation processes allow individuals to retain the meaning and importance of their lost relationship and maintain a symbolic bond with the departed person? Do deactivation processes allow individuals to detach more easily from their former partner and keep painful thoughts, memories, and feelings associated with their prior relationship at bay? What factors ensure a successful balance between hyperactivation and deactivation processes as people move through the stages of grief and mourning? (4) How do repeated losses of attachment figures (e.g., parents, close friends, siblings) across the life course influence how people react when their adult romantic relationships end due to separation or death of a partner? and (5) Are attachment patterns (in children) and attachment orientations (in adults) prospectively related to prolonged grief disorder? If so, what are the mechanisms that explain these connections? We look forward to the next generation of attachment scholars responding to these critical questions.

Attachment-Based Interventions

Bowlby based attachment theory in part on his experience as a clinician, making it somewhat ironic that the systematic design and evaluation of attachment-based interventions emerged relatively late in the development of the attachment field as a whole, beginning in the late 1980s (e.g., Barnett, Blignault, Holmes, Payne, & Parker, 1987; Lieberman, Weston, & Pawl, 1991). At the same time, foundational research defining the nature of attachment security and its strongest precursor, parental sensitivity, laid necessary groundwork for attachment-based interventions by portending key intervention targets and processes. Thirty years later, it is fair to say that attachment-based interventions have "caught up," not only demonstrating impressive positive effects for both children and adults (Steele & Steele, 2018), but also raising questions important to refining attachment theory itself.

The five chapters on attachment-based interventions addressed two interrelated questions: *How do attachment-based interventions work?* and *What are the key processes and mechanisms involved?* Three chapters focus on attachment-based interventions for infants and young children (Bakermans-Kranenburg & Oosterman, Dozier & Bernard, and Toth, Alto, & Warmingham). Two chapters focus on attachment-based interventions for adults (Talia & Holmes and Johnson). As a whole, these chapters illustrate several characteristics common to both child- and adult-oriented interventions. The first is a relational focus such that "the patient is the relationship" (Lieberman & Van Horn, 2008). In this regard, attachment-based interventions for children target the quality of the developing child–parent attachment. Attachment-informed psychotherapeutic models for adults, of which Johnson's emotionally focused therapy is one, view psychological disorders as manifestations of "disruptions" in adults' capacities to trust themselves and others (Talia & Holmes), resulting in emotional isolation and helplessness (Johnson). Attachment-informed therapies are thus designed to provide corrective relational and emotional experiences that "reactivate" clients' abilities to trust both themselves and others.

A second common characteristic concerns an emphasis on the relationship between the interventionist or therapist and client(s) as a key engine of therapeutic change. This emphasis follows from Bowlby's (1988) explicit recommendations and from attachment research demonstrating the critical role of parental sensitivity in infant attachment quality (Fearon & Belsky, 2016). Child-oriented attachment-based interventions highlight the role of the interventionist as an engaged and empathic secure base from which a mother or father can safely explore new parenting behaviors. Likewise, in the context of attachment-based interventions for adults, the therapist provides a secure base from which an adult can consider new working models of self and other. In short, as Johnson notes, "the therapist emulates parenting behaviors associated with attachment security."

A third characteristic common to child and adult attachment-based interventions centers on their careful attention to *how* the intervention is delivered. For example, in Dozier's Attachment and Biobehavioral Catch-up (ABC) program, the chief indicator of intervention fidelity is the frequency and quality of parent coaches' "in-the-moment" comments that connect the parent's behaviors to the intervention's substantive foci. Similarly, Bakermans-Kranenburg and Oosterman delineate six deliberately employed strategies through which the VIPP-SD program may increase parental sensitivity (e.g., "focus on positive fragments"). Similarly, in the realm of attachment-informed psychotherapeutic models for adults, Talia and Holmes emphasize the therapist's meta-communication and Johnson identifies the therapist's discovery of emotional triggers and the depth of the client's emotional processing as a therapeutic linchpin. Many of these intervention processes have been fruitfully operationalized and tested, for example through Dozier and colleagues' analysis of parent coaches' in-the-moment comments (Caron, Bernard, & Dozier, 2018) and Talia and colleagues' (2017) Patient Attachment Coding System. Continued study of the most active ingredients of attachment-based interventions ought to improve their effectiveness and efficiency and facilitate deeper insights into central issues in attachment theory and research, such as the conditions that promote stability and change in attachment security and working models.

These chapters also suggest several important next steps for the design and evaluation of attachment-based interventions, three of which we highlight here. First, whereas both theory and research suggest that changes in maternal sensitivity mediate intervention effects on infant attachment, only a few studies have tested this mediated pathway. While their findings illustrate maternal sensitivity as an underlying driver of intervention effects, more studies are required. Ideally, such studies will include large samples and the measurement of mediators that take place *prior* to the measurement of outcomes so that the temporal precedence of the mediator is confirmed (Dozier & Bernard; Toth et al.). Another hypothesized but infrequently tested mediator is the parent's IWMs and/or reflective functioning. Further study of these proposed mediators will not only illuminate intervention mechanisms, but also help clarify the antecedents of attachment security and organization.

Second, whereas theory and research suggest that changes in attachment security mediate intervention effects on downstream child outcomes, there has been surprisingly little investigation into this mediated pathway. This is an area in which attachment-informed psychotherapeutic models for adults could provide guidance to attachment-based interventions for children. Specifically, in response to the "dire need" in the field of adult psychotherapy for "a coherent unifying vision of . . . what it means to be human," Johnson offers an attachment-informed definition of adult health that includes a sense of connection to others, a coherent inner world, and "full, flexible engagement with the world." To the extent that the developers and evaluators of early attachment-based interventions hypothesize and examine intervention effects beyond infant attachment security, it will be helpful to delineate specific expectations about exactly which downstream outcomes attachment-based interventions should and should *not* affect and why, as well as which longer-term outcomes might be best promoted directly, rather than indirectly via effects on attachment security. More precisely rendered findings can then be applied not only to improve the interventions but also to address the boundary conditions of the influence of early attachments on later developmental outcomes. Greater precision and standardization in outcomes at both conceptual and operational levels will also fuel a more unified and generative translation of early intervention research findings to U.S. child and family policies (Shonkoff, 2010).

Third, a fuller understanding of attachment-based interventions will require better explicating "what works for whom?" Future studies might build on the differential susceptibility model (Belsky & Pleuss, 2009), testing both parents' and children's susceptibility to attachment-based interventions (Bakermans-Kranenburg & Oosterman). Another valuable avenue would center on defining the ideal fit between the attachment orientation of an adult client and that of his or her therapist (Talia & Holmes).

We look forward to attachment researchers tackling these and other next steps in the design and evaluation of attachment-based interventions. Such efforts will, in turn, help illuminate the nature of attachment, writ large.

Attachment, Systems, and Services

Galvanized in part by attachment theory and research, supporting early child development has become an increasingly prominent goal of practitioners and policymakers. The six chapters on attachment, systems, and services addressed two questions: *How are attachment theory and research relevant to systems and services for children and families?* and *What lessons can we learn from these programs?* Together, these chapters illustrate how attachment theory and research have influenced the design, implementation, and evaluation of many policies, service systems, and programs for children and families. These include widely used services such as child care (Owen & Frosch) and early childhood education (Hamre & Williford), as well as more specialized systems, such as those serving children of separated and divorced parents (Lamb), those designed to protect children when their primary caregivers cannot (Manly, Smith, Toth, & Cicchetti; Zeanah & Dozier), and more preventive programs, such as home visiting (Berlin, West, & Jones Harden). Such services typically reflect a patchwork of federal mandates and state- and locally implemented initiatives. Whereas it can be advantageous for services to vary according to community characteristics and needs, it is also the case that inconsistencies in program implementation create confusion and compromise service quality. The chapters in this section of the book point to numerous ways in which attachment theory and research could be more rigorously applied in order to increase service consistency and quality.

In the domain of child care and early childhood education, attachment theory and research have focused attention on the importance of the quality of the relationships between young children and their caregivers and teachers, especially with respect to these adults' sensitive and supportive caregiving behaviors. Owen and Frosch argue that child care systems and services could be improved through greater consideration of (1) the relationships between child care providers and parents (i.e., "parent–caregiver partnerships") and (2) children's transitions between caregivers, especially in light of relatively high rates of staff turnover among child care providers (see also Ahnert). Both Owen and Frosch and Hamre and Williford encourage greater use of evidence-based curricula and interventions that target the quality of the caregiver–child or teacher–child relationship. Hamre and Williford also urge more widespread use of Quality Rating and Improvement Systems (QRISs), federally coordinated, and state-level initiatives to regulate the quality of preschools and related programs. Many QRISs to date have fruitfully employed the observational Classroom Assessment Scoring System (CLASS; Pianta, La Paro, & Hamre, 2008), which includes an assessment of teachers' emotional supportiveness, an important attachment-informed aspect of classroom quality. QRISs evaluate data and these evaluations are then systematically fed back to inform service improvements.

Systems and services for children of separated and divorced parents are arguably the least systematically implemented of those considered here, with many critical decisions about child custody and visitation often decided by a single judge. In this domain, Lamb encourages shared parenting arrangements that include overnight visits in order to provide both parents ample opportunities, via hands-on caregiving and nurturance, to continue to serve as attachment figures to their child.

In the domain of child protection and home visiting services, all chapters call for greater application of attachment theory, research, and attachment-based interventions. Resonating with Owen and Frosch's concerns about sensitively handling children's child care transitions, both Manly and colleagues and Zeanah and Dozier highlight the need for better understanding of attachment and better appreciation of the potential for traumatic loss in very young children among those who work in or with the child protection system, including Child Protective Services (CPS) staff, lawyers, and judges. More comprehensive training, provided as part of educational programs in social work, law, and other professions; continuing educational workshops; and expert consultations are recommended, as is wider use of the Safe Babies Court Teams (Osofsky & Lieberman, 2011; Zero to Three, 2020), a model that integrates child protective decision making with training in attachment and attachment-based interventions. Such trainings may not only improve services but also clarify important issues pertaining to attachment and loss, which in turn may help clarify what kind of relationships constitute attachments per se (see also Ahnert). Greater use of attachment-based interventions in the context of (1) services for maltreated children and their biological parents, (2) promoting secure attachments of foster children to their foster parents, and (3) preventive home visiting services is also recommended by Manly and colleagues; Zeanah and Dozier; and Berlin and coauthors. In this regard, the ABC program is a strong candidate, having demonstrated positive effects with caregivers and their infants and toddlers receiving both CPS and foster care and with low-income families receiving home-based federal Early Head Start services (Dozier & Bernard; Zeanah & Dozier). In addition, both Manly and coauthors and Zeanah and Dozier call for supporting the often-ongoing relationships between biological and foster parents through initiatives such as the Quality Parenting Initiative (Shauffer, 2012). Finally, Manly and colleagues and Berlin and colleagues call for more program evaluation, especially using attachment-based measures such as observational assessments of parent/caregiver sensitivity.

In summary, despite the somewhat fragmented and uncoordinated nature of U.S. systems and services for children and families, all of those discussed in this section reflect the beneficial influence of attachment theory and research, and all arguably stand to benefit from a greater infusion of both. As a whole, these chapters uniquely call attention to the importance of a child's multiple attachments and to their "networks of attachment relationships" (Fearon & Schuengel). These chapters also highlight the value of supporting such networks, such as by nurturing partnerships between the important adults in a young child's life (e.g., between child care providers and parents, between biological and foster parents). Provocative questions raised by these chapters include (1) whether a secure attachment with a child care provider can buffer the effects of an insecure child–parent attachment (Owen & Frosch) and (2) what a child carries forward from relationships that are disrupted (Zeanah & Dozier). Carefully constructed studies that address these and other questions concerning the quality and outcomes of children's multiple early relationships, especially under unusually challenging (e.g., foster care) and unusually supportive (e.g., high-quality child care, home visitation) circumstances, stand to improve our understanding of the touchstone issues raised by these chapters as well as the lifespan development of IWMs.

Concluding Thoughts

In the opening of this chapter, we reflected on some of the reasons for the enduring contributions of attachment theory to psychological science. In the pages that followed, we highlighted what we've learned and some of the cross-cutting themes of the field, as well as the research questions that remain, based on our contributors' insightful discussions of the nine fundamental questions that they addressed. We are left hopeful about the future of attachment theory and research, the number of interesting issues beckoning for further study, and the further potential of this field to address even more fundamentally important questions within the social and behavioral sciences, with their implications for therapeutic intervention, public policy, and public understanding.

However, we also note some of the more critical voices among the contributors to this volume. Roisman and Groh, for example, use the term *exhaustion* to describe the current era of attachment work, questioning whether it is a period of theoretical and methodological rigidity with limited scientific and translational advances. In a similar vein, Mesman reflects on the vulnerability to confirmation bias among attachment researchers who need (but often fail) to ask the "uncomfortable questions" that would be more generative and help improve and advance attachment theory and research. Moreover, Keller claims that attachment theory is weak due to conceptually fuzzy concepts and explanatory processes. These criticisms, from both within and outside the community of attachment scholars, caution against undue self-congratulations and underscore the continuing need for clear thinking and self-criticism, both hallmarks of good scientific inquiry. Indeed, someone perusing the table of contents of this book might wonder how a theory that has stood the test of time so well requires a volume like this to discuss—and only partially resolve—such fundamental questions as what kinds of relationships constitute attachment relationships, how to assess the security of attachment, and the nature and function of IWMs. Are these unresolved issues indicators of theoretical generativity or ambiguity?

Therefore, we close this chapter with two challenges for the future of attachment theory and research. They derive from our own reflections after writing the forgoing pages, recognizing that there are many other challenges and important questions contained in both our preceding comments and in the 46 chapters that future researchers should also consider. We believe that these two challenges, however, are uppermost in what is needed to ensure the continued generativity of attachment theory and research.

First, we believe that the field needs an integrated lifespan view of attachment and its development, one that has a central theoretical focus on IWMs and their development. By "integrated" we mean a view that synthesizes attachment scholarship as it is being conducted by developmental, social/personality, clinical, and other researchers into a more coherent, consolidated perspective. We emphasize IWMs because this construct is central to definitional and measurement issues, understanding the correlates and outcomes of attachment as well as stability and change over time, and the nature and effectiveness of clinical interventions. It is thus central to creating a more coherent view of the development of attachment throughout life. Simply stated, it is impossible to understand the development of attachment without a systematic understanding of the development of IWMs.

Most attachment scholars would agree that, from infancy through adulthood, attachment becomes an increasingly individual (trait-like) orientation at the same time that experience in multiple relationships with different attachment figures produce different representational models of relationships. This developmental process begins in infancy with attachments to mothers and fathers (and often with certain other caregivers) and continues to unfold with the development of other close relationships, including romantic affiliations and close friendships in adolescence and beyond. Over the life course, the relationships that are considered "primary" attachments change developmentally from parents to adult life partners, even though primary attachments from early life leave a continuing representational legacy. Here is where the pivotal questions emerge. How do IWMs become elaborated, refined, and/or generalized with relational experience? Do the IWMs associated with early attachments become integrated over time, refined by further relational experiences, and develop into a single, inclusive working model that shapes behavior and relationships in different contexts? Or do individuals gradually develop multiple, relationship-specific working models that, over time, differentially affect attachment-relevant thoughts, feelings, and behavior based on the relevance of different models to different situations? What determines when and how IWMs become evoked or activated and, in turn, influence responses and actions? Currently, we do not have a coherent theoretical view of the processes leading from multiple attachments to IWMs to individual attachment orientations to behavior. Greater collaboration between researchers who study attachment in childhood and those who focus on adult attachment could contribute to a more integrated lifespan view.

Central to this theoretical task is the empirical challenge of measuring IWMs better and more directly. The field currently uses several methods to measure IWMs, and these are models on which to build. But another approach is suggested by Waters and colleagues, who offer script-based approaches as one illustration of how researchers might build on modes of representation and information processing that are well studied in psychology and are currently incorporated into broad conceptualizations of IWMs. Script approaches can thus explain processes associated with IWMs in a conceptually refined manner that links to research literatures within and outside attachment theory. So also would approaches that examine attachment-related processes of emotion regulation, memory and information-processing, attributional biases, and the behavioral strategies (minimizing/deactivating and maximizing/hyperactivating) discussed by Cassidy and other contributors. Such processes can be measured throughout the lifespan along with assessments of attachment security and its behavioral correlates with the potential of offering a clearer formulation of how IWM processes develop and mediate the influence of attachment.

To summarize, we propose that a more coherent view of the development of IWMs is needed to advance a lifespan theory of the development of attachment, and that this task is *essential* to advancing attachment theory on a variety of issues. An important component of this task will be to create measures of IWMs that are developmentally appropriate and can be embedded within a theoretical view of how IWMs evolve across the lifespan. We recognize that this will be a major challenge to accomplish, but we believe it is a truly necessary and potentially highly rewarding endeavor.

The second challenge is more easily described. Attachment theorists must devote more effort to defining the boundary conditions of attachment principles and processes. In other words, we must identify not only what attachment is and what it should influence, but what it is *not* and what it should *not* influence. Attachment researchers have long been more attentive to convergent validity in their studies than to discriminant validity. This has yielded a research literature in which the correlates of attachment patterns have expanded almost exponentially. This issue connects to the forgoing, insofar as unmeasured IWMs have provided an extremely flexible explanatory device for novel (and potentially unexpected) correlates of attachment security and insecurity. If attachment theory is to maintain fidelity to Bowlby's formulations, we must clarify what attachment orientations should predict, and what they should not predict, especially because identifying the latter would facilitate the exploration and perhaps discounting of alternative explanations. These efforts may also sensitize the field to deal better with unanticipated "Black Swan" findings, some of which may require revisions to certain propositions, tenets, or hypotheses associated with attachment theory.

In the chapters of this volume, there are a handful of contributors who sought to clarify these boundary conditions. Szepsenwol and Simpson, for example, discuss how far life history theory goes in identifying the association of attachment security with later behavior, including variability in reproductively related behavior, but explicitly excluding variables like life satisfaction and religiosity. Ehrlich and Cassidy connect early attachment to diseases and chronic conditions that are clearly tied to health behaviors, stress, and coping, but not to those that have a strong genetic basis, except insofar as how attachment may be related to disease progression rather than disease onset. These examples illustrate the benefits of considering the boundary conditions of attachment. Doing so provides greater clarity to the hypotheses underlying and guiding attachment research and motivates more incisive exploration of unexpected research findings, which might merit alternative explanations. Ideally, as attachment researchers explore both expected and unexpected findings, they will be able to more precisely define which attachment-related outcomes, which currently include such wide-ranging phenomena as reproductive fitness, physiological biomarkers, and marital satisfaction, should be anticipated by attachment theory in which specific conditions.

The next generation of attachment scholars is faced with several remarkable, compelling, and exciting challenges, the solutions to which will likely advance our understanding and appreciation of people and relationships in important and unique ways. We look forward to what the next decades of attachment research will offer.

REFERENCES

Ainsworth, M. D. S. (1967). *Infancy in Uganda.* Baltimore: Johns Hopkins Press.

Ainsworth, M. D. S. (1991). Attachment and other affectional bonds across the life cycle. In C. M. Parkes, J. Stevenson-Hinde, & P. Marris (Eds.), *Attachment across the life cycle* (pp. 33–51). New York: Routledge.

Arriaga, X. B., Kumashiro, M., Simpson, J. A., & Overall, N. C. (2018). Revising working models across time: Relationship situations that enhance attachment security. *Personality and Social Psychology Review, 22,* 71–96.

Barnett, B., Blignault, I., Holmes, S., Payne, A., & Parker, G. (1987). Quality of attachment in a sample of 1-year-old Australian children. *Journal of the American Academy of Child and Adolescent Psychiatry, 26,* 303–307.

Belsky, J., & Cassidy, J. (1994). Attachment: Theory and evidence. In M. Rutter & D. Hay (Eds.), *Development through life* (pp. 373–402). Oxford, UK: Blackwell.

Belsky, J., & Pluess, M. (2009). Beyond diathesis stress: Differential susceptibility to environmental influences. *Psychological Bulletin, 135*(6), 885–908.

Bowlby, J. (1973). *Attachment and loss: Vol. 2. Separation.* New York: Basic Books.

Bowlby, J. (1979). *The making and breaking of affectional bonds.* London: Tavistock.

Bowlby, J. (1980). *Attachment and loss: Vol. 3. Loss, sadness and depression.* New York: Basic Books.

Bowlby, J. (1982). *Attachment and loss: Vol. 1. Attachment* (2nd ed.). New York: Basic Books. (Original work published 1969)

Bowlby, J. (1988). *A secure base: Parent–child attachment and healthy human development.* New York: Basic Books.

Bretherton, I., & Munholland, K. A. (2016). The internal working model construct in light of contemporary neuroimaging research. In J. Cassidy & P. R. Shaver (Eds.), *Handbook of attachment: Theory, research, and clinical applications* (3rd ed., pp. 63–88). New York: Guilford Press.

Caron, E. B., Bernard, K., & Dozier, M. (2018). In-vivo feedback predicts parent behavior change in the Attachment and Biobehavioral Catch-up intervention. *Journal of Clinical Child and Adolescent Psychology, 47,* S35–S46.

Collins, N. L., Guichard, A. C., Ford, M. B., & Feeney, B. C. (2004). Working models of attachment: New developments and emerging themes. In W. S. Rholes & J. A. Simpson (Eds.), *Adult attachment: Theory, research, and clinical implications* (pp. 196–239). New York: Guilford Press.

Cortes Hidalgo, A. P., Muetzel, R., Luijk, M. P. C. M., Bakermans-Kranenburg, M. J., El Marroun, H., Vernooij, M. W., . . . Tiemeier, H. (2019). Observed infant–parent attachment and brain morphology in middle childhood: A population-based study. *Developmental Cognitive Neuroscience, 40,* 100724.

Del Giudice, M., Gangestad, S. W., & Kaplan, H. S. (2016). Life history theory and evolutionary psychology. In D. M. Buss (Ed.), *The handbook of evolutionary psychology* (2nd ed., Vol. 1, pp. 88–114). Hoboken, NJ: Wiley.

Duschinsky, R., Bakkum, L., Mannes, J. M. M., Skinner, G. C. M., Turner, M., Mann, A., . . . Beckwith, H. (in press). Six attachment discourses: Convergence, divergence and relay. *Attachment and Human Development.*

Dykas, M. J., & Cassidy, J. (2011). Attachment and the processing of social information across the life span: Theory and evidence. *Psychological Bulletin, 137,* 19–46.

Fearon, R. P., & Belsky, J. (2016). Precursors of attachment security. In J. Cassidy & P. R. Shaver (Eds.), *Handbook of attachment: Theory, research, and clinical applications* (3rd ed., pp. 291–313). New York: Guilford Press.

Fearon, R. P., & Roisman, G. I. (2017). Attachment theory: Progress and future directions. *Current Opinion in Psychology, 15,* 131–136.

Feeney, J. A. (2016). Adult romantic attachment: Developments in the study of couple relationships. In J. Cassidy & P. R. Shaver (Eds.), *Handbook of attachment: Theory, research, and clinical applications* (3rd ed., pp. 434–463). New York: Guilford Press.

Feldman, R. (2017). The neurobiology of human attachments. *Trends in Cognitive Sciences, 21,* 80–99.

Fletcher, G. J. O., Simpson, J. A., Campbell, L., & Overall, N. C. (2015). Pair-bonding, romantic love, and evolution: The curious case of *Homo sapiens. Perspectives on Psychological Science, 10,* 20–36.

Fraley, R. C. (2019). Attachment in adulthood: Recent developments, emerging debates, and future directions. *Annual Review of Psychology, 70,* 401–422.

Grossmann, K. E. (1999). Old and new internal working models of attachment: The organization of feelings and language. *Attachment and Human Development, 1,* 253–269.

Hazan, C., & Shaver, P. (1987). Romantic love conceptualized as an attachment process. *Journal of Personality and Social Psychology, 52,* 511–524.

Hinde, R. (1988). Continuities and discontinuities: Conceptual issues and methodological considerations. In M. Rutter (Ed.), *Studies of psychosocial risk* (pp. 367–383). Cambridge, UK: Cambridge University Press.

Hinde, R. A. (1997). *Relationships: A dialectical perspective.* Hove, UK: Psychology Press.

Hrdy, S. B. (2009). *Mothers and others.* Cambridge, MA: Harvard University Press.

Keller, H., Bard, K., Morelli, G., Chaudhary, N., Vicedo, M., Rosabal-Coto, M., . . . Gottlieb, A. (2018). The myth of universal sensitive responsiveness: Comment on Mesman et al. (2017). *Child Development, 89,* 1921–1928.

Keller, H., & Kärtner, J. (2013). Development: The cultural solution of universal developmental tasks. In M. J. Gelfand, C.-Y. Chiu, & Y.-Y. Hong (Eds.), *Advances in culture and psychology* (Vol. 3, pp. 63–116). New York: Oxford University Press.

Kerns, K. A., & Brumariu, L. E. (2016). Attachment in middle childhood. In J. Cassidy & P. Shaver (Eds.), *Handbook of attachment: Theory, research, and clinical applications* (3rd ed., pp. 349–365). New York: Guilford Press.

Knee, C. R., & Petty, K. N. (2013). Implicit theories of relationships: Destiny and growth beliefs. In J. A. Simpson & L. Campbell (Eds.), *Oxford handbook of close relationships* (pp. 183–198). New York: Oxford University Press.

Kochanska, G., & Kim, S. (2012). Toward a new understanding of legacy of early attachments for future antisocial trajectories: Evidence from two longitudinal studies. *Development and Psychopathology, 24,* 783–806.

Kok, R., Thijssen, S., Bakermans-Kranenburg, M. J., Jaddoe, V. W. V., Verhulst, F. C., White, T., . . . Tiemeier, H. (2015). Normal variation in early parental sensitivity predicts child structural brain development. *Journal of the American Academy of Child and Adolescent Psychiatry, 54,* 824–831.

Lieberman, A. F., & Van Horn, P. (2008). *Psychotherapy with infants and young children: Repairing the effects of stress and trauma on early attachment.* New York: Guilford Press.

Lieberman, A. F., Weston, D. R., & Pawl, J. H. (1991). Preventive intervention and outcome with anxiously attached dyads. *Child Development, 62,* 199–209.

Main, M. (1990). Cross-cultural studies of attachment organization: Recent studies, changing methodologies, and the concept of conditional strategies. *Human Development, 33,* 48–61.

Main, M., & Goldwyn, R. (1984). *Adult attachment scoring and classification system.* Unpublished manuscript, University of California, Berkeley.

Main, M., Kaplan, N., & Cassidy, J. (1985). Security in infancy, childhood, and adulthood: A move to the level of representation. In I. Bretherton & E. Waters (Eds.), Growing points of attachment theory and research. *Monographs of the Society for Research in Child Development, 50*(1–2, Serial No. 209), 66–104.

Meehan, C. L., & Hawks, S. (2013). Cooperative breeding and attachment among the Aka foragers. In N. Quinn & J. M. Mageo (Eds.), *Attachment reconsidered: Cultural perspectives on a Western theory* (pp. 85–113). New York: Palgrave Macmillan.

Mesman, J., Minter, T., Angnged, A., Ciccé, I. A. H., Salali, G. D., & Migliano, A. B. (2017). Universality without uniformity: A culturally inclusive approach to sensitive responsiveness in infant caregiving. *Child Development, 89,* 837–850.

Mesman, J., van IJzendoorn, M. H., & Sagi-Schwartz, A. (2016). Cross-cultural patterns of attachment: Universal and contextual dimensions. In J. Cassidy & P. R. Shaver (Eds.), *Handbook of attachment: Theory, research, and clinical applications* (3rd ed., pp. 852–877). New York: Guilford Press.

Mikulincer, M., & Shaver, P. R. (2016). *Attachment in adulthood: Structure, dynamics, and change* (2nd ed.). New York: Guilford Press.

Osofsky, J. D., & Lieberman, A. F. (2011). A call for integrating a mental health perspective into systems of care for abused and neglected infants and young children. *American Psychologist, 66*(2), 120–128.

Pianta, R. C., La Paro, K., & Hamre, B. K. (2008). *Classroom Assessment Scoring System (CLASS).* Baltimore: Brookes.

Raikes, H. A., & Thompson, R. A. (2008). Attachment security and parenting quality predict children's problem-solving, attributions, and loneliness with peers. *Attachment and Human Development, 10*(3), 1–26.

Shauffer, C. (2012, May/June). The Quality Parenting Initiative: Fostering in the 21st century. *Fostering Families Today,* pp. 24–25.

Shonkoff, J. (2010). Building a new biodevelopmental framework to guide the future of early childhood policy. *Child Development, 81,* 357–367.

Simpson, J. A., & Belsky, J. (2016). Attachment theory within a modern evolutionary framework. In J. Cassidy & P. R. Shaver (Eds.), *Handbook of attachment: Theory, research, and clinical applications* (3rd ed., pp. 91–116). New York: Guilford Press.

Simpson, J. A., Rholes, W. S., Eller, J., & Paetzold, R. (2021). Major principles of attachment theory: Overview, hypotheses, and research ideas. In P. van Lange, A. W. Kruglanski, & E. T. Higgins (Eds.), *Social psychology: Handbook of basic principles* (3rd ed., pp. 222–239). New York: Guilford Press.

Simpson, J. A., Rholes, W. S., Oriña, M. M., & Grich, J. (2002). Working models of attachment, support giving, and support seeking in a stressful situation. *Personality and Social Psychology Bulletin, 28,* 598–608.

Sroufe, L. A., Egeland, B., Carlson, E., & Collins, W. (2005). *The development of the person: The Minnesota Study of Risk and Adaptation from birth to maturity.* New York: Guilford Press.

Sroufe, L. A., & Waters, E. (1977). Attachment as an organizational construct. *Child Development, 48,* 1184–1199.

Steele, H., & Steele, M. (Eds.). (2018). *Handbook of attachment-based interventions.* New York: Guilford Press.

Talia, A., Miller-Bottome, M., & Daniel, S. I. (2017). Assessing attachment in psychotherapy: Validation of the Patient Attachment Coding System (PACS). *Clinical Psychology and Psychotherapy, 24*(1), 149–161.

Thompson, R. A. (2016). Early attachment and later development: Reframing the questions. In J. Cassidy & P. R. Shaver (Eds.), *Handbook of attachment: Theory, research, and clinical applications* (3rd ed., pp. 330–348). New York: Guilford Press.

Thompson, R. A. (2017). Twenty-first century attachment theory: Challenges and opportunities. In H. Keller & K. A. Bard (Eds.), *The cultural nature of attachment* (pp. 301–319). Cambridge, MA: MIT Press.

Thompson, R. A. (2020). Eyes to see and ears to hear: Sensitivity in research on attachment and culture. *Attachment and Human Development, 22,* 85–89.

Zeifman, D. M. (2019). Attachment theory grows up: A developmental approach to pair bonds. *Current Opinion in Psychology, 25,* 139–143.

ZERO TO THREE. (2020). The Safe Babies Court Team approach. Retrieved from *www.zerotothree.org/resources/services/the-safe-babies-court-team-approach.*

Author Index

Subject Index

Note. *f* or *t* following a page number indicates a figure or a table.